Prediction of
Tumor Treatment Response

Pergamon Titles of Related Interest

Bragg/Rubin/Youker   ONCOLOGIC IMAGING

Kallman   RODENT TUMORS IN EXPERIMENTAL CANCER THERAPY

Mizer/Scheller/Deye   RADIATION THERAPY SIMULATION WORKBOOK

Bentel/Nelson/Noell   TREATMENT PLANNING & DOSE CALCULATION IN RADIATION ONCOLOGY, FOURTH EDITION

Related Journals*

International Journal of Radiation Oncology/Biology/Physics

Journal of Cancer Education

European Journal of Cancer & Clinical Oncology

Medical Oncology and Tumor Pharmacotherapy

Journal of Free Radicals in Biology & Medicine

Advances in Free Radical Biology and Medicine

Current Advances in Cancer Research

*Free sample copies available on request.

PREDICTION OF TUMOR TREATMENT RESPONSE

Edited by

J. Donald Chapman, Ph.D.
Cross Cancer Institute
Edmonton, Alberta, Canada

Lester J. Peters, M.D.
University of Texas M. D. Anderson Cancer Center
Houston, Texas

H. Rodney Withers, M.D., D.Sc.
UCLA Medical Center
Los Angeles, California

PERGAMON PRESS
NEW YORK · OXFORD · BEIJING · FRANKFURT
SÃO PAULO · SYDNEY · TOKYO · TORONTO

U.S.A.	Pergamon Press Inc., Maxwell House, Fairview Park, Elmsford, NY 10523, U.S.A.
U.K.	Pergamon Press plc, Headington Hill Hall, Oxford OX3 0BW, England
PEOPLE'S REPUBLIC OF CHINA	Pergamon Press, Room 4037, Qianmen Hotel, Beijing, People's Republic of China
FEDERAL REPUBLIC OF GERMANY	Pergamon Press GmbH, Hammerweg 6, D-6242 Kronberg, Federal Republic of Germany
BRAZIL	Pergamon Editora Ltda, Rua Eça de Queiros, 346, CEP 04011, Paraiso, São Paulo, Brazil
AUSTRALIA	Pergamon Press Australia Pty Ltd, P.O. Box 544, Potts Point, N.S.W. 2011, Australia
JAPAN	Pergamon Press, 5th Floor, Matsuoka Central Building, 1-7-1 Nishishinjuku, Shinjuku-ku, Tokyo 160, Japan
CANADA	Pergamon Press Canada Ltd., Suite No. 271, 253 College Street, Toronto, Ontario, Canada M5T 1R5

First edition 1989

Library of Congress Cataloging-in-Publication Data
Prediction of tumor treatment response.
Revised and expanded versions of papers originally presented at a conference held in Banff, Alta. on April 21–24, 1987.
Includes bibliographies and index.
1. Cancer—Treatment—Evaluation—Technique.
2. Cancer cells. 3. Tumors—Pathophysiology.
I. Chapman, J. Donald. 1941– . II. Peters, Lester J., 1942– . III. Withers, H. Rodney (Hubert Rodney), 1932– . [DNLM: 1. Neoplasms—therapy—congresses. 2. Prognosis. QZ 266 P9235]
RC267.P74 1988   616.99'406   88–9986

British Library Cataloguing in Publication Data
Prediction of tumor treatment response.
1. Man. Tumors. Therapy
I. Chapman, J. Donald II. Peters, Lester J.
III. Withers, H. Rodney
616.99'206

ISBN 0–08–034689–8

Printed in Great Britain by A. Wheaton & Co. Ltd, Exeter

Contents

Preface and Acknowledgments

The concept of this monograph arose in parallel with the planning for an international conference to present and review modern laboratory assays which might predict tumor treatment response. We, the editors, first discussed the merits of such a conference during the annual meeting of the American Society of Therapeutic Radiology and Oncology in Miami, Florida, in the fall of 1985. A symposium at that meeting, entitled "Radiobiology's Contribution to Radiotherapy in A.D. 2000," had forced participants to think in a futuristic mode. We were aware that several new procedures and technologies were providing information about cells from individual tumors which might predict response to specific treatments. To our knowledge, no previous meeting had addressed this specific theme, especially emphasizing the treatment response of solid tumors. It took eighteen months—in hindsight what appears to be a relatively short time—to organize proper sponsorship, funding, and a program for the conference entitled "Prediction of Tumor Treatment Response" held in Banff, Alberta, on April 21–24, 1987.

Over those eighteen months we had the expert assistance of an international Program Committee, which included Drs. Robert F. Kallman, Edmond P. Malaise, Luka Milas, G. Gordon Steel, Christian Streffer, Herman D. Suit, Robert M. Sutherland, Ian F. Tannock, Ralph R. Weichselbaum, and Gordon F. Whitmore. The conference was structured into an introductory lecture and five half-day sessions, each devoted to a specific theme of predictive assays, and included presentations by invited keynote speakers along with proffered papers presented in poster format. Two hours of each session was devoted to poster viewing and general discussion of the keynote lectures and proffered posters. The conference was considered by most attendees as a great success and certainly focused attention on new laboratory assays which may have future use in predicting the response of individual tumors to specific therapies.

Early in the planning, it became clear that one meeting could not cover all of the current research and development into laboratory assays which might relate to cancer prognosis and treatment outcome. Five broad themes were chosen for the conference focus: Tumor Histology and Molecular Pathology, Tumor Cell Kinetics and Cytogenetics, Tumor Cell Responses *In Vitro*, Tumor Cell Responses *In Vivo*, and Tumor Physiology and Metabolic Imaging. It became obvious that a three-day conference could not comprehensively cover all of the current research within any one of these broad themes of predictive assays. Nevertheless, the keynote lectures constituted many of the "near future" techniques which might be available for clinical research.

The Program Committee was concerned that the information presented and discussed at this conference should be available to the larger cancer research community and not only to those who were present to participate and enjoy the grandeur of Western Canada's Rocky Mountains. The concept of developing a monograph which addressed the specific themes of this conference was discussed and approved by the Program Committee and Pergamon Press. All keynote speakers were invited to prepare a chapter for this monograph which, in many cases, is broader than their specific lecture presentation. In some cases, the conference speaker declined this invitation, and an alternate scientist, equally versed in the specific field, has contributed a chapter to the monograph. Each of the five sections in the monograph concludes with a commentary chapter on the whole theme, developed by members of the Conference Program Committee. These summary chapters refer to information presented in the keynote addresses as well as information presented in poster format, which is not published as part of this monograph. At the end of each commentary chapter, the title, authorship, and address of each presented poster is listed. This will assist the reader with specific references in the summary chapters to information presented in poster format. All poster presentations should be considered as preliminary information and the specific authors should be contacted to determine if and where their research has been published.

This monograph could not have been developed without the cooperation of the various authors of each specific chapter. We trust that it will serve a useful role in the rapidly changing field of cancer research. We wish to thank Karen Brown and Gina Kennedy for their dedicated assistance in typing and assembling this monograph.

The conference and monograph would not have materialized without the generous assistance of the following organizations:

Alberta Cancer Board
Alberta Heritage Foundation for Medical Research
American College of Radiology
M.D. Anderson Hospital and Tumor Institute
National Cancer Institute, U.S.A.
Pergamon Press

J. Donald Chapman
Lester J. Peters
H. Rodney Withers

List of Contributors

Fraser L. Baker. Department of Experimental Radiotherapy, M.D. Anderson Hospital and Tumor Institute, Mail Slot 66, 1515 Holcombe Boulevard, Houston, Texas 77030

William A. Brock. Department of Experimental Radiotherapy, M.D. Anderson Hospital and Tumor Institute, Mail Slot 66, 1515 Holcombe Boulevard, Houston, Texas 77030

Truman R. Brown. Fox Chase Cancer Center, 7701 Burholme Avenue, Philadelphia, Pennsylvania 19111

Ronald N. Buick. Biology Division, Ontario Cancer Institute and Department of Medical Biophysics, University of Toronto, 500 Sherbourne Street, Toronto, Ontario M4X 1K9

Raymond S. Bush. Department of Radiation Oncology, Ontario Cancer Institute, 500 Sherbourne Street, Toronto, Ontario M4X 1K9

James Carmichael. Newcastle General Hospital, Regional Radiotherapy Center, Heaton, Newcastle upon Tyne, England NE7 8AL

J. Donald Chapman. Radiobiology Program, Cross Cancer Institute, 11560 University Avenue, Edmonton, Alberta, Canada T6G 1Z2

Martin J. Cline. Department of Medicine, University of California, Los Angeles, California 90024

Freidrich-Wilhelm Eigler. Abteilung fur Allgemeine Chirurgie, Universitatsklinikum Essen, Hufelandstr. 55, D4300-Essen 1, Federal Republic of Germany

Fuad S. Freiha. Division of Urology, Stanford University Medical Center, Stanford, California 94305

Michael L. Friedlander. Department of Medical Oncology, Royal Prince Alfred Hospital, Missenden Road, Camperdown, New South Wales 2050, Australia

James Fuscoe. Biomedical Sciences Division, Lawrence Livermore National Laboratory, P.O. Box 5507, Livermore, California 94550

Adi F. Gazdar. National Cancer Institute, Navy Medical Oncology Branch, Naval Hospital, Building 8, Room 5101, Bethesda, Maryland 20814

Eli Glatstein. Radiation Biology Section, Radiation Oncology Branch, National Cancer Institute, Bethesda, Maryland 20892

Joe W. Gray. Biomedical Sciences Division, Lawrence Livermore National Laboratory, P.O. Box 5507, Livermore, California 94550

Eberhard Gross. Abteilung fur Allgemeine Chirurgie, Universitatsklinikum Essen, Hufelandstr. 55, D4300-Essen 1, Fed. Rep. of Germany

Carina Henningsson. Department of Immunology, University of Alberta, Edmonton, Alberta, Canada T6G 2H7

Gloria H. Heppner. The E. Walter Albachten Department of Immunology, Michigan Cancer Foundation, 110 E. Warren Avenue, Detroit, Michigan 48201

Richard P. Hill. Ontario Cancer Institute, 500 Sherbourne Street, Toronto, Ontario M4X 1K9

Daniel Ihde. National Cancer Institute and Naval Hospital, and Uniformed Services University of the Health Sciences, Bethesda, Maryland 20814

Friedrich Kallinowski. Department of Applied Physiology, University of Mainz, D-6500 Mainz, Fed. Rep. of Germany

Robert F. Kallman. Department of Therapeutic Radiology, Division of Radiation Biology, Stanford University Medical Center, Stanford, California 94305

Kenneth A. Krohn. Division of Nuclear Medicine, University of Washington, Seattle, Washington 98195

B. Michael Longenecker. Department of Immunology, University of Alberta, Edmonton, Alberta, Canada T6G 2H7

Grant D. MacLean. Department of Medicine, Cross Cancer Institute, 11560 University Avenue, Edmonton, Alberta, Canada T6G 1Z2

Edmond P. Malaise. Laboratoire de Radiobiologie Cellulaire, Institute Gustave-Roussy, 94805 Villejuif Cedex, France 050

Alexander J. B. McEwan. Department of Nuclear Medicine, Cross Cancer Institute, 11560 University Avenue, Edmonton, Alberta, Canada T6G 1Z2

Nicholas J. McNally. Gray Laboratory, Northwood, England HA6 2RN

John E. McNeal. Division of Urology, Stanford University Medical Center, Stanford, California 94305

Luka Milas. Department of Experimental Radiotherapy, M.D. Anderson Hospital and Tumor Institute, 1515 Holcombe Boulevard, Houston, Texas 77030

Bonnie E. Miller. The E. Walter Albachten Department of Immunology, Michigan Cancer Foundation, 110 E. Warren Avenue, Detroit, Michigan 48201

Fred R. Miller. The E. Walter Albachten Department of Immunology, Michigan Cancer Foundation, 110 E. Warren Avenue, Detroit, Michigan 48201

John D. Minna. National Cancer Institute and Naval Hospital, and Uniformed Services University of the Health Sciences, Bethesda, Maryland 20814

James B. Mitchell. Radiation Biology Section, Radiation Oncology Branch, National Cancer Institute, Building 10, Room B3B69, Bethesda, Maryland 20892

Wolfgang F. Mueller-Klieser. Department of Applied Physiology, University of Mainz, Saarstrasse 21, D-6500 Mainz, Federal Republic of Germany

James Mullikin. Biomedical Sciences Division, Lawrence Livermore National Laboratory, P.O. Box 5507, Livermore, California 94550

James Mulshine. National Cancer Institute and Naval Hospital, and Uniformed University of the Health Sciences, Bethesda, Maryland 20814

Antoine A. Noujaim. Faculty of Pharmacy and Pharmaceutical Sciences, University of Alberta, Edmonton, Alberta, Canada T6G 2H7

Maria G. Pallavicini. Biomedical Sciences Division, Lawrence Livermore National Laboratory, P.O. Box 5507, Livermore, California 94550

Jae-Gahb Park. National Cancer Institute and Naval Hospital, and Uniformed Services University of the Health Sciences, Bethesda, Maryland 20814

Tamara Pelzer. Institut fur Medizinische Strahlenbiologie, Universitatsklinikum Essen, Hufelandstr. 55, D4300-Essen 1, Federal Republic of Germany

Lester J. Peters. Division of Radiotherapy, M.D. Anderson Hospital and Tumor Institute, 1515 Holcombe Boulevard, Houston, Texas 77030

Daniel Pinkel. Biomedical Sciences Division, Lawrence Livermore National Laboratory, P.O. Box 5507, Livermore, California 94550

Elise Redwine. Division of Urology, Stanford University Medical Center, Stanford, California 94305

Einar K. Rofstad. Institute for Cancer Research and The Norwegian Cancer Society, The Norwegian Radium Hospital, Montebello, 0310 Oslo 3, Norway

Angelo Russo. Radiation Biology Section, Radiation Oncology Branch, National Cancer Institute, Bethesda, Maryland 20892

S. Selvaraj. Faculty of Pharmacy and Pharmaceutical Sciences, University of Alberta, Edmonton, Alberta, Canada T6G 2H7

Rosella Silvestrini. Oncologia Sperimentale C, Istituto Nazionale per lo Studio e la Cura dei Tumori, Via Venezian 1, 20133 Milan, Italy

Thomas A. Stamey. Division of Urology, Stanford University Medical Center, Stanford, California 94305

G. Gordon Steel. Radiotherapy Research Unit, Institute of Cancer Research, Sutton, Surrey, England SM2 5PX

Christian Streffer. Institut fur Medizinische Strahlenbiologie, Universitatsklinikum Essen, Hufelandstr. 55, D4300-Essen 1, Federal Republic of Germany

Herman D. Suit. Massachusetts General Hospital, Harvard School of Public Health, Harvard University, Boston, Massachusetts 02114

Mavanur R. Suresh. Faculty of Pharmacy and Pharmaceutical Sciences, University of Alberta, Edmonton, Alberta, Canada T6G 2H7

Robert M. Sutherland. University of Rochester Cancer Center, 601 Elmwood Avenue, Box 704, Rochester, New York 14642

Tom R. Sykes. BIOMIRA, Inc., Edmonton, Alberta, Canada, T6N 1E5

James E. Talmadge. Preclinical Screening Laboratory, Program Resources, Inc., National Cancer Institute Frederick Cancer Research Facility, Frederick, Maryland 21701

Ian F. Tannock. Departments of Medicine and Medical Biophysics, Ontario Cancer Institute, 500 Sherbourne Street, Toronto, Ontario M4X 1K9

Paul J. Tofilon. Department of Experimental Radiotherapy, M.D. Anderson Hospital and Tumor Institute, Mail Slot 66, 1515 Holcombe Boulevard, Houston, Texas 77030

Barbara J. Trask. Biomedical Sciences Division, Lawrence Livermore National Laboratory, P.O. Box 5507, Livermore, California 94550

Chun-Ming Tsai. National Cancer Institute and Naval Hospital, and Uniformed Services University of the Health Sciences, Bethesda, Maryland 20814

Dirk van Beuningen. Institut fur Medizinische Strahlenbiologie, Universitatsklinikum Essen, Hufelandstr. 55, D4300-Essen 1, Federal Republic of Germany

Herman van Dekken. Radiobiological Institute TNO, Rijswijk, The Netherlands

Ger van den Engh. Biomedical Sciences Division, Lawrence Livermore National Laboratory, P.O. Box 5507, Livermore, California 94550

William P. Vaughan. University of Nebraska Medical Center, Omaha, Nebraska 68105.

Peter W. Vaupel. Department of Applied Physiology, University of Mainz, D-6500 Mainz, Federal Republic of Germany

Stefan M. Walenta. Department of Applied Physiology, University of Mainz, D-6500 Mainz, Federal Republic of Germany

Alexander M. Walker. Massachusetts General Hospital, Harvard School of Public Health, Harvard University, Boston, Massachusetts 02114

Ralph Weichselbaum. Michael Reese/University of Chicago Center for Radiation Therapy, 5841 South Maryland Avenue, Box 440, Chicago, Illinois 60637

Gordon D. Whitmore. Physics Division, Ontario Cancer Institute, 500 Sherbourne Street, Toronto, Ontario M4X 1K9

H. Rodney Withers. Department of Radiation Oncology, University of California— Los Angeles, Center for Health Sciences, Los Angeles, California 90024

INTRODUCTION

1

Predictors of Radiation Response in Use Today: Criteria for New Assays and Methods of Verification

Herman D. Suit and Alexander M. Walker

INTRODUCTION

The ninety year history of radiation therapy has witnessed dramatic increases in our understanding of the nature of cancer and the effectiveness of our ability to manage the cancer patient. Even so, there remains the formidable problem of failure of the best standards of radiation treatment to achieve control of the primary and regional disease and to do so without treatment-related morbidity. There are four general research strategies designed to improve the efficacy of radiation therapy. These are to: (1) employ superior dose distributions, viz., reduce treatment volume towards target volume and yet be certain that the target volume is totally encompassed by the treatment volume on each session; (2) increase the differential response between tumor and normal tissue so as to favor the latter; (3) expand our knowledge of the natural history of tumors with particular reference to patterns of local and regional spread to aid in defining the distribution of clonogens in tissues and hence plan dose distribution more rationally; and (4) develop the capability of predicting the responses of tumor and normal tissue to standard radiation treatment and to predict the change in response probability by modifying treatment strategy. Success in these research programs would not only increase the frequency of control of the primary tumor but also improve survival rate.

From the early period of radiation therapy, efforts have been mounted to develop clinical information of predictive value. There has been and is an obvious need to assist the physician in deciding on the plan of management of the individual patient, e.g., (1) should radiation alone be employed and if so, to what dose level (i.e., the degree of aggressiveness); (2) should radiation be combined with surgery and/or drugs; or (3) should treatment be by modalities other than radiation. Recently interest in predictors of radiation response has expanded substantially, as evidenced by this monograph. This has resulted from a vast augmentation of our ability to study physiological, biochemical, and radiobiological characteristics of individual tumors. Further, there is the realization that efforts to evaluate the efficacy of new strategies of treatment, (e.g., combination of radiation and hypoxic cell sensitizers, accelerated fractionation patterns) are, almost certainly, being confounded by heterogeneity of tumors with reference to the tumor characteristic with which the new treatment is designed to deal. In a clinical trial of a new treatment strategy, patients should be stratified not only on the basis of the clinically proven predictors but also on the basis of the physiological or other characteristics which defeat standard treatment. Some of the failures of clinical trials to demonstrate gains by highly promising new treatment strategies have stemmed directly from this category of heterogeneity.

There are now under laboratory and clinical investigation an imposing array of new treatment strategies and a formidable spectrum of potential predictors of radiation response which are pertinent to the rationale underlying the new strategies. These new predictors include *in vitro* assays for identification of tumors whose cells are inherently less radiation-sensitive; demonstration of regions of hypoxia or of metabolic deprivation within tumors; measurements of proliferative activity within the tumor cell population; identification of patients who are immune-deficient, and quantification of oncogene products among others.

RESPONSE PREDICTORS EMPLOYED IN 1988

Several valuable predictors of response of human tumors to fractionated irradiation are in regular use. These have been discussed previously [7,8,9,11] and are only mentioned here. The most established predictor is, of course, the histopathologic type. For example, the dose to achieve a 90% local control rate (TCD_{90}) for testicular seminomas is 30 Gy (2 Gray per fraction given over a 3 week period). For Hodgkin's disease, such a success rate would require dose levels of 40–55 Gy. For small squamous cell carcinomas of vocal cord (T1) the TCD_{90} would be ~67 Gy, and the TCD_{90} for squamous cell carcinomas of 5–6 cm diameter is 72–75 Gy. In contrast, the maximum dose feasible for external beam photon irradiation of glioblastoma multiforme is ~70 gy. This probably corresponds to less than the TCD_5.[11]

For tumors of a specified histological type, size is the most important predictor of response now available. The dose required to achieve a specified tumor control probability (TCP) increases with tumor size.[12] This is true for virtually all solid tumors which have been investigated. Further, tumor size has been well documented as an important parameter for TCP in the radiation treatment of spontaneous tumors and early generation isotransplants of spontaneous tumors in laboratory animals.[13,14] The clinical presentation of the tumor also affects the TCP for a given dose fractionation schedule. For example, non-necrotic tumors of the anterior faucial pillar, retromolar trigone, and base of the tongue are more likely to be controlled than are necrotic lesions.[15] Tumors of the head and neck region of a particular size and type treated by a specified protocol are more likely to be controlled if occurring in females rather than in male patients.[16] Hemoglobin level modifies tumor control probability for carcinomas of the head and neck region and uterine cervix[16-18] *vide infra.*

Recently, there has been an impressive demonstration of the value of determining the parameters of radiation sensitivity of normal tissue in deciding radiation dose level. Reference is made here to the report by Hart *et al.*,[19] who determined the radiation sensitivity of bone marrow cells of a patient with ataxia telangectasia being planned for irradiation of a medulloblastoma and found it to be three times that for bone marrow cells from normal patients. Accordingly, they reduced the administered dose by about one-third of that which would be employed in the treatment of a normal patient. Reactions of normal tissues were comparable to that expected following standard dose levels administered to normal patients. The result has thus far been judged by those clinicians to be satisfactory; at 1 year, computed axial tomography (CAT) reveals no tumor at the posterior fossa.[20]

Regression of tumor during treatment has been widely accepted as a reliable predictor of the efficacy of chemotherapy. However, for a population of tumors of a well-defined category, e.g., histological type, size, etc., and treated to a specified radiation dose-fractionation protocol, regression during treatment has been evaluated by retrospective analyses of data[21-23] and judged not to be clinically useful.[23] This is probably due to the fact that local control demands inactivation of all tumor cells. The number of clonogenic cells which survive in tumors which *recur* following definitive radiation therapy, yielding a TCP ≥ 0.1, is in the range of 1–5.[24] Hence, at completion of unsuccessful treatment the number of viable clonogens is far below the detection level of experienced clinicians or sophisticated radiographic procedures.

There are also other clinical parameters used as predictors, viz., Karnovsky status, immune competence of the host among others.

FUTURE PROSPECTS

In deciding upon treatment strategy for a patient today, the clinician obviously knows the histopathological type, size of tumor, anatomic size, Hgb level, patient's sex, Karnovsky status, and can observe regression during the first part of treatment. Based upon these clinical factors the clinician can approximate the TCP for a particular patient problem following standard treatment. The available data do not provide a basis for close estimates of TCP. A large body of data is needed to establish the relationship between TCP and each of these parameters for several dose levels. Fortunately, data are accumulating in many centers on local control and local morbidity in patients for whom the tumor size is well-defined (clinical, CAT, MRI measurements) and many other clinical features have been recorded in detail. The consequence will be a rich accretion of data from which those relationships can be derived.

REQUIREMENTS FOR A PREDICTOR

For a predictor to be of practical clinical value, the test or measurement should pose little or no hazard to the patient. Importantly, the procedure should not complicate or prejudice the subsequent definitive treatment, be this radiation, surgery, or chemotherapy. The results of the predictor test should be available either at the start of definitive treatment or not later than at mid-point during the course of treatment. The true value of the predictors should be established and the circumstances or clinical conditions for which the predictor has practical value clearly defined.

There are several constraints on the utility of physiological or biochemical measurements designed to serve as predictors of TCP following radiation treatment. First, clonogens comprise only a portion of the cells in tumor tissue. Clonogen here refers to cells with the capacity to produce a continuously expanding progeny. The measurements must reflect the physiological or biochemical status of the clonogens. For virtually all physiological or biochemical parameters there are broad distributions of values in tumor tissues. Available techniques for measuring these parameters yield only mean values, e.g., of glutathione, creatine phosphate, ATP, pO_2, blood flow, among others. The resolution of all measurement techniques applicable to living tissue is largely relative to cell size. Hence, the relationship between measured value of a parameter and its actual level in clonogens is not necessarily one to one. Secondly, there are errors in measurement of all parameters. Thirdly, there may be an absolutely false positive result, in that the measured value may correctly reflect the status of the clonogens but other processes (e.g., physiologic) may negate the impact of the parameter being studied. Fourthly, there cannot be a predictor which yields a yes/no statement as to the treatment outcome in any individual patient. The predictive data, at best, allow the physician to assign the patient to a well-characterized category for which there would be a known *probability* of local control for the particular treatment. Thus, the position of the patient's tumor on a dose response curve might be determined as a probability, but not as an actual outcome. This differs from many diagnostic tests in medicine where yes/no answers are provided.

A predictive assay requires heterogeneity amongst tumors with respect to the tested parameter. This is a statement of the obvious. Nonetheless, heterogeneity amongst tumors of a well-defined category must be obtained if a physiological or other test is to be predictive of response.

The slope of the dose response curve for control of tumor reflects the inherent slope due to the stochastic processes of cell inactivation and heterogeneity between tumors with respect to the relevant parameters of radiation response. Among the tumors in the population of tumors being studied, heterogeneity within individual tumors is not important in this context; it is only the heterogeneity *between* tumors which is significant. The maximal steepness of a dose response curve would be obtained for: (1) a population of tumors uniform with respect to the number of clonogens and distribution of cellular radiation sensitivity amongst those clonogens; (2) constant radiation treatment protocol; and (3) defined and consistently applied criteria for scoring of results. There have been numerous publications giving dose response data for human tumors treated by fractionated radiation. Three recent reviews of dose response data include estimates of slopes for the dose response relationships.[25-27] Brahme[25] has proposed a gamma factor as a descriptor of slope. This is the increase in tumor control probability in percent points for a 1% increase in dose. We use the symbol $\gamma\,50$ to represent the slope at a TCP of 0.5, where the dose response curve is at or near maximal steepness. Figure 1.1 presents the cumulative distribution of

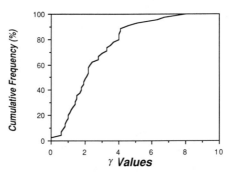

FIG. 1.1 Cumulative distribution of γ_{50} factors for dose response relationships for human tumors. This curve is derived from analyses published in three reviews of the literature. See text.

γ_{50}s derived from the three reports[25–27] and represents 54 slope estimates for various epithelial tumors (lymphoma and melanoma not included). Where there was more than one estimate for the same reported study, a mean of the values was taken. The result is an estimate of gamma factors for 45 reported series. This plot indicates that 50% of the gamma factors were less than 2, and 90% were less than 4.8.

For a better understanding of the upper limit on slope, we have calculated γ factors for model tumors treated with 35 equal radiation doses. We stipulate that all tumors are identical in terms of the various parameters of radiation response, i.e., there is no heterogeneity between tumors. Tumor control probabilities were calculated assuming Poisson statistics of cell inactivation and that regrowth always occurs when one or more clonogenic cells survive.

$$TCP = e^{-SF^{v}M}$$

SF = survival fraction

v = number of equal doses

M = number of clonogens

For computation of cell inactivation we employed a modification of the multitarget and single hit model that includes a term for cell killing by non-reparable damage or single hit mechanism(s).[28]

$$SF = e^{-aD/Do}[1-(1-e^{-(1-a)D/Do})]^n$$

a = the proportion of energy absorbed in the production of non-reparable damage

D = dose

D_0 = mean lethal dose

n = extrapolation number

To estimate the γ_{50}, the following relationship was utilized: $\gamma_{50} = TCD_{50} \times \cdot01[(TCD_{60}-TCD_{40}).20]$. The resulting γ_{50} factors for

35 fraction irradiation are 6.7–9.2 for clonogen numbers of 10^6–10^8. This means that the dose response curves for this model tumor are substantially steeper than Figure 1.1 would suggest for most human tumors, assuming that clonogen numbers in clinical tumors would be >10^6. The slope of the response curve becomes progressively less steep as the number of clonogens decreases (see Table 1.1). Namely, γ_{50} factors decrease from 6.6 to 1.9 as clonogen numbers are reduced from 10^6 down to 10^2. At this time, clonogen numbers in human tumors are not known. Hence, a firm statement as to the slope of a dose response curve for a perfectly uniform population of human tumors cannot be made. Human tumors contain some 10^9–10^{10} cells. A true clonogen number of only 10^6 would mean that the ratio of clonogens to total cells would be 10^{-3}–10^{-4}. A relatively flat dose response curve could be obtained where a small number of resistant clonogens dominated the observed response.

TABLE 1.1 γ_{50} *Factors for model tumors*
[n = 4, ω = .3, q = 1.00, v = 35]

Log M	γ_{50}
2	1.9
4	4.1
6	6.6
8	9.2

An examination of the slopes of curves of TCP vs. dose of tumors of experimental animals is pertinent in this context. Ramsay and Suit[29] have performed dose response assays on early generation isotransplants of a spontaneous fibrosarcoma (FSaII) and on a spontaneous squamous cell carcinoma (SCCVII) with allocation of tumors to dose so as to increase the efficiency of estimation of slopes. Treatment was administered to 6mm tumors in 10 equal doses on a BID basis using clamp hypoxia. This should yield a nearly homogeneous population of tumors and result in curves of near maximal steepness. γ_{50} factors for these experiments were 3.8 and 4.2, respectively. Assays on 8mm FSaII irradiated under normal or AIR conditions in 20 equal doses on a BID schedule yielded a γ_{50} factor of 3.9. Experiments have been performed on rat rhabdomyosarcoma by Fischer and Moulder[30]; the slopes of the dose response curves were less steep than that for the FSaII and SCCVII. Also, the slopes were approximately the same for single and for fractionated dose irradiation (v = 1–22).

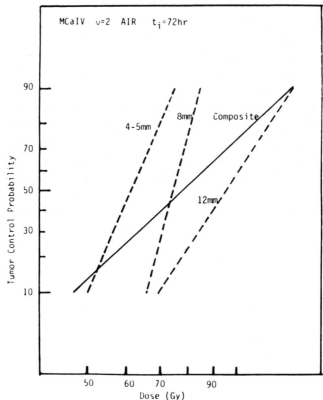

FIG. 1.2   Dose response curves for local control of early generation isotransplants of MCaIV in C3Hf/Sed mice irradiated at 4, 8, and 12mm sizes. Radiation was administered in two equal doses separated by 72 hours. The mice were anesthetized and respired AIR. The solid line represents the dose response curve for the data pooled from the three separate assays.

The impact of heterogeneity on dose response curves can be readily appreciated by examination of Figure 1.2. Here dose response curves are shown for 4–5, 8, and 12mm diameter isotransplants of C3H mouse mammary carcinoma irradiated in two equal doses separated by 72 hours under AIR breathing conditions. The solid line represents the dose response curve for the pooled data from the three assays. Its lesser slope directly reflects the heterogeneity among the subject tumors with respect to size. Heterogeneity amongst tumors for one or more parameters affecting tumors response would result in flattening of the dose response curve.

The very shallow slopes of dose response curves for local control of human tumors (γ_{50} values of <2) almost certainly reflect heterogeneity amongst the patients and their tumors in the study. Specifically, the tumors were not randomly allocated to the different dose levels. Nor were they stratified as to size or pattern of clinical presentation. Additionally, the patients were not stratified as to hemoglobin or sex. Further, the ranges of doses employed were quite limited.

Clinical studies are based upon a population of spontaneous autochthonous tumors, with unique parameters of radiation response. Accordingly, a clinical study of the dose response relationship for tumor control will be based on a population of tumors which are to some degree heterogeneous. The observed slope of the dose response curve for such a population of tumors would not, of course, be the slope for one of the tumors. If a dose response assay for local control were performed on 100 tumors cloned from one human tumor (e.g., isotransplants of the same size and subjected to exactly the same treatment), the dose response curve should be steep. This concept is illustrated in Figure 1.3, which shows a series of dose response curves—each of which is based upon clones from an individual spontaneous tumor (the thin lines). The thick and flatter line would result were the assay based on the parent tumors.

Analyses of slopes of dose response curves do not permit definition of the degree of heterogeneity. That the observed γ_{50} values are, in many instances, so very low, points to the existence of substantial heterogeneity. This should mean that there is a realistic basis for expecting that research to develop predictors will be fruitful.

REQUIREMENTS OF A TRIAL OF A PREDICTOR

In planning the trial of a predictor of radiation response, there are several parameters which must be controlled. First, the dose to each tumor must be known and constant from one patient to the next for each dose level employed. Secondly, to be certain that geographic misses do not confound the analysis of tumor control probability, there must be assurance that the treatment volume covers the target volume on all treatment sessions. Thirdly, the trial should employ a patient stratification scheme which makes full use of available predictors. For example, tumors should be of a single histological type; the size (volume) should be carefully determined and of a narrow range (in addition to designating T stage); and the clinical presentation should be of defined categories. Further, there should be stratification as to Hgb level and sex. Fourthly, there must be a well-defined protocol for follow-up observation of the treated site and scoring for local control of tumor and of various levels of treatment-related morbidity.

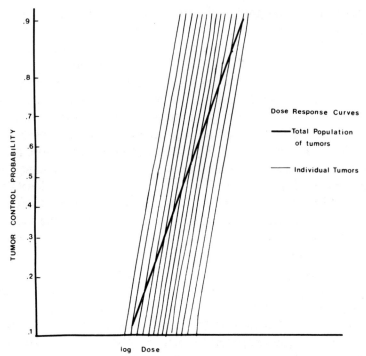

FIG. 1.3   Theoretical consideration of heterogeneity amongst individual spontaneous tumors on the observed dose response curve for tumor control. The fine lines represent the slopes of dose response curves which would be obtained by irradiating 100 clones from an individual tumor. The result is a series of relatively steep curves reflecting the actual sensitivity of a series of individual tumors. The thick line is the curve which would result from irradiating the original spontaneous tumors.

Quite clearly, the preferred strategy to test the efficacy of an assay as a predictor should be a prospective study designed to examine for a correlation between the value of the parameter measured and the outcome. This procedure is being employed now for a broad range of predictors; many of these are discussed later in this monograph.

However, there are rich opportunities to utilize retrospective analyses of clinical records and biological materials. This is true for those centers where detailed records have been maintained. Most of our knowledge of the value of histological type, etc., has come from retrospective studies of patient records. Investigations have been reported on the vascular density and outcome using histological material and patient records.[31,32] Currently, tissue is being retrieved from paraffin blocks containing the biopsy sample to analyze for aneuploidy.[33] The value of such retrospective analyses should have validity provided complete clinical records are kept. In this way, the outcome of treatment

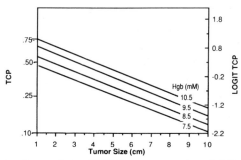

FIG. 1.4   Regression lines relating TCP (tumor control probability) and tumor size amongst 332 male patients treated in Denmark by radiation alone for squamous cancer of the supraglottis and pharynx according to pre-treatment hemoglobin.[18]

can be analyzed in terms of well-defined clinical stratification and in terms of the particular test of interest. Further, this type of study could be interinstitutional.

With few exceptions, the values of parameters (Hgb, tumor size, pO_2, labelling index, etc.) to be studied as predictors are continuously variable. We consider here two studies on hemoglobin level and tumor size as determinants of TCP.

STUDY OF Hgb AND TUMOR RESPONSE

A Danish Cooperative Group has determined Hgb and tumor size in 332 male patients treated by radiation alone for squamous carcinoma of the supraglottis and pharynx by a constant radiation treatment protocol. Those data and the two-year local control results were generously provided by J. Overgaard.[18]

Patients were divided into groups on the basis of both hemoglobin concentration and tumor size. The failure fractions in these groups were analyzed with respect to hemoglobin concentration and with respect to size using a logistic regression procedure. Logistic regression functions fit predicted failure probabilities, whose logit is a linear combination of terms incorporating the various predictor terms. The regression showed substantial and independent contribution of both hemoglobin and tumor size to failure probability. The equation was:
Logit (failure) = 1.884 + 0.2346 (size in cm) – o.2915 (Hgb in mM).

This relationship between TCP and tumor size for four values of hemoglobin are presented in Figure 1.4. An important increment in TCP is predicted as Hgb increases from 7mM (11.2gm%) to 10.5mM(16.8gm%). The greatest number of patients were in the range

8–9 and 9–10mM. The curve for 9.5mM was significantly higher than that for 8.5mM with stratification for size (p = 0.02).

Blitzer et al.[34] have examined local control results in 122 patients with T3 and T4 squamous carcinomas of oro-pharynx who were treated by radiation alone (<55 Gy) at the Massachusetts General Hospital (MGH). They controlled for ethanol abuse, sex, N status, QD or BID, and dose. Using the Cox proportional hazard, the effect of Hgb can be modeled as:

$$H(t) = HO(t) \, e^{-0.156(Hgb-14)}$$

where $H(t)$ = hazard or instantaneous failure rate

$HO(t)$ = hazard at time t_1 for patient with Hgb = 14gm%.

In this series, as in the Danish series, as Hgb goes up, failure rate goes down. However, in patients with cancer of the urinary bladder Hgb level has been found to be a predictor of response only for certain stages.[35] Hence, the importance of Hgb as a predictor will need further study employing tumors at various sites.

Predictive equations such as the ones derived from the Danish and the MGH head and neck data might be used to great advantage in future trials. Provided the values of the predictive factors are known at the outset, the allocation of treatment could be balanced according to the levels of the predictive factors individually, or collectively, via the predictive equation. The latter technique would involve allocating patients to strata of predicted tumor control rates and then ensuring a balanced treatment allocation within strata. Whether patients are allocated in strata determined by each of the known predictors separately or by predictors taken together, an appropriate analysis would take the predictors into account. Statistical adjustment for known predictors of disease will tend to increase the precision of treatment evaluation and will permit a rational search for subgroups within which given therapies might be particularly effective. The total number of patients needed to demonstrate a difference is likely to be less for highly stratified protocols (even with smaller numbers of subjects per cell) combined with a predictive equation than for the conventional relatively unstratified protocols.

The efficacy of a predictor can be readily described in terms of true positivity (TP), false positivity (FP), and false negativity (FN). The true positivity rate (TP) indicates the proportion of subjects correctly identified as having the specific characteristic determined by a test. For example, if the predictor of a high local failure rate were a measured tissue pO_2 < 20mm Hg, then the TP rate would be the proportion of tumors with a pO_2 < 20mm which were read as having pO_2 < 20mm

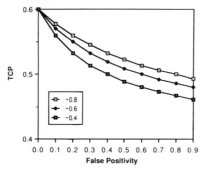

FIG. 1.5   Curves relating TCP for patients identified by a predictor to be treated by a new method and false positivity. The TCP is 0.6 and 0.4 for the true positive and false positive tumor populations.

Hg. FP would be the proportion of tumors with a pO_2 of >20mm Hg for which measurement gave an erroneous reading <20mm. FN represents the proportion of tumors whose pO_2 is <20mm Hg which were mistakenly measured to have a $pO_2 > 20$mm Hg.

Predictor tests are expected to be employed to identify subjects who would be predicted to experience a high failure rate following conventional therapy and would accordingly be advised to accept a more radical, complex, hazardous, or costly treatment. The power of a predictor test depends primarily on the TP and FP rates. The new treatment would presumably be performed on all patients reading positive, i.e., TP and FP patients. The TP determines the subjects upon which the new treatment would be employed with an expectation of a clinical gain. The false positivity specifies the proportion of patients subjected to the non-standard treatment *without* expected benefit. A high FN rate reduces the number of patients who should be accessed into the trial of new treatment.

The impact of FP on the observed TCP is illustrated in Figure 1.5. A model population of tumors is comprised of tumors of two types, A and B, in equal proportions. Both A and B tumors have a TCP of 0.4 if treated by the standard method. Type B tumors exhibit a TCP of 0.4 whether treated by the conventional or by the new method, whereas type A tumors have a TCP of 0.6 if treated by the new method. Consider that a predictive assay has been developed to identify patients with tumors of type A and is being employed to select patients for accession into a trial of the new treatment method. For FP of 0.0, all of the tumors in the study would be type A, and accordingly, the TCP of the tested group would be 0.6. The observed TCP decreases as the FP increases, and to a lesser extent, as TP decreases. Thus, demonstrating a gain by employing the new method might be feasible if FP were zero, i.e., a 20 percentage point gain (a TCP increases from 0.4 to 0.6). However, the likelihood of demonstrating a true gain becomes increasingly small as FP increases above zero.

The gain from utilization of two predictors may be considered by the example in Table 1.2. For each, the TP and FP are 0.8 and 0.2, respectively. The observed TCP increases from 0.50 to 0.56 to 0.59 for use of none, one, or two predictors. The advantage in using multiple predictors is the reduction of FPs. However, the total number of subjects for the test also decreases. No allowance in these models has been made for FN. In biological reality, the tests are not likely to be totally independent.

TABLE 1.2 *Number of Predictors and TCP Observed in Test Population of Tumors*

A and B each comprise 50% of tumors.
New Treatment Yields TCP of 0.6 for A Tumors and 0.4 for B Tumors.
Predictors are Designed to Identify A Tumors. Predictors yield TP of 0.8 and FP of 0.2.

	No. Subjects	
No. Predictors	*Identified (TP & FP)*	*TCP*
0	100	0.50
1	50	0.56
2	34	0.59

For the physiological, biochemical, or radiobiological parameters being considered, the TP is not likely to exceed 0.8. Nor is FP likely to be less than 0.2. In contrast, the predicitive power of many serological tests is high, e.g., TP of to 0.99 and FP of 0.01. This is particularly true for some of the modern tests using monoclonal antibodies.

SUMMARY

There is a twofold need for quantitative predictors of response of human tumors to radiation therapy. First, predictors should provide the clinician with improved estimates of TCP for standard treatment given to patients fitting well-defined and narrow strata. These strata should include at least the currently employed predictors: histological type, tumor size, Hgb, sex, and clinical presentation. Other parameters which may be considered include histological grade, Karnovsky status, and regression pattern during the initial phase of treatment. Secondly, predictors based upon physiological, biochemical, or radiobiological determinations are likely to prove of great value in identifying patients most likely to benefit from new treatment strategies. Trials of the new treatments should be based upon patients so identified. Further, predictors may be of value in deciding the appropriate dose level.

A requirement for a physiological, biochemical, or radiobiological assay to have predictive value is that there be heterogeneity amongst the population of tumors being studied with reference to the particular characteristics being measured. Heterogeneity within a tumor is unimportant in this context. An indicator of heterogeneity in a population of tumors is the slope of the dose response curve for tumor control (Logit TCP vs. ln dose), i.e., less steepness means more heterogeneity. There is probably sufficient heterogeneity even within well-defined clinical strata to make the search for new classes of predictors an important venture.

ACKNOWLEDGMENTS

The authors are pleased to acknowledge the excellent work by Claire Hunt in preparation of the manuscript. Further, we happily acknowledge the fine effort by Michael Stracher in performing many of the computations required in this manuscript and in the preparation of the figures. Finally, we appreciate the computation of gamma factors and slope of the model tumors by Michael Goitein for the fractionated irradiation.

This work was supported by a research grant from DHHS, National Cancer Institute, CA13311.

REFERENCES

1. Suit, H. D., Statement of the problem pertaining to dose fractionation and total treatment time on response of tissue to x-irradiation. In: *Time Dose Relationships in Radiation Biology as Applied to Radiotherapy*. NCI-AEC Conference, Carmel, California, 1969. BNL 50203(C57), 1970, vii–x.
2. Cox, J. D., Chairman, Workshop on Patterns of Failure after Cancer Treatment. *Cancer Treatment Symposia*, Vol. 2, 1983.
3. The Third Rome International Symposium, "The Challenge of Local Tumor Control and Its Impact on Survival. *Int. J. Radiat. Oncol. Biol. Phys.* 12(1), 1986.
4. Suit, H. D., Modification of Radiation Response. *Int. J. Radiat. Oncol. Biol. Phys.* **10**: 101–108, 1984.
5. Coleman, C. N., Hypoxic cell radiosensitizers: Expectations and Progress in Drug Development. *Int. J. Radiat. Oncol. Biol. Phys.* **11**: 323–329, 1985.
6. Suit, H. D. and Westgate, S. J., Impact of Improved Local Control on Survival. *Inst. J. Radiat. Oncol. Biol. Phys.* **12**: 453–548, 1986.
7. Peters, L. J., Brock, W. A., Johnson, T., Meyen, R. E., Tofilon, P. J. and Milas, L., Potential Methods for Predicting Tumor Radiocurability. *Int. J. Radiat. Oncol. Biol. Phys.* **12**: 459–467, 1986.

8. Peters, L. J., Hopwood, L. E., Withers, H. R. and Suit, H. D., Predictive Assays of Tumor Radiocurability. *Cancer Treatment Symposia*, Vol. 1: 67–74, 1984.
9. Trott, K. R., *In Vivo* Measurements on the Tumour Predicting Response. In *Cancer Treatment: End Point Evaluation*. Ed. B. A. Stoll., John Wiley & Sons, Ltd., New York, 1983. 303–319.
10. Brock, W. A., Maor, M. H. and Peters, L. J., Predictors of tumor response to radiotherapy. *Radiation Research* **104**: 290–296, 1985.
11. Suit, H. D., Prediction of Response of Tumours to Radiation Treatment. In *Proceedings of the Third International Meeting on Progress in Radio-Oncology*. Ed: K. H. Karcher., In press, 1987.
12. Fletcher, G. H., Basic Principles of Radiotherapy. In *Textbook of Radiotherapy*. Third Edition. Lea and Febiger, Philadelphia, 1980. 180–228.
13. Suit, H. D., Shalek, R. J., Wette, R., Radiation response of C3H mouse mammary carcinoma evaluated in terms of cellular radiation sensitivity. In *Cellular Radiation Biology*. Williams & Wilkins, Baltimore, 1965. 514–530.
14. Todoroke, T. and Suit, H. D., Therapeutic Advantage in Preoperative Single Dose Radiation Combined with Conservative and Radical Surgery in Different Size Murine Fibrosarcomas. *J. Surg. Oncol.* **29**: 207–215, 1985.
15. Gelinas, M. and Fletcher, G. H., Incidence and causes of local failure of irradiation in squamous cell carcinoma of the faucial arch, tonsillar fossa, and base of tongue. *Radiology* **108**: 383–387, 1973.
16. Overgaard, J., Hansen, H. S., Jorgensen, K. and Hansen, M. H., Primary Radiotherapy of Larynx and Pharynx Carcinoma—An Analysis of Some Factors Influencing Local Control and Survival. *Int. J. Radiat. Oncol. Biol. Phys.* **12**: 515–521, 1986.
17. Bush, R. S., Conference Summary. Comments and conclusions from clinical studies. *Brit. J. Cancer* **41** (Suppl.IV): 323–331, 1980.
18. Overgaard, J., Unpublished data. 1987.
19. Hart, R. M., Evans, R. G., Kimler, B. F. and Park, C. H., Radiotherapeutic Management of Medulloblastoma in a Pediatric Patient with Ataxia Telangiectasia. *Int. J. Radiat. Oncol. Biol. Phys.* 12 Suppl. 1: 114, 1986.
20. Evans, R. G., Personal communication. 1987.
21. Suit, H. D., Lindberg, R. D. and Fletcher, G. H., Prognostic significance of extent of tumor regression at completion of radiation therapy. *Radiology* **84**: 1100–1107, 1965.
22. Barkley, H. T. and Fletcher, G. H., The significance of residual disease after external irradiation of squamous cell carcinoma of the oropharynx. *Radiology* **124**: 493, 1977.
23. Suit, H. D and Walker, A. M., Assessment of the response of tumours to radiation: Clinical and experimental studies. *Brit. J. Cancer* **41** (Suppl. IV): 1–10, 1980.
24. Suit, H. D., Sedlacek, R., Fagundes, L., Goitein, M. and Rothman, K., Time distribution of recurrences of an immunogenic and non-immunogenic tumor following local irradiation. *Radiation Research* **73**: 251–266, 1978.
25. Brahme, A., Dosimetric precision requirements in radiation therapy. *Acta Radiol. Oncol.* **23** (Fasc.5): 379–391, 1984.
26. Williams, M. V., Denekamp, J. and Fowler, J. F., Dose-response relationships for human tumors: Implications for clinical trials of dose modifying agents. *Int. J. Radiat. Oncol. Biol. Phys.* **10**: 1703–1707, 1984.
27. Mijnheer, B. J., Battermann, J. J. and Wambersie, A., What degree of accuracy is required and can be achieved in photon and neutron therapy? Submitted to *Radiotherapy and Oncology*, 1987.
28. Suit, H. D., Radiation biology: A basis for radiotherapy. In *Textbook of Radiotherapy*, G. H. Fletcher, 2nd Edition, Lea & Febiger, Philadelphia, 1973, 75–121.

29. Ramsay, J. and Suit, H. D., Unpublished data.
30. Fischer, J. J. and Moulder, J. E., The steepness of the Dose-response curve in radiation therapy. *Radiology* 117: 179–184, 1975.
31. Siracka, E., Siracky, J., Pappova, N. and Revesz, L., Vascularization and radio-curability in cancer of the uterine cervix. *Neoplasma* 29: 183–188, 1982.
32. Awwad, H. K., El Naggar, M., Mocktar, N. and Barsoum, M., Intercapillary distance measurement as an indicator of hypoxia in carcinoma of the cervix uteri. *Int. J. Radiat. Onco. Biol. Phys.* In press, 1986.
33. Hedley, D. W., Friedlander, M. L., Tayler, I. W., Rugg, C. A. and Musgrove, E. A., Method for analysis of cellular DNA content of paraffin-embedded pathological material for flow cytometry. *J. Histochem. Cytochem.* 31: 1333–1335, 1983.
34. Blitzer, P., Wang, C. C., Suit, H. D. and Stracher, M. A., 1987. Unpublished data.
35. Quilty, P. M. and Duncan, W., The influence of hemoglobin level on the regression and long term local control of transitional cell carcinoma of the bladder following photon irradiation. *Int. J. Radiat. Oncol. Biol. Phys.* 12: 1735–1742, 1986.

PART I

TUMOR HISTOLOGY AND MOLECULAR PATHOLOGY

2

Morphometric Indices of Tumor Progression and Response to Treatment in Prostatic Carcinoma

John E. McNeal, Thomas A. Stamey, Fuad S. Freiha, and Elise Redwine

INTRODUCTION

Adenocarcinoma of the prostate has long been regarded as a cancer whose natural history and response to treatment are highly unpredictable.[1,2] Uniquely among malignant tumors, the frequency of incidentally discovered prostate carcinoma at autopsy is on the order of 100-fold higher than the prevalence of clinically recognized disease.[2] It has accordingly been proposed that the vast majority of prostate cancers are biologically "latent", that is incapable of behaving aggressively, and that latent cancers are morphologically indistinguishable from the few aggressive carcinomas.[3] This concept leads to the conclusion that it is impossible to identify which patients need treatment, and extremely difficult to evaluate treatment response since all but a small fraction of patients will have a favorable clinical course independent of any intervention.

The concept of latent carcinoma has been partly refuted by the successful use of clinical staging by rectal examination and histologic grading of biopsy samples to predict prognosis.[4] The uniquely broad range of histologic differentiation seen in prostatic carcinoma has facilitated the development of reliable grading systems, but the range of variation in prognosis about the mean average for any grade has weakened the value of this information for the individual patient. In part, this broad range of prognosis about the mean may result from the fact that tumor areas of different histologic grade often coexist in a single prostate cancer, and biopsy samples may not be representative.

The difficulty of evaluating prognostic indices and therapeutic modalities is compounded by the fact that in prostate cancer, distant metastases may not be detectable for a number of years following treatment of the primary tumor. For example, in a recent study, it was reported that a series of patients having the most favorable clinical stage of prostate cancer showed no evidence of distant metastases after four years with no treatment.[5] Subsequently, it was reported that after a few additional years of follow up, 16% of these patients *had* developed metastases.[6] The appearance of delayed matastasis has made it difficult to compare the relative value of radiation therapy versus radical prostatectomy as definitive treatments for this malignancy.

It has been our conviction that the apparent unpredictability of prostate carcinoma stems in large part from the inadequacy of rectal examination to estimate tumor volume and from the inability of small biopsy samples to forecast the histologic grade of the entire tumor. These inaccuracies have continued to give some credence to the concept of "latent carcinoma", though this concept has never been proven and was based on the assumption that deviation of prostate cancer from the behavior of other malignancies was equivalent to unpredictability.

We have sought to discover the determinants of biologic behavior in prostatic carcinoma through detailed quantitative morphologic analysis of entire tumors in radical prostatectomy specimens coupled with careful long-term clinical follow-up.[7] The primary morphologic variables quantiated were tumor volume and histologic grade. The primary biologic endpoint was the appearance of distant metastasis facilitated by the use of serum prostate-specific antigen as an early index of recurrent disease. The presence of lymph node metastases at time of surgery was taken as a secondary biologic endpoint, and the extent of capsule penetration and seminal vesicle invasion were also quantitated for comparison with other predictive variables.

The hypothesis that tumor volume is a determinant of biologic behavior is derived from the concept of "tumor progression" as defined by Foulds.[8] Using evidence from a variety of human and animal tumors, Foulds concluded that cancers do not express their full biologic malignant potential at inception but acquire many of their aggressive features with the passage of time. Recent evidence for the common spontaneous evolution of cell heterogeneity in populations of malignant cells provides support for this concept.[9,11] Goldie and Coldman[12] have derived a mathematical model which relates the rate of evolution of cell heterogeneity to the time of development of drug resistance or metastatic capability. The time scale is the number of tumor cell population doublings, which should be roughly proportional to the volume of the cancer.

In addition, we hypothesized that the wide range of histologic differentiation expressed in prostatic carcinoma is a morphologic reflection of evolving cell heterogeneity. It has never been established whether poorly differentiated prostatic cancers are high grade malignancies at inception or whether they evolve from better differentiated neoplasms. If evolution to poor differentiation is the rule, then there are two morphologic indices of stage of progression in this neoplasm which can be used to establish the phase of the disease at which metastatic potential first appears.

In this model, it is not expected that the relationship between volume and differentiation should be invariant. In the concept of evolving cell heterogeneity, the development of any given malignant characteristic depends on a mutational event or a series of such events. At each cell division there is a small and probably constant probability of occurrence, which depends on the inherent degree of genetic or epigenetic instability in the cell population. Based on these assumptions, the mathematical formulations proposed by Goldie and Coldman show that a biologic alteration first appears in a few of a large series of tumors after a definite number of cell doublings. With each successive doubling, the proportion of tumors showing biologic alteration increases along a sigmoid curve until, after a relatively small number of tumor mass doublings, nearly all tumors show the change in biologic (or morphologic) features. If the alteration is a shift to higher histologic grade, it would be expected to appear in an increasing percentage of cancers across a range of volume. However, once the shift to higher grade appears in a given tumor and, assuming that it has a higher proliferation rate, the volume of higher grade cancer should represent a larger proportion of total tumor volume after each successive mass doubling.

THE EXPERIMENT AND RESULTS

A preliminary study was performed on 100 prostates with carcinoma in a series of unselected autopsies at Herrick Memorial Hospital, Berkeley, California.[7] In four of these patients, carcinoma was diagnosed during life, but none had prostatectomy. Evidence of distant metastasis was sought in clinical and autopsy records, but lymph nodes were not studied. In this portion of the study, the relationship between tumor volume and differentiation across the entire volume range was investigated, and criteria were established to relate capsule penetration to other variables.

The main portion of the study consisted of 100 radical prostatectomies with lymph node dissections performed for clinically-diagnosed and biopsy-confirmed prostate cancer. Patients with nodal metastases discovered at laparotomy did not have prostatectomy, but some cases with microscopic nodal metastases were found after prostatectomy. Quantitative criteria for capsule penetration established in the preliminary study were applied to these cases. Refined grading criteria established during the preliminary study were also used.

In both series, the prostates were serially blocked at 3mm intervals, and the areas of tumor on each slide were outline in ink and transferred by tracing to maps showing the extent and contour of each cancer. Where more than one cancer was indentified, only the largest was considered. The tumor areas measured from each slide were summed and multiplied by the section thickness and a factor of 1.5 to correct for tissue shrinkage during processing. This value was recorded as the tumor volume.

In each series, cancers were graded by the Gleason system[4] based on inspection of all tumor areas. In the preliminary study, Gleason primary and secondary grades were recorded, and the higher of these two numbers were used in final tabulation. In the main study, all grades seen were recorded, and the percent contribution of each grade to total tumor area was estimated. In the final tabulation, the percent of the tumor composed of Gleason grades 4 and 5 was the only parameter used.

In the preliminary study, depth of capsule penetration of the tumor was quantitated at three levels; tumor in contact with capsule (level I), tumor penetrating into capsule (level II) and tumor completely through capsule (level III). At each level, the extent of penetration was measured as the sum of centimeter lengths of penetration at that level on all slides. In the main study only the extent of penetration at level III was measured.

All patients were entered into an extensive follow up program, including periodic serum PSA measurement. We have determined that PSA elevation is reliably the earliest indication of disease progression.[13] Where disease progression consisted of recurrent tumor in the pelvis, radiation therapy was administered, and patients continued to be followed for evidence of distant metastases. Local recurrences were tabulated in a different category from distant metastases. The follow up program has been in operation for over three years.

In the preliminary study, 100 autopsy carcinomas were divided into five consecutive volume ranges, and the number of tumors of each Gleason grade was tabulated for each range (Figure 2.1). Grades 1 and 2 were combined and Grade 3 was subdivided into tumors with

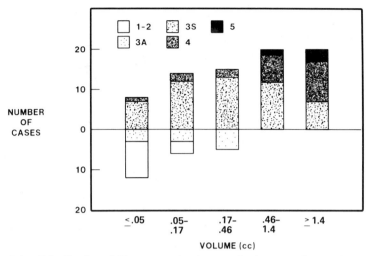

FIG. 2.1.   Distribution of Gleason grades (worse of primary and secondary grades) among five consecutive volume ranges (cubic centimeters) of 20 cases each in 100 prostate cancers at autopsy.

relatively large, well-formed glands (3A) and those with very small, poorly-formed glands (3S). Highly differentiated cancers (Grades 1–2) were found only in the two smallest volume ranges (under 0.17cc), and poorly differentiated carcinomas (Grades 4 and 5) were common only in the two largest volume ranges (over 0.46cc). The findings were consistent with the hypothesis that the great majority of prostatic carcinomas are highly differentiated or moderately differentiated at inception and become poorly differentiated with time and increasing volume.

The four carcinomas in this series which were clinically recognized and had distant metastases were among the largest ten cancers of the series; the smallest was 5.4cc in volume. All four cancers which had metastasized were either Grade 4 or Grade 5. It was concluded that both grade and volume were valid measures of biologic progression and that the evolution of Grade 4 carcinoma probably represented a strong morphologic marker for acquisition of metastatic capability.

In the main series of prostatectomy cases, the 100 cancers were divided into four consecutive volume ranges and degrees of histologic differentiation was compared between tumors of different volumes (Figure 2.2). Rather than using the entire range of Gleason grades, the estimated percent of tumor area which was poorly differentiated (Grade 4 and 5) was tabulated for each cancer. A progressive trend to greater numbers of poorly differentiated carcinomas and larger percent of

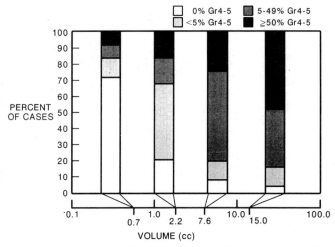

FIG. 2.2.   Proportion of poorly differentiated areas (Gleason grades 4–5) in 100 prostate cancers from radical prostatectomies as a function of tumor volume (cubic centimeters). Comparison between four consecutive volume ranges of 25 cases each.

poorly differentiated areas was found across all volume ranges. The trend was similar to that shown in Figure 2.1, although 90 of the 100 prostatectomy cancers were in the volume range occupied by the largest 40 of the autopsy carcinomas (< 0.46cc).

We hypothesized that the appearance of Grade 4 areas represents a mutational event with a constant probability of occurrence at each cell division. Following Goldie's model, we drew a hypothetical sigmoid curve of the percent of tumors showing Grade 4–5 areas as a function of increasing tumor volume (Figure 2.3). We further hypothesized that Grade 4–5 areas would have a proliferation rate higher than that of the better differentiated areas, so that once Grade 4–5 areas had appeared they would comprise a larger proportion of the cancer at each tumor mass doubling. This progression is represented by a series of sigmoid curves to the right of the initial curve in Figure 2.3. Such a hypothetical model predicts that at successive volume increments there will be a progressive shift in the number of tumors having any given percent of Grade 4–5 areas, as illustrated by the vertical bars. Figure 2.4 illustrates the fit of our data from Figure 2.2 to this set of hypothetical curves.

The intercorrelations between cancer volume, differentiation, capsule penetration and seminal vesicle invasion are shown in Figure 2.5. The correlations are almost identical to those for the autopsy carcinomas larger than 0.46cc. Thus, it would appear that clinically evident carcinomas simply represent the higher end of the volume range in the

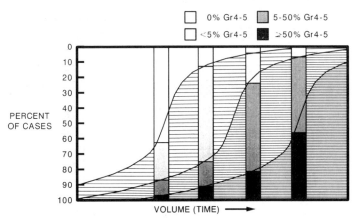

FIG. 2.3. Hypothetical increase in proportion of Gleason grade 4–5 cancer with volume, assuming that Grade 4–5 cancer is a more rapidly growing mutation with a constant probability of occurrence at each cell division (sigmoid curve). Growth rate of Grade 4–5 cancer is presumed constant (space between curves).

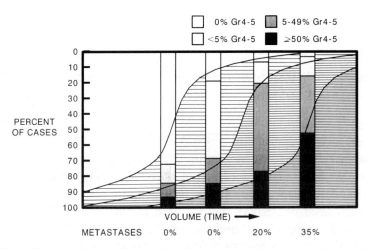

FIG. 2.4. Correspondence of actual data from prostatectomy cancers (Figure 2.2) to hypothetical curves of Figure 2.3.

same population of cancers which is identified incidentally at autopsy. There are many prostate cancers which are clinically innocuous because there are many prostate cancers which are very small. The above data do not indicate a need to propose the existence of a group of "latent carcinomas".

The patients who had lymph node metastases at surgery or subsequently developed distant metastases are also identified in Figure

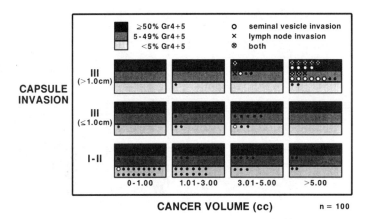

FIG. 2.5.   Relationship of cancer volume and capsule penetration to differentiation, seminal vesicle invasion, and lymph node involvement in 100 prostate cancers at prostatectomy. Fourteen cases designated as lymph node positive include two cases with distant metastases and no lymph node involvement. Level III capsule penetration is complete penetration of capsule. Extent of level III measured in length of capsule segment penetrated.

2.5. They are all high volume, high grade cancers emphasizing a high degree of predictability in the natural history of prostatic carcinoma which is supported logically by the concept of tumor progression.

DISCUSSION

Rational therapy of cancer and accurate prediction of response to therapy depend on an understanding of the natural history and biologic features of the neoplasm under study. Attempts to extrapolate from the behavior of other neoplasms to that of carcinoma in the prostate have failed, leading to an underserved reputation of unpredictability. Ours is the first attempt to define the biologic behavior of prostate cancer through a detailed study of the morphology of prostate cancer. Though our clinical follow-up program is still in an early phase, our evidence to date suggests that prostate cancer may well be among the most predictable of malignant tumors. The strong correlation of both volume and differentiation with stage of progression have not been reported for other cancers. Their evaluation requires examination of the entire carcinoma removed at prostatectomy, as demonstrated by shortcomings of estimating volume at rectal examination and grade through biopsy sampling. The possibility remains that volume can be reliably estimated by *in vivo* imaging techniques such as ultrasound and that tissue culture behavior and immunohistochemistry may reveal important cell biology parameters on small samples.

At present, prostatectomy provides not only the surest definitive therapy for smaller prostate cancers but also the only way to evaluate prognosis. The possibility that radiation therapy might produce comparable results probably cannot be tested until there are better ways of determining the stage of biologic progression of any given cancer without removing the prostate.

The next frontier in therapy of prostatic carcinoma will be the effective treatment of distant metastasis. Chemotherapy and hormonal therapy have not shown much promise in the treatment of demonstrable metastatic disease. However, our results to date suggest that we will be able to identify a group of patients who are at exceptionally high risk of having undetectable microscopic metastases at the time of prostatectomy. We currently believe that only Grade 4 and Grade 5 carcinoma have a substantial ability to metastasize and that risk of metastasis is proportional to the absolute volume of Grade 4–5 rumor. By multiplying total tumor volume by estimated percent Grade 4–5, we have found that only two of 14 patients with nodal metastasis or subsequent distant metastasis have less than 3cc of Grade 4–5 cancer.

Once better defined, this high risk group is a logical target for efforts to develop effective adjuvant chemotherapy and/or hormonal therapy. The failure of these modalities in patients with large volume metastatic disease may not accurately predict poor responsiveness of microscopic disease. Our contribution in this area is therefore toward the precise definition of the problem, which is prerequisite to finding its solution.

REFERENCES

1. Whitmore, W. F., The natural history of prostatic cancer. *Cancer* **32**: 1104–12 1973.
2. Stamey, T. A., Cancer of the prostate: an analysis of some important contributions and dilemmas. *Monogr. Urol.* **3**: 67–94 1982.
3. Franks, L. M., Latent carcinoma of the prostate. *J. Pathol. Bacteriol* **68**: 603–16 1954.
4. Gleason, D. F., Histologic grading and clinical staging of prostatic carcinoma. In *Urologic Pathology: The Prostate* (M. Tannenbaum, Ed.), Lea & Febiger, Philadelphia, 1977.
5. Cantrell, B. B., DeKlerk, D. P., Eggleston, J. C., Boitnott, J. K., and Walsh, P. C., Pathological factors that influence prognosis in stage A prostatic cancer: the influence of extent versus grade. *J. Urol.* **125**: 516–20 1981.
6. Epstein, J. I., Paull, G., Eggleston, J. C. and Walsh, P. C., Prognosis of untreated stage A1 prostatic carcinoma: a study of 94 cases with extended follow-up. *J. Urol.* **136**: 837–39 1986.

7. McNeal, J. E. Bostwick, D. G., Kindrachuk, R. A., Redwine, E. A., Freiha, F. S. and Stamey, T. A., Patterns of progression in prostate cancer. *Lancet* **1**: 60–63 1986.
8. Foulds, L., The Experimental study of tumor progression: a review. *Cancer Res.* **14**: 327–39 1954.
9. Nowell, P. C., The clonal evolution of tumor cell populations. *Science* **194**: 23–28 1976.
10. Fidler, I. J. and Hart, I. R., Biologic diversity in metastatic neoplasms: origins and implications. *Science* **217**: 998–1003 1982.
11. Poste G. and Greig, R., On the genesis and regulation of cellular heterogeneity in malignant tumors. *Invas. Metast.*, **2**: 137–76 1982).
12. Goldie, J. H. and Coldman, A. J., A mathematical model for relating the drug sensitivity of tumors to their spontaneous mutation rate. *Cancer Treat. Rep.* **63**: 1727–31 1979).
13. Stamey, T. A., Unpublished data.

3

Proto-Oncogenes in Human Cancer: Implications for Treatment

Martin J. Cline

INTRODUCTION

Proto-oncogenes were originally defined as normal genes similar in structure to cancer-inducing genes of certain retroviruses. A better definition for proto-oncogene is a normal cellular gene with the potential to contribute to the induction or progression of a malignant tumor when its structure or expression is altered.[1,2]

TABLE 3.1 *Classes of Proto-oncogenes*

I.	*Protein Kinases* src fgr abl ros yes fps fes met pim-l kit
II.	*Growth Factor Related* erbB1. erbB2(neu) fms sis erbA
III.	*GTP-Binding* ras-Ha ras-Ki N-ras
IV.	*Nuclear Localization* myc N-myc L-myc myb fos

Proto-oncogenes can be grouped according to their function, including genes for growth factors or their receptors, for guanosine triphosphate (GTP)-binding proteins, for protein kinases, and for DNA-binding proteins (Table 3.1). Although we do not understand the functions of most oncogene proteins in detail, there is evidence that many oncogenes are involved in controlling cell proliferation. The best understood proto-oncogenes are those that encode growth factors or receptors for growth factors. Examples include the c-erb B1, c-erb B2,

33

and c-sis oncogenes.[1,3–5] Many other proto-oncogenes encode proteins which reside at or near the cell membrane and have protein kinase activity (Table 3.1).[6] This activity is presumed to phosphorylate critical intracytoplasmic proteins and thereby modify their structure and function. The membrane-associated protein kinases thereby act as a system for signal transmission from the surface to the interior of the cell. Another class of proto-oncogenes also involves a signal transduction system. These encode proteins which reversibly bind GTP. These proteins are also located near the cell surface and are related to proteins which mediate the cellular responses to various hormones. Another class of proto-oncogenes, including *c-myc* and *c-myb*, encodes proteins which bind to DNA.

PROTO-ONCOGENE ACTIVATION

Proto-oncogenes can be activated to become cancer-inducing genes by a variety of circumstances. Several mechanisms of activation have been identified, including chromosomal translocation, genetic mutation, and gene amplification. In some animal tumors, a fourth mechanism of promoter insertion has been identified.

Chromosomal rearrangements are frequent in human cancers, and non-random chromosomal rearrangements are the rule in particular types of cancer. These rearrangements may alter the structure of a proto-oncogene or alter the controls of expression of a proto-oncogene—which, in turn, result in qualitative or quantitative abnormalities of the protein products of the proto-oncogenes. Oncogenes thus far identified in such chromosomal translocations are *c-myc* in B cell lyphomas and *c-abl* in chronic myeloid leukemia.

Mutation within the coding sequence of an oncogene can also activate the gene with production of an altered protein. Such mutations can arise from chemical mutagens or ionizing irradiation.

Amplification is another means of proto-oncogene activation. Most proto-oncogenes occur as single copy genes (i.e., one copy of the gene on a single chromosome). In some tumors, many copies of an oncogene occur. This phenomenon is known as gene amplification. Amplified proto-oncogenes allow cancer cells to make more oncoproteins and are presumed thereby to endow cells with a proliferative advantage or altered growth characteristics. Many examples of proto-oncogene amplification have been found in human cancers.[8]

TABLE 3.2 *Proto-oncogene Alterations in Human Cancer*

Alteration	Tumor Type	Approximate Frequency
Tumor Specific		
N-*myc* amplification	Neuroendocrine	20%
N-*ras* mutation	Acute myeloid leukemia	10–50%
c-*abl* translocation	Chronic myelocytic leukemia	> 90%
c-*myc* gene translocation	Burkitt's lymphoma	> 80%
c-*erbB1* amplification	Squamous carcinomas	10–20%
c-*erbB2* amplification	Adenocarcinomas	10–20%
p53 rearrangement	Osteosarcomas	?
Tumor Non-specific		
c-*myc* amplification	Adeno- and squamous-carcinomas and sarcomas	10–20%
c-*myb* allelic deletion	Adeno- and squamous-carcinomas and sarcomas	10–30%
c-*ras-Ha* allelic deletion	Adeno- and squamous-carcinomas and sarcomas	10–30%
c-*ras-Ha* and c-*ras-Ki* mutations	Carcinomas	10%

PROTO-ONCOGENE ALTERATION IN HUMAN CANCER

A number of proto-oncogene alterations occur in human cancers (Table 3.2). Some alterations are frequent, others are rare. Some proto-oncogenes are altered in a variety of tumors, whereas others are altered only in specific tumor types. For example, c-*myc* is amplified in a variety of adenocarcinomas, squamous carcinomas, and sarcomas, whereas the same gene is translocated to the region of an immunoglobulin gene in B cell lymphomas. Mutation of the 13th codon of the N-*ras* proto-oncogene has been identified only in acute myeloid leukemias.

c-*erbB1* encodes the epidermal growth factor receptor. It is amplified only in squamous carcinomas and brain tumors where increased copies of the receptor are apt to convey a proliferative advantage. c-*erbB2* also encodes a protein that probably functions as a growth factor receptor on glandular epithelium, since c-*erbB2* has been found to be amplified only in adenocarcinomas.[5]

ONCOGENE ACTIVATION AND TUMOR BEHAVIOR

Some proto-oncogene changes, such as amplification of c-*myc* in carcinomas and of c-*erbB2* in adenocarcinomas are more frequent in metastases than in primary tumors, suggesting a correlation between gene amplification and tumor progression or metastatic potential.

There is evidence that certain oncogene alterations correlate with the stage and behavior of certain human cancers. The most thoroughly studied example is N-myc amplification in neuroblastomas,[9] although amplification of this proto-oncogene occurs in only about 20% of these tumors.

Changes in several oncogenes correlate with clinical behavior of breast cancer. We have found proto-oncogene alterations in about 60% of primary breast cancers. These involve the *c-myc, c-myb, c-ras-Ha, c-rasKi,* and *c-erbB2* proto-oncogenes. In a study of 53 primary breast cancer cases operated upon in 1983 and 1984, we found alterations were more frequent in large tumors and in stage III and IV tumors. For example, the frequency of amplified *c-erbB2* in lymph node negative and positive primary breast cancers was, respectively, 0 of 14 and 8 of 35 (P < 0.05). Similarly, proto-oncogene abnormalities were more frequent in those tumors which recurred within two years of modified radical mastectomy than in those which did not recur (14 of 15 vs. 10 of 26). These data suggest that analysis of proto-oncogenes may provide prognostic information about tumor behavior and may shape therapeutic strategy in breast cancer.

IMPLICATIONS FOR THERAPY

Knowledge about proto-oncogene alterations in hhuman cancer may have an impact on current treatment programs and in ddevising new therapies. The neuroblastoma/N-myc story illustrates one application of molecular analysis of proto-oncogenes to cancer treatment.[9] As noted above, amplification of this gene generally occurs in poor prognostic tumors of stages III and IV.. When *N-myc* amplification occurs in an early sttage tumor, it probably means that this tumor will behave in an unusually aggressive manner. Therefore, more aggressive treatment of stage I and II tumors with *N-myc* amplification is being considered. Similarly, the identification of certain proto-oncogene alterations in primary breast cancers with negaative axillary lymph nodes could ultimately be an indication for adjuvant chemotherapy. It seems likely, therefore, that proto-oncogene analysis will be used to identify subsets of tumors requiring particular treatment, much as we now use antigenic analysis to identify particular subsets of leukemias and lymphomas.

Most of this information has been included in another recently published review by the author.[10]

REFERENCES

1. Bishop, J. M., Cellular oncogenes and retroviruses. *Ann. Rev. Biochem.* **52**: 301–354, 1983.
2. Cooper, G. M., Cellular transforming genes. *Science* **218**: 801, 1982.
3. Downward, J., Yarden, Y., Mayes, E., Scrace, G., Totty, N., Stockwell, P., Ullrich, A., Schlessinger, J. and Waterfield, M. D., Close similarity of epidermal growth factor receptor and v-erb-B oncogene protein sequences. *Nature* (London) **307**: 521–527, 1984.
4. Klein, G. and Klein, E., Evolution of tumors and the impact of molecular oncology. *Nature* (London) **315**: 190–195, 1985.
5. Yokota, J., Teroda, M., Togoshima, K., Sugimura, T., Yamamoto, T., Battafora, H. and Cline, M. J., Amplification of the *c-erbB2* oncogene in human adenocarcinomas *in vivo*. *Lancet* **1**: 765–767, 1986.
6. Hunter T., The proteins of oncogenes. *Scientif. Amer.* **248**: 70, 1984.
7. Hurley, J. B., Simon, M. I., Teplow, D. B., Robinshaw, J. K. and Gilman, A. F., Homologies between signal transducing G protein and ras gene products. *Science* **226**: 860–862, 1984.
8. Yokota, J., Tsunetsugu-Yokota, Y., Battafora, H., Lefevre, C. and Cline, M. J., Alterations of the myc, myb, and Harvey-ras proto-oncogenes are frequent in human cancers and show clinical correlation. *Science* **231**: 261–265, 1986.
9. Seeger, R. C., Brodeur, G. M., Sather, H., Dalton, A., Siegel, S. E., Wong, K. Y. and Hammond, D., Association of multiple copies of the N-myc oncogene with rapid progression of neuroblastomas. *New Engl. J. Med.* **313**: 1111–1116, 1985.
10. Cline, M. J., Keynote address: The role of proto-oncogenes in human cancer: Implications for diagnosis and treatment. *Int. J. Radiat. oncol. Biol. Phys.* **13**: 1297–1301, 1987.

4

Tumor-Associated Carbohydrate Antigens as Developmentally Regulated and Prognostic Markers: A Novel Integrated Approach Using Synthetic Antigens and Corresponding Monoclonal Antibodies

B. Michael Longenecker, Grant D. MacLean, Alexander J. B. McEwan, Carina Henningsson, Tom R. Sykes, S. Selvaraj, Mavanur R. Suresh, and Antoine A. Noujaim

INTRODUCTION

The diagnosis and management of cancer remains a major problem for the medical community at this time. CAT scanning enabled detection of lesions as small as 5–10mm, but the findings are often nonspecific. Certain tumor markers (e.g., beta HCG and AFP) have dramatically altered the management of germ cell malignancies, but for the majority of cancers there are no sensitive and specific serodiagnostic markers.

The histology of "adenocarcinoma" gives no indication of its behavioral characteristics. It may be a relatively indolent cancer or an aggressive malignancy. It may be drug sensitive or resistant and it may have come from any one of a number of different primary sources. Considering three common examples of adenocarcinoma illustrates these points.

In 1985, in Alberta, there were 910 new patients diagnosed with breast cancer, 852 new cases of colorectal cancer, and 155 new cases of ovarian cancer. During the same year there were 278, 368, and 66 deaths from these same three cancers, respectively. Despite similar histological characteristics, these cancers may have different patterns of metastasis and different sensitivities to systemic therapy. Nearly three quarters of patients receiving chemotherapy for breast cancer respond to treatment. However, there is conflicting evidence that this response conveys survival advantage. In contrast, less than one quarter of patients with colorectal cancer respond to chemotherapy. Smith and co-workers failed to find any survival advantage conferred to these patients by chemotherapy.[1] More than two thirds of patients with adenocarcinoma of the ovary respond to aggressive chemotherapy, with significant survival advantage for many.[2] Nevertheless, we cannot determine which patients with metastatic ovarian cancer will benefit from aggressive combination chemotherapy. A response rate of 60–80% is encouraging[2], but early relapses and failures to respond, resulting in nearly 40–50% mortality at two years, motivate us to attempt to identify those patients for whom current therapy is either inadequate or inappropriately aggressive.

All three of these common cancers can be widely disseminated without symptoms, clinical signs, or definite abnormalities on scans or X-rays. For most cancers, there are no sensitive or specific serodiagnostic markers which enable detection of early relapse or disease progression. For none of these common cancers is there a reliable prognostic marker which indicates which patients are likely to benefit from aggressive interventional therapy. Jacobs and co-workers examined the morphologic parameters of histologic differentiation, mitotic activity, and cellular pleomorphism in ovarian cancer and found that none of these was associated with response to therapy or survival.[3]

The hybridoma technology[4] created the possibility of designing new tests for detection of new serum tumor markers by monoclonal antibodies (MAbs) and the possibility of radioimmunodetection of metastatic cancer. In this monograph, we will focus our discussion on cancer-associated carbohydrate markers of potential diagnostic and especially prognostic significance. In particular, we will present some of the data summarizing our recent experience using synthetic tumor-associated carbohydrate antigens of the Thomsen-Freidenreich (TF) and Tn series. This novel integrated approach emphasizes serodiagnosis, immunohistology, radioimmunoimaging, and therapy.

The Thomsen-Freidenreich (TF) antigenic determinant is revealed on human erythrocytes by neuraminidase treatment, and is described as part of the MN blood group antigens. TF has been characterized as β-D-Gal-$(1\rightarrow3)$-α-GalNAc attached to glycophorin or other proteins through O-serine or O-threonine-linkages.[5] Tn, the TF precursor, is reported to be α-GalNAc-O-serine/threonine. TF is normally cryptic, due to the presence of a terminal sialic acid residue while Tn is exposed only in individuals with a recessive genetic disorder.[6] Springer[5] has claimed expression of TF and Tn determinants on over 90% of cancers of the breast, lung, and pancreas—although the molecular nature of the determinants was not clear.

Our group was the first to generate MAbs against TF-like antigens expressed on human cancer cells.[7,8] Recently, we reported the successful use of synthetic tumor-associated glycoconjugates (S-TAGs) to derive MAbs with human cancer specificity[9] and to directly stimulate T cells which display anti-cancer reactivity.

THE COMBINED USE OF SYNTHETIC TUMOR-ASSOCIATED GLYCOCONJUGATES AND THEIR CORRESPONDING MAbs

Our main objective was to develop clinically useful MAbs, using S-TAGs as immunogens and S-TAGs themselves, not only for tumor detection and monitoring but also for enabling assessment of tumor invasiveness or aggressiveness. These reagents may be useful in assessing prognosis and in planning therapy. Figure 4.1 illustrates the structures of the various S-TAGs and control antigens used in these studies. Figure 4.2 illustrates the various applications of the S-TAGs and their corresponding specific MAbs. Because S-TAGs can be conveniently synthesized in relatively large amounts (hundreds of mgs) and as they are >99% pure as judged by NMR, it is possible to precisely predefine the specificities of the MAbs produced against them. Furthermore, it is possible to choose from among hundreds of clones those with the highest affinity and desired specificity. Table 4.1 illustrates this principle, using MAbs generated against TF and Tn S-TAGs. We were able to generate several MAbs which react specifically with TF-α and Tn. None of the MAbs made against TFβ reacted with Tn, but all cross-reacted with TF-α.

TABLE 4.1 *Specificity of MAbs Generated Against TF or Tn S-TAGs*

Immunogen	No. of Clones	No. of clones positive[a] with:		
		TFα	TF-β	Tn
TF-α	55	55	11	8
TF-β	36	36	36	0
Tn	22	0	0	22

[a]As judged by ELISA using immobilized S-TAGs

STRUCTURE OF TERMINAL IMMUNODOMINANT GROUPS	NAME	TRIVIAL NAME
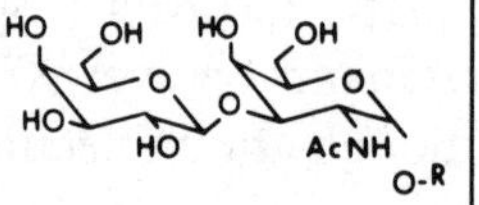	β-D-Gal-(1-3)-αGalNAc-O-(CH$_2$)$_8$-R	TF(α)
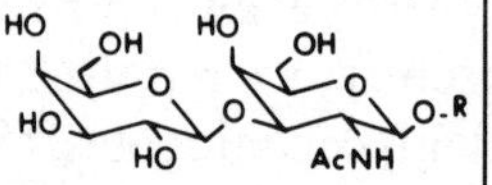	β-D-Gal-(1-3)-βGalNAc-O-(CH$_2$)$_8$-R	TF(β)
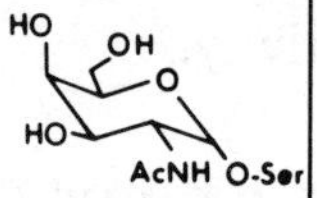	GalNAc-O-Ser-R	Tn
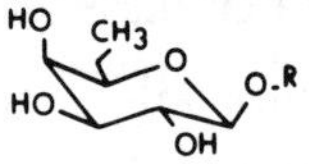	6-deoxy-D-Gal-O-R	Fuc.
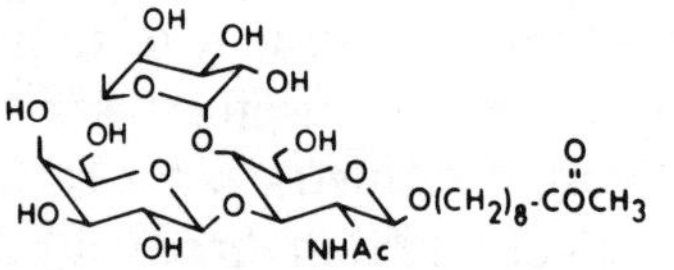	β-Gal-(1-3)-β-GlcNAc-O-(CH$_2$)$_8$-COCH$_3$ $\uparrow$ 1,4 α-Fucose	Lewis^a (Le^a)

FIG. 4.1.   The chemical structure of the synthetic antigens is shown along with the nomenclature. The Thomsen-Freidenreich (TF) haptens used in these studies were of both the TF alpha and TF beta conformation, referring to the linkage between the sugar ring and the carbohydrate spacer arm. Tn (GalNAc-O-serine) is the immediate precursor to TF alpha. Denoted as "R" is the carrier protein—in this case either HSA or KLH.

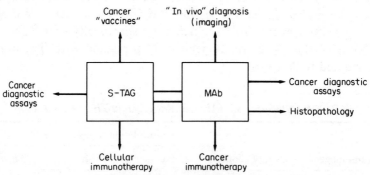

FIG. 4.2.   Schematic description of the various applications proposed for S-TAGs and corresponding MAbs.

IMMUNOHISTOCHEMISTRY: AN IMPORTANT TOOL FOR
DETERMINING THE CANCER SPECIFICITY OF ANTI-S-TAG MAbs

We routinely screen our anti-S-TAG MAbs on frozen sections of human tumors using an immunoperoxidase technique in an avidin biotin system. We have found that this technique provides important information on tumor specificity of MAbs which is not available using established human cell lines. In fact, we have found that many of our most promising anti-S-TAG MAbs for cancer diagnosis react strongly with frozen sections of appropriate cancers, but show little or no consistent reactivity with cancer cell lines of the same histological type. For example, MAb 155H.7, which reacts with approximately 90% of frozen sections of human adenocarcinomas[9] as well as with most human adenocarcinomas *in vivo* does not react consistently with any human adenocarcinoma cell line we have tested.

The immunoperoxidase technique on frozen sections can also be used to screen for specific changes in carbohydrate expression in "preneoplastic" lesions. For example, Yuan and co-workers[10] have used our MAb 49H.8[7] to document the early appearance of TF antigen in preneoplastic atypical areas in colon adenocarcinomas. Others have also noted that 49H.8 shows better cancer specificity when compared with PNA or polyclonal anti-TF antibodies[11]. We have also noted strong marking of 49H.8 in cell membrane structures in colon adenomas which were considered possibly "premalignant" by the pathologist reporting the routine histological (H & E) specimen. No marking was seen of "obviously benign adenomas".[10]

TABLE 4.2 *Summary of Radioimmunoimaging Results With MAb 155H.7*

Dose	Uptake			
	0	1	2	3
4mg	4	1	–	–
8mg	4	–	1	–
16mg	2	–	1	2
32mg	–	1	–	4

0 = no uptake
1 = equivocal uptake, less than liver activity
2 = uptake equal to liver activity
3 = uptake greater than liver activity

IN VIVO DIAGNOSIS: RADIOIMMUNOIMAGING WITH MAb 155H.7

The demonstration of uptake *in vitro* by about 90% of adenocarcinomas[9] and consistent tumor uptake *in vivo* in animal models[12] has led to the development of an extended Phase I clinical trial to evaluate possible toxicity and to determine if a dose effect was apparent.

Twenty patients have been imaged at doses of 4mg (five patients), 8mg (five patients), 16mg (five patients) and 32mg (five patients). The antibody was labelled with 80–120 MBq ^{131}I and injected by slow intravenous infusion in patients with prior negative patch testing with 155H.7. Anterior and posterior images of thorax and abdomen were obtained immediately after the infusion and at 24, 48, 72, and 96 hours post injection. The images were acquired over 10 minutes, and data were stored in a gamma camera computer. Patients were entered into the study if they had demonstrable metastatic disease from adenocarcinoma of the large bowel (nine patients), breast (seven patients), ovary (two patients), and endometrium (two patients). Informed consent was obtained from all patients.

No adverse reaction was noticed in any patients following injection of antibody at any dose level. Uptake of monoclonal antibody was graded by comparison with liver uptake. Equivocal uptake was noted in only one patient at a dose level of 4 and 8mg. As the dose of antibody was increased, uptake became increasingly evident, and at the 32mg dose level, four of the five patients showed unequivocal uptake (Table 4.2).

Uptake and retention data are currently being calculated from stored data to assess half-life of antibody in tumor and in normal tissues. Uptake has been noted in soft tissue and in bone metastases. Figure 4.3 demonstrates uptake in a palpable pelvic mass in the right iliac fossa in a patient with ovarian carcinoma. Uptake was evident 24 hours post injection and increased in intensity over the period of the study. Figure 4.4 shows uptake in the superior mediastinum in a patient with metastatic endometrial carcinoma.

The results clearly indicate a dose effect, and show that increasing doses of 155H.7 are associated with improvements in imaging efficacy. The images are unique, in that they are the first scintigraphic demonstration that tumor localization is possible using monoclonal antibodies generated against synthetic carbohydrate antigens. Uptake and kinetic data will be correlated with tumor vascularity and with clinical course to attempt to define prognostic indicators. The generation of monoclonal

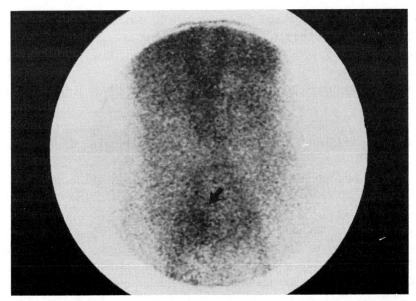

FIG. 4.3.   Radioimmunoimaging with ^{131}I-155H.7.
Uptake in a palpable pelvic mass (arrow) in an ovarian carcinoma patient is noted.

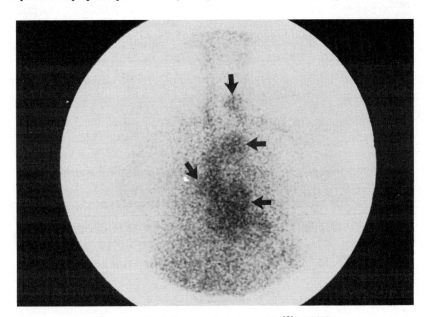

FIG. 4.4.   Radioimmunoimaging with ^{131}I-155H.7.
Uptake in lymph nodes in superior mediastinum (arrows) in a patient with metastatic endometrial carcinoma is noted. Heart uptake is also noted, which may be due to blood pool.

antibodies against TF and Tn antigens will offer the opportunity for assessing, *in vivo*, the ratio of TF/Tn uptake in tumors, to further refine these indicators, and to establish a role for radioimmunoimaging—not in the enumeration of metastatic sites but for the *in vivo* staging of primary and metastatic carcinoma.

IN VITRO DIAGNOSTIC ASSAYS: MEASUREMENT OF CIRCULATING ANTIGEN

As will be discussed later, a great deal of evidence indicates that the degree of expression of TF and/or Tn antigens on a tumor may relate to the stage of differentiation of that tumor, tumor aggressiveness, and perhaps prognosis. As it is not always possible to obtain appropriate tumor biopsies to estimate antigen expression using immunohisto-chemical techniques, our approach has been to develop novel methods to estimate relative degrees of carbohydrate epitope expression on glycoproteins shed from tumors. Using this approach we have demonstrated elevated serum levels (micrograms equivalents/ml) of TF in breast cancer:[13]

Normal Controls (n = 107)	19.2 ± 9.4
Metastatic Breast Ca (n = 45)	51.5 ± 23.2 (p<0.001)
Disease-Free Breast Ca Pts (n = 19)	28.0 ± 12.6 (p<0.005)
Benign Breast Disease (n = 90)	11.3 ± 14.0 (p<0.025)

TABLE 4.3 *Reactivity of Human MAb's with S-TAGs*[a]

Reactivity Patterns			Number of H-MAb Producing Clones
TFα	TFβ	Tn	
+	−	−	7
−	+	−	5
−	−	+	1
+	+	−	7
+	−	+	1
−	+	+	0
+	+	+	2

[a]As determined by ELISA on immobilized S-TAGs

MEASURING THE IMMUNE RESPONSE TO TF/Tn ANTIGENS—
THE HUMORAL RESPONSE

High titres of naturally occurring anti-TF antibodies pre-exist in all humans tested[5], and these titres have been reported to decrease in adenocarcinoma patients,[5,14] presumably due to the formation of antigen-antibody complexes. It has been reported that natural anti-TF antibodies are a heterogeneous mixture of carbohydrate-specific antibodies.[15] We established human B-cell clones secreting human anti-TF-like MAbs from lymph nodes draining human colon cancer in order to further characterize such antibodies. Table 4.3 illustrates the S-TAG specificity of 23 clones producing human monoclonal antibody produced by EBV-transformed B-cell lines.[16] It is noteworthy that we found all possible patterns of reactivity with TFα, TFβ, and Tn S-TAGs—with the exception of MAbs, which reacted with TFβ and Tn but not TFα. In contrast to our results obtained with murine MAbs (Table 4.1), we did detect five human MAbs which reacted specifically with TFβ. In Table 4.4 we illustrate the specificity of 55V.8, an IgM human MAb which reacts strongly with TFα and TFβ with some crossreactivity with Tn. This MAb reacts with neuraminidase-treated human RBC and WBC as well as with all human carcinoma cell lines examined to date—strongly suggesting that it reacts with natural TF-like determinants on human cells. Unlike most human MAb-producing clones, the 55V.8 clone is extremely stable, having been in culture for over three years and consistently producing about 50μg of MAb/ml of culture fluid.

TABLE 4.4 *Specificity of Human MAb 55V.8*

S-TAGs	Tumor Cell Lines	Human Blood Cells
HSA 0.02±0.01[a]	209.D6[c] 0.76±0.06	RBC 0.21±0.32
TFα 1.98±0.40	209.D7[d] 0.74±0.07	N'-RBC[i] 1.12±0.10
TFβ 1.76±0.21	LoVo[e] 0.74±0.10	PBL 0.04±0.01
Tn 0.58±0.09	SKLu.1[f] 0.69±0.09	N'-PBL 0.64±0.05
Epi[b] 0.99±0.08	SKOV.3[g] 0.32±0.06	
	CAOV.3[h] 0.67±0.08	

[a] OD±S.D. determined using an ELISA
[b] Epiglycanin—a tumor-associated glycoprotein which carries multiple TF and Tn determinants
[c] Human small cell lung cancer line
[d] Human small cell lung cancer line
[e] Human colorectal adenocarcinoma cell line
f Human lung adenocarcinoma cell line
[g] Human ovarian adenocarcinoma cell line
[h] Human ovarian adenocarcinoma cell line
[i] N' = Neuraminidase-treated cells

MEASURING THE IMMUNE RESPONSE TO TF/Tn ANTIGENS— THE CELL MEDIATED IMMUNE RESPONSE

A great deal of literature amassed over the past two decades demonstrates the overwhelming importance of T-cell mediated immunity (CMI) as an anti-cancer mechanism. Unfortunately, no method exists to measure CMI specific for any human cancer-associated antigen. Such measurements could be extremely important prognostic indicators, as they might estimate the degree of CMI directed against actual cancer-associated antigens.

Numerous reports demonstrate that the T-cell mediated delayed-type hypersensitivity (DTH) reaction is a potent anti-tumor rejection mechanism.[17-19] Certain cancer patients may develop a DTH-like reaction following intradermal injection of crude preparations containing natural TF antigen.[5,20] Prompted by this observation, we attempted to investigate whether T cells which mediate a DTH reaction could specifically recognize TF and Tn carbohydrate determinants. These experiments were primarily designed to examine the specificity of T cell-mediated DTH induced by various antigens. DTH reactions were estimated by measuring footpad swelling following intradermal injection of antigen-primed T cells mixed with the appropriate natural or synthetic antigen. Natural antigens which carry TF or Tn determinants used in this study included a mouse mammary adenocarcinoma (TA3–Ha), epiglycanin (epi), the TA3–Ha–associated tumor glycoprotein similar to a glycoprotein found in human cancer sera which carries multiple TF and Tn determinants, and neuraminidase-treated human RBC (N^1-RBC).[5,7,21-23] Synthetic antigens were TF, Tn, and related control haptens, conjugated to an appropriate carrier molecule.

Mice were immunized with irradiated TA3-Ha cells, killed 10 days later, and the spleens removed. 10^7 primed spleen cells were mixed with cells known to express cell surface TF determinants (irradiated TA3-Ha or neuraminidase-treated human RBC = N^1-RBC), or with cells which do not express detectable TF determinants (irradiated L1210 tumor cells[7] or untreated RBC), and injected subcutaneously into the footpads of normal unimmunized mice. Figure 4.5 shows that the DTH response was elicited only by cells which are known to have cell surface TF determinants (TA3-Ha and N'-RBC).

In order to determine the fine antigen specificity of the DTH effector cells, purified epi, S-TAGs (Tn, TF(α), TF(β)) or fucose linked to HSA were immobilized on sepharose microspheres and injected together with primed spleen cells in a local footpad assay. Epi-primed DTH effector cells were triggered by epi as well as by Tn, TF(α) or

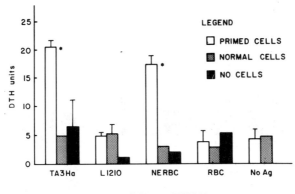

ANTIGEN IN FOOTPAD

FIG. 4.5.   Cell Specificity of the *In Vivo*-Primed DTH Response
Locally bred (Balb×A/J) F_1 mice were injected with 10^6 irradiated (10,000rads) Ta3Ha cells emulsified in CFA (50%) i.p. After 7–10 days the animals were killed, the spleens removed, and a single cell suspension was made by passing the spleen cells through a metal mesh. 10^7 primed cells were mixed with the indicated irradiated (TA3Ha or L1210 tumor cells) or non-irradiated (RBC or neuraminidase-treated human RBC (NERBC)) cells and injected into one hind footpad of syngeneic non-immunized mice. Twenty-four hours later the thickness of the right and the left footpads were measured with an oditest (0–10mm, 0.01mm increments) thickness gauge (obtained from H. C. Kroplin, W. Germany), and the DTH swelling estimated by subtracting the thickness of the uninjected footpad from that of the injected one.
Estimate of DTH:
= [swelling of injected foot]—[swelling of uninjected foot]
   Net DTH:
= [Ave DTH (primed cells+antigen)]—[ave DTH (primed cell only)]
The unit of swelling is 10–2mm. ⋆$p < 0.005$

TF(β) haptens conjugated to HSA, but not by fucose conjugated to HSA nor by HSA alone (see Fig. 4.6a) nor was it elicited by glucose absorbed to BSA (data not shown).

Similarly, cells primed with Tn-HSA were tested for the ability to produce a local DTH reaction in response to TA3-Ha as well as the various S-TAGs. As shown in Figure 4.6b, the anti-Tn DTH reaction was triggered by TA3-Ha, Tn-HSA, TF(α)-HSA, and TF(β)–HSA, but not by Fuc-HSA, nor by BSA alone. Several attempts to generate a carbohydrate-specific response with HSA as the immunogen were unsuccessful. Effector cell populations generated with TF(α) or TF(β) S-TAGs had recognition specificities essentially identical to those generated to Tn (data not shown).

To determine if the carrier molecule affects the recognition specificity of the epi-primed effector cell population, the TF(α) hapten was conjugated to KLH instead of HSA. Epi-primed cells plus the indicated antigen (Fig. 4.6c) were injected into the footpads of normal

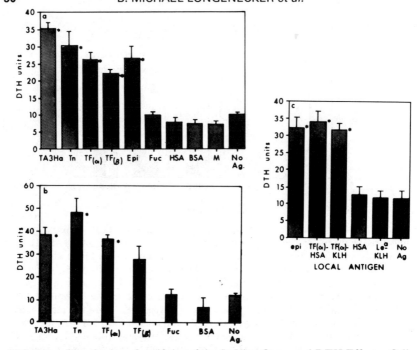

FIG. 4.6.   Fine Antigen Specificity of the *In Vitro*-Generated DTH Effector Cells.
(*a*) 10^7 cells primed to epi *in vitro* were injected together with the indicated antigens
in a local DTH assay. Soluble antigens were linked to sepharose-microspheres. DTH
was measured 24 hours later. *p <0.005

(*b*) 10^7 cells primed to Tn-HSA *in vitro* were injected together with the indicated
antigens in a local DTH assay. Soluble antigens were linked to sepharose- microspheres. DTH was measured 24 hours later. *p < 0.005

(*c*)   Contribution to the Specificity by the Carrier. Protein 10^7 epi primed cells plus
(a) epi, (b) TF(d) conjugated to HSA, (c) TF(d) conjugated to KLH, (d) HSA alone,
(e) Le^a conjugated to KLH or (f) no antigen were injected into a local DTH assay.
DTH was measured 24 hours later. *p < 0.005.

mice. Figure 4.6c shows that the epi-primed cell population recognized
and responded equally well to both TF(α)-HSA and TF(α)-KLH. The
response was not elicited by HSA alone, nor by the unrelated Lewis[a]
blood group antigen (see Fig. 4.1) coupled to KLH.

Several experiments (data not shown) confirm that the DTH reactions elicited by epi and appropriate S-TAGs were mediated by T cells
which bear the phenotype expected of DTH effector cells (Thy-1[+],
Lyt-1[+], Lyt-2[−]) and demonstrate that the response is genetically restricted by the H-2 complex. These experiments provide the first conclusive
demonstration that T cells can recognize carbohydrate determinants.
We then questioned whether or not this specific T-cell response to

tumor carbohydrate determinants has functional significance with regard to anti-cancer immunity.

TABLE 4.5

| Dose: | EPI | Immunizing Antigen | | |
		TF-HSA	Glu-BSA	HSA
0.1μg	1/20[a]	4/15	0/10	0/12
0.5μg	5/20[b]	7/15[c]	0/10	0/12
1.0μg	8/20[c]	5/15[b]	0/10	0/12
5.0μg	8/15[c]	6/15[c]	0/10	0/12
10 μg	7/20[c]	3/15	0/10	0/12
cont.	0/20	0/15	0/10	0/12

Effect of pre-immunization using various defined antigens for systemic protection against a challenge with live TA3Ha cells. Mice (Balb×A/J) F_1 were immunized with varying doses of epi, S-TAG, HSA, or Glu-BSA emulsified in 50% CFA and injected i.p. Ten days later the immunized animals were challenged with $3×10^3$ TA3Ha cells i.p. and survival was monitored.

[a] Number of mice alive at four weeks over total mice inoculated
[b] $P < .025$
[c] $P < .01$
[d] $P < .005$

AUGMENTING THE ANTI-TF/Tn T CELL DTH RESPONSE AS A MEANS OF IMPROVING THE PROGNOSIS

The characteristic amplification of the DTH reaction and the involvement of activated macrophages makes it a particularly effective anti-tumor response, especially against cancers with associated mucins.[24] Many types of tumors contain mucins which may mask cell surface antigens and shield cancer cells from some forms of immune destruction, such as complement-mediated lysis and cytotoxic lympho-cyte-mediated killing.[25-32] As mucins have characteristically very high carbohydrate contents,[24] T-DTH cellular recognition of carbohydrate determinants may be important for the initiation of anti-tumor DTH reactions. In support of this notion, Table 4.5 demonstrates that mice which had been pre-immunized with epi or with the appropriate S-TAG were protected against a TA3-Ha tumor transplant. Furthermore, Table 4.6 shows that a Thy-1$^+$, Lyt-1$^+$, Lyt-2$^-$ T cell population, which was generated using epi and S-TAGs as immunogens, specifically inhibited the growth of TA3-Ha cells. This leads not only to the question of whether augmentation of the anti-TF/Tn T cell DTH response in humans may have therapeutic benefit, but also to the question of whether measurement of this response is useful for prognostic determination.

TABLE 4.6 *Cell Surface Phenotype of Anti-Tumor Effector Cells Primed In Vitro With S-TAG*

Group	Cell Treatment	Tumor Size ± S.D.
1	Untreated	21 ± 3
2	Complement (C')	40 ± 10
3	Anti-Thy-1+c'	129 ± 11
4	Anti-Lyt-1+c	120 ± 10
5	Anti-Lyt-2+c'	60 ± 18

Cells primed with TF S-TAG were treated with anti-Thy-1, anti-Lyt-1, or anti-Lyt-2 antibody in the presence of complement or with complement alone. The treated cells were mixed with 2×10^5 live tumor cells and the mixture injected into the footpads of normal mice. The tumor growth was measured six days later. Tumor size was measured in units of 10^{-2}mm. Groups three and four differ from the other groups. ($p < 0.001$).

DISCUSSION

In this manuscript we have summarized our integrated approach to cancer diagnosis, prognosis, and therapy using the combination of S-TAGs and their corresponding specific MAbs. The concept that we are developing is; as certain carbohydrate antigens are developmentally regulated, they are sequentially expressed as a function of cell differentiation on both embryonic as well as neoplastic cells and thus may be good prognostic indicators. A brief review of the literature in this area follows and we conclude with a clear enunciation of our working hypothesis.

CARBOHYDRATE ANTIGENS AS DEVELOPMENTALLY-REGULATED MARKERS

A good deal of evidence[33,34] indicates that carbohydrate recognition may play a role in a number of cellular interactions, such as: (1) cellular differentiation during development; (2) homing of cells to specific organs; (3) cell-cell adhesion; (4) contact inhibition; and (5) fertilization. Certain toxins, (e.g. tetanus and cholera) have been found to bind carbohydrate determinants and may mediate *in vivo* effects through a process initiated by a carbohydrate recognition event.

Oncogenic transformation of cells also appears to be accompanied by changes in the expression of cell-surface glycolipids and glycoproteins,[5,33,34] including tumor-associated mucins.[24] These changes can be sufficiently different from adjacent normal and progenitor cells to be recognized by the body's immune system. This aberrant surface carbohydrate expression may be related to the invasive properties of tumor cells and may provide the key to failure of the tumor cell to express normal "functional cell contact" and "cell communication".[33,34]

Structural changes in surface carbohydrate expression may be the result of: (a) blocked synthesis, sometimes accompanied by accumulation of precursor oligosaccharides; (b) loss of crypticity by membrane conformational change; (c) activation of glycosyltransferases in progenitor cells resulting in carbohydrate neosynthesis; (d) accelerated degredation of cell surface glycoconjugates; or (e) switch in qualitative expression pattern of certain glycoconjugates.[5,24,33-35] As a result of these changes in carbohydrate content, particularly glycolipids, the tumor cell membrane may result in an altered fluidity, which in turn may affect the function of receptors, membrane enzymes, and cellular metabolism.

There is sufficient scientific evidence which confirms that many diverse carbohydrate structures present on the cell surface are developmentally regulated and correlate with the stage of cell differentiation.[33,34] Briefly: (1) there is an ordered, sequential appearance of certain CHO determinants which correlates with the stage of embryonic development; (2) MAbs directed against these stage-specific structures can profoundly disrupt development; and (3) various carbohydrate structures appear to serve as receptors or regulators of cell growth and differentiation.

Developmental biologists were among the first to apply the MAb technology to study cell surface carbohydrate antigens, discovering that many different carbohydrate antigen systems are developmentally regulated and stage-specific (e.g., Lewis, Forssman, and SSEA antigenic systems). Further studies[36] have suggested that the activation of highly specific glycosyl transferases might be a major mechanism for the appearance, disappearance, and reappearance of CHO antigens during various stages of embryogenesis and differentiation. Many MAb-defined differentiation antigens of hemopoetic origin are also carbohydrates.[34,37] Thus, carbohydrate antigens are surface markers that can distinguish immature from mature cells.

SPECIFIC ALTERATIONS IN CHO METABOLISM MAY BE AN EARLY EVENT IN NEOPLASTIC TRANSFORMATION

Several recent studies have described specific changes in carbohydrate antigen expression and glycosyltransferase enzyme expression in preneoplastic lesions,[10,36,38] Holmes and Hakomori[36] described the induction of a specific fucosyltransferase in premalignant lesions and hepatomas of rats fed chemical carcinogens. This led to the accumulation of the tumor-associated glycolipid fucosyl-GM_1, which has been described as a human tumor marker. Several groups have demonstrated a remarkable dependency of the expression of Lewis determinants and their sialylated forms on differentiation of several embryonic organ systems and cancer.[39–45] Whereas cell morphology by light microscopy may not correlate with prognosis, expression on cancer cells of developmentally regulated antigens, defined by specific MAbs, may correlate with tumor aggressiveness and prognosis.

CARBOHYDRATE CHANGES ON TUMORS AS PROGNOSTIC MARKERS

As more aggressive behavior of some cancers appears associated with alteration of certain CHO differentiation antigens,[5,46–48] it is important to identify CHO antigents expressed as a function of development or cell differentiation. From our discussion of the "ordered expression" of certain carbohydrate differentiation antigens during embryonic development and evidence for their role in cell differentiation, we believe that precursor-product CHO relationships may relate to prognosis.

In elegant studies, Yogeeswaran and co-workers[46,47] demonstrated that the degree of sialylation of cell surface glycoproteins shows an excellent positive correlation with cancer metastasis using animal model systems. Arends *et al.*[49] found that sialylated Lewis[a] (SLA, CA 19.9) positive human colorectal carcinomas tend to behave more aggressively than CA 19.9 negative tumors, although they found no statistically significant survival differences. Several authors[50–52] have claimed a correlation exists between the degree of differentiation of colon adenocarcinomas and the expression of Ca 19.9. This suggests that a study with synthetic SLA precursor-product sequences may provide useful markers for prognosis of colon cancer.

Previous studies have set a precedent in the correlation of the expression of certain gangliosides with histological grading and prognosis of patients with astrocytomas[53] or neuroblastomas.[54]

The system we are focusing on in this manuscript is TF/Tn. Several studies have suggested a correlation of expression of Tn:TF ratios with tumor aggressiveness and/or prognosis. Investigators studying the expression of TF and Tn in human bladder tumors have shown that invasive recurrence was less likely where TF antigen was cryptic.[55,56] On the other hand, the vast majority of patients with a cancer phenotype of TF^+, Tn^+, or cryptic TF^-, showed poor prognosis with cancer recurrence within two years of diagnosis. These studies suggest that TF-series expression may have prognostic significance.

Perhaps the best evidence for a functional role of the TF-system in malignancy is provided by a genetic disorder which results in a selective loss of 3-β-D-galactosyltransferase activity and the appearance of Tn positive RBCs and hematopoietic stem cells (the Tn syndrome). This disorder is associated with a high incidence of leukemia and other hematopoietic disorders. This suggests that the structure of the Tn antigen might play a crucial role in the regulation of pluripotent stem cells, and its expression may be related to a proliferative advantage of Tn^+ cells.[6]

Springer and colleagues have extensively studied TF and Tn antigen expression on human breast carcinomas[5,20,57] and claim that Tn expression is increased on highly invasive anaplastic carcinomas, while well-differentiated carcinomas express more TF than Tn. Howard and Batsakis[58] found that of 22 breast carcinomas, 17 were well-differentiated tumors expressing TF antigen. The remaining five were undifferentiated tumors lacking TF antigen. Yuan and co-workers[10] used one of our TF MAbs[7] to study the early expression of TF antigens on premalignant polyps and colon adenocarcinoma (normal adult mucosa was not marked by the MAbs). We have also confirmed this finding. This MAb marked fetal colon tissue, suggesting that TF may be an oncodevelopmental antigen in human colon cancer.

MUCIN-TYPE GLYCOPROTEINS AS TUMOR MARKERS

Mucins are high mw glycoproteins (>500kd), containing an unusually high carbohydrate content of 60–80%, normally secreted by seroviscous tissues functioning primarily as biological lubricants and providing a barrier to protect cells against physical and chemical trauma. Mucins are also secreted by the vast majority of adenocarcinomas. Recent evidence strongly suggests that mucins may function to protect the tumor from the host immune system.[26,27,59] This observation prompted our interest in cancer-associated mucins and their associated oligosaccharide side chains.

Many human tumors display altered production of mucins with different carbohydrate antigens from those in normal mucins. These antigenic changes associated with malignancy have also been described in preneoplastic lesions.[60–64] Carbohydrate antigens found on mucins are also commonly present on glycolipids associated with cell membranes.[24,33,34,65] Elevated levels of mucins in the serum of cancer patients may result not only from increased transcription and an increased number of tumor cells, but also from mechanisms which alter the structure, density, or molecular organization of mucins. Suppressed transcription of normally active glycosyl-transferases or enhanced transcription of normally quiescent glycosyl-transferases can result in the expression of aberrant oligosaccharides on mucins. Enhancement of glycosidase activity may also account for the expression of new tumor-associated carbohydrate epitopes on mucins. All of these factors may lead to considerable diversity of carbohydrate antigen expression on mucins. Numerous monoclonal antibodies which recognize tumor-associated carbohydrate epitopes on mucins have been described, including: CA 19.9, CA 50, DU-PAN-2, and Sialylated LE^x for pancreatic and colorectal cancer; CA 125 and MoV^2 for ovarian cancer, and F36/22, B72.3, DF3, 115D8, M18, $HMFG_1$, and $HMFG_2$ for breast cancer.[24] Serologic assays developed with several of these MAbs may prove promising in the monitoring of tumor burden in certain cancer patients. Most of these assays are based on the use of a single MAb used in a sandwich assay of sufficient sensitivity for detection due to the polyvalency of carbohydrate epitopes usually found on single mucin molecules. We hypothesize that much more information about the state of differentiation of the tumor might be derived when using several MAbs, recognizing more than one CHO epitope derived from a specific biochemical sequence on the same mucin molecule. The development of assays based on the use of such MAbs in combination might provide better specificity and sensitivity than assays using either MAb alone.[24,66,67] Additional evidence that specific carbohydrate changes on cancer cells may have predictive or prognostic significance are provided in Table 4.7.[68–78]

HYPOTHESIS

Our hypothesis is that the expression of specific carbohydrate antigens should reflect the stage of cell differentiation and hence tumor aggressiveness, which may be significant in cancer management and in planning therapy.

TABLE 4.7   Evidence that Specific Carbohydrate Changes on Cancer Cells May Have Predictive and/or Prognostic Significance

Antigen	Tumor	Reagent	Prognostic Parameter	Immunohistochemical Data	References
TF	Bladder	Rabbit Polyclonal anti-TF, PNA	Cancer recurrence	Vast majority of patients lacking cryptic TF or expressing TF reoccurred. Very few tumors with normal phenotype (= cryptic TF$^+$) reoccurred	(55,56,68)
TF	Prostate	PNA	Cancer grade and metastasis	Higher cancer grade and metastasis correlated with presence of TF or lack of cryptic TF	(38)
TF	Colon adeno Colon polyps	MAb 49H.8, Polyclonal Aby, PNA	"Premalignant" lesions	MAb 49H.8–100% specific for colon Ca And stained colon polyps with highest "premalignant" potential based on size, dysplasia, and villous type	(10)
TF and Tn	Breast Ca	Human anti-TF	Well diff. Ca vs. anaplastic	87% well diff. Br Ca TF > Tn but in only 8% anaplastic, "highly invasive"	(5,57)
TF	Colon	Rabbit anti-T, PNA	"Morphologically altered" crypts	STRONG T-Ag expression in altered crypts and mucin adjacent to malignant tissue	(69)
TF	Colon	PNA	"Premalignant polyps"	Mucin alteration (PNA$^+$) in "premalignant" polyps	(61)
TF	Colon	PNA, other lectins	Cellular differentiation, malignant transformation	MUCIN-CHO antigen changes indicative of goblet cell differentiation, TF-Ag on mucin of malignant cells; altered mucin in transitional mucosa suggests early transformation	(62)
TF	Colon (ulcerative colitis)	PNA, other lectins	Dysplasia, carcinoma development	TF-Ag expression in goblet cell mucin in ulcerative colitis predictive of development of dysplasia/carcinoma	(63)
TF	Colon polyps	PNA	"Premalignant" adenomas	TF-Ag expression on adenomas	(70)
TF	All	PNA	Relapse	>15% PNA$^+$ cells predictive of relapse	(71)
SLA	Breast	MAb	Breast tissue and carcinoma differentiation	Increased expression in poorly differentiated carcinomas	(72)

SLA	Colonic	MAb	Premalignant polyps	Increased expression in polyps with highest "premalignant" potential	(50)
SLA	Pancreatic	MAb	Staining of well vs. poorly diff. tumors	No. of positive cells and intensity of staining much less in poorly differentiated and anaplastic Ca	(51)
CA-50	Pancreatic	MAb	Staining well vs. poorly diff. tumors	No. of positive cells less in poorly differentiated adenomas and rare in anaplastic Ca	(52)
Le^x(SSEA-1)	Colorectal	MAb	Preferential staining of atypical adenomas; and differentiation	Le^x is a marker for immature cells in normal colon and stains all atypical and malignant lesions	(50)
Le^x (SSEA-1)	Embryonal carcinoma cells	MAb	Tumor cell adhesion	Anti-SSEA-1 inhibits cell-substratum adhesion	(73)
Le^x; mono, di, tri, and sialyted derivatives	Renal	MAb	Tumor and embryonic differentiation	Expression of various Le^x structures indicate degree of tumor differentiation and correlates with embryonic development	(39)
LeY	Breast, Colon, Gastric	MAb	Relationship to cellular differentiation	Presence on epidermal growth factor receptor, CEA, and in urine of lactating women	(74–76)
LeY	Colon	MAb	Relationship to cellular differentiation	Presence on immature cells of crypt base and 100% of colorectal adenocarcinomas	(77)
Mucin	Colorectal	MAb	Survival, recurrence-free period	Shorter survival and recurrence-free period, less tumor perivascular lymphocytic cuffing, and paracortex lymph node response in highly mucinous tumors	(59)
GD_3	Acute myeloid leukemia	MAb	Degree of myeloid differentiation	Marker for immature cells and acute leukemia	(78)
GD_3	Astrocytoma	MAb	Grade of malignancy	Increase in GD_3 concentration with increasing grades of malignancy	(53)
GT1b	Neuroblastoma	Chemical Analysis	Presence of disease or survival	Absence of GT1b in vast majority of patients who died of disease	(54)

An excellent precedent exists in the leukemia field in which leukemia cells are thought to be "frozen" in a state of differentiation followed by clonal expansion. Thus leukemia and lymphoma cells are generally classified according to the normal lymphoid or myeloid cells to which they are morphologically and functionally related. This approach has led to the identification of leukemia and lymphoma subtypes, using specific antibodies with implications for prognosis and therapy. As we know that many of the specific CHO markers on solid tumors are functionally related to development, cell interaction, receptor function, etc., it is reasonable to expect that they will turn out to be excellent prognostic markers.

ACKNOWLEDGMENTS

Supported by the Alberta Heritage Savings Trust Fund (AHSTF-ARC) and the National Cancer Institute of Canada. Dr. Longenecker is a Terry Fox Research Scientist of the National Cancer Institute of Canada.

REFERENCES

1. Smith, F. P., Byrne, P. J., Cambareri, R. C. and Schein, P. S., Gastrointestinal Cancer. In *Cancer Chemotherapy* (H.M. Pinedo, Ed.), *The EORTC Cancer Chemotherapy Annual* 1: pp. 292–316. *Excerpta Medica*, Amsterdam–Oxford, 1979.
2. Sausville, E. A. and Young, R. C., Gynecologic malignancies. In *Cancer Chemotherapy* (H. M. Pinedo and B. A. Chabner, Eds.), Annual 7, pp. 366–395. Elsevier Science Publishers, New York–Amsterdam–Oxford, 1985.
3. Jacobs, A. J., Deligdisch, L., Deppe, G. and Cohen, C. J., Histologic correlates of virulence in ovarian adenocarcinoma I. Effect of differentiation. *Am. J. Obstet. Gynecol.* **143**: 574–580 (1982).
4. Kohler, G. and Milstein, C., Continuous cultures of fused cells secreting antibody of predefined specificity. *Nature* **256**: 495–497 (1975).
5. Springer, G. F., General carcinoma autoantigens. *Science* **224**: 1198–1203 1984.
6. Vainchenker, W., Vinci, G., Testa, U., Henri, A., Tabilio, A., Fache, M., Rochant, H. and Cartron, J., Presence of the Tn antigen on hematopoietic progenitors from patients with the Tn syndrome. *J. Clin. Invest.* **75**: 541–546 1985.
7. Longenecker, B. M., Rahman, A. F. R., Barrington-Leigh, J., Purser, R. A., Greenberg, A. H., Willan, D. J., Keller, O., Petrik, P. K., Thay, T. Y., Suresh, M. R. and Noujaim, A. A., Monoclonal antibody against a cryptic carbohydrate antigen of murine and hyman lymphocytes. I. Antigen expression in non-cryptic or unsubstituted form on certain murine lymphomas, on a spontaneous murine mammary carcinoma, and on several human adenocarcinomas. *Int. J. Cancer* **33**: 123–129 1984.
8. Rahman, F. R. and Longenecker, B. M., A monoclonal antibody specific for the Thomsen-Freidenreich cryptic T antigen. *J. Immunol.* **129**: 2021–2023 1982.
9. Longenecker, B. M., Willans, D. J., Maclean, G. D., Selvaraj, S., Suresh, M. R. and Noujaim, A. A., Monoclonal antibodies and synthetic tumor-associated glycoconjugates in the study of the expression of Thomsen-Freidenreich-like and Th-like antigens on human cancers. *J. Natl. Cancer Inst.* **78**: 489–496 1987.

10. Yuan, M., Itzkowitz, S. H., Boland, C. R., Kim, Y. D., Tomita, J. T., Palekar, A., Bennington, J. L., Trump, B. F. and Kim, Y. S., Comparison of T-antigen expression in normal, premalignant, and malignant human colonic tissue using lectin and antibody immunohistochemistry. *Cancer Res.* **46**: 4841 1986.

11. Wolf, M. F., Koerner, U. and Schumacher, K., Specificity of reagents directed to the Thomsen-Freidenreich antigen and their capacity to bind to the surface of human carcinoma cell lines. *Cancer Res.* **46**: 1779–1782, 1986.

12. Noujaim, A. A., Longenecker, B. M., Suresh, M. R., Maclean, G. D., Tamer, C. J. and Sykes, T. R., Tumor markers and their relevance in the design of radioimmunoimaging experiments. *NATO Advance Study Institutes Proceedings* (in press).

13. Suresh, M. R., Baker, D. A., Bray, J. and Noujaim, A. A., *Abstracts of the Third International Symposium on Radiopharmacology*, Freiburg, Fed. Rep. of Germany, 1983.

14. Bray, J., Maclean, G. D., Dusel, F. J. and McPherson, T. A., Decreased levels of circulating lytic anti-T in the serum of patients with metastatic gastrointestinal cancer: a correlation with disease burden. *Clin. Exp. Immunol.* **47**: 176–182, 1982.

15. Hoppner, W., Fischer, K., Poschmann, A. and Paulsen, H., Use of synthetic antigens with the carbohydrate structure of asialoglycophorin A for the specification of Thomsen-Freidenreich antibodies. *Vox Sang* **48**: 246–253, 1985.

16. Winger, L., Winger, C., Shastry, P., Russel, A. and Longenecker, B. M., Efficient generation *in vitro*, from human peripheral blood mononuclear cells, of monoclonal Epstein-Barr virus-transformants producing specific antibody to a variety of antigens, without prior deliberate immunizations. *P.N.A.S.* **80**: 4484–4488, 1983.

17. Fujiwara, H., Takai, Y., Sakamoto, K. and Hamaoka, T., The mechanism of tumor growth inhibition by tumor-specific Lyt 1^+2^- cells. I. Antitumor effect of Lyt 1^+2^- T cells depends on the existence of adherent cells. *J. Immunol.* **135**: 2187–2191, 1985.

18. Economou, G. C., Takeichi, N. and Boone, C. W., Common tumor rejection antigens in methylcholanthrene-induced squamous cell carcinomas of mice detected by tumor protection and radioisotopic footpad assay. *Cancer Res.* **37**: 37–41, 1977.

19. Nelson, M. and Nelson, D. S., Thy and Ly markers on lymphocytes initiating tumor rejection. *Cell. Immunol.* **60**: 34–42, 1981.

20. Springer, G. F., Desai, P. R., Marthy, M. S., Tegetmeyer, H. and Seanlon, E. F., Human carcinoma-associated precursor antigens of the blood group MN system and the host's immune responsed to them. *Prog. Allergy* **26**: 42–69, 1979.

21. Friberg, S. Jr., Comparison of an immunoresistant and an immunosusceptible ascites subline from murine tumor TA3. I. Transplantability, morphology and some physiocochemical characteristics. *J. Natl. Cancer Inst.* **48**: 1463–1471, 1972.

22. Schmit, A., Codington, J. F. and Slayter, H. S., Epiglycanin as a membrane glycoprotein. Isolation of plasma membrane from the TA3-Ha tumor cell. *Carbohydrate Res.* **151**: 173–184, 1986.

23. Codington, J. F., Bhavanandan, V. P., Bloch, K. J., Nikrui, N., Ellard, J. V., Wang, P. S. and Jeanloz, R. W., Antibody to epiglycanin and radioimmunoassay to detect epiglycanin-related glycoproteins in body fluids of cancer patients. *J. Natl. Cancer Inst.* **73**: 1029–1038, 1984.

24. Rittenhouse, H. G., Manderino, G. L. and Hass, G. M., Mucin-type glycoproteins as tumor markers. *Lab. Med.* **16**: 556–560, 1985.

25. Van Den Eijden, D., Evans, N. A., Codington, J. F., Reinhold, V., Silber, C. and Jeanloz, R. W., Chemical structure of epiglycanin, the major glycoprotein of the TA3Ha ascites line. *J. Biological Chem.* **254**: 12153–12159, 1979.

26. Miller, S. C., Hay, E. D. and Codington, J. F., Ultrastructural and histochemical differences in the cell surface properties of strain-specific and non-strain-specific TA3 adenocarcinoma cells. *J. Cell. Biol.* **72**: 511–529, 1977.

27. Gately, C. L., Muul, M., Greenwood, M. A., Papazoglou, S., Dick, S. J., Kornbrith, D. L., Smith, B. H. and Gately, M. K., *In vitro* studies on the cell-mediated immune response to human brain tumors. II. Leukocyte-induced coats of gycosaminoglycan increases the resistance of glioma cells to cellular immune attack. *J. Immunol.* **133**: 3387–3395, 1984.

28. Sherblom, A. P., Buck, R. L. and Carraway, K. L., Purification of the major sialoglycoproteins of 13762 MAT-B1 and MAT-C1 rat ascites mammary adenocarcinoma cells by density gradient centrifugation in cesium chloride and guanidine hydrochloride. *J. Biol. Chem.* **255**: 783–790, 1980.

29. Bhavanandan, V. P., Umemoto, J., Banks, J. R. and Davidson, E. A., Isolation and partial characterization of sialoglycopeptides produced by a murine melanoma. *Biochem.* **16**: 4426–4437, 1977.

30. Funakoshi, I. and Yamishina, I., Structure of O-glycosidically-linked sugar units from plasma membranes of an ascites hepatoma, AH 66: *J. Biol. Chem.* **257**: 3782–3787, 1982.

31. Chandrasekaran, E. V. and Davidson, E. A., Sialoglycoproteins of human mammary cells: Partial characterization of sialoglycopeptides. *Biochemistry* **18**: 5615–5620, 1979.

32. Codington, J. F., Linsley, K. B. and Jeanloz, R. W., Immunochemical and chemical investigations of the structure of glycoprotein fragments obtained from epiglycanin, a glycoprotein at the surface of the TA3-Ha cancer cell. *Carbohydrate Res.* **40**: 171–182, 1975.

33. Hakomori, S., Tumor-associated carbohydrate antigens. *Ann. Rev. Immunol.* **2**: 103–126, 1984.

34. Feizi, T., Demonstration by monoclonal antibodies that carbohydrate structures are glycoproteins and glycolipids are onco-developmental antigens. *Nature* **314**: 53–55, 1985.

35. Yogeeswaran, G., Surface glycosphingolipids and glycoprotein antigens. In *Cancer Markers: Development and Diagnostic Significance* (S. Sell, Ed.), pp. 371–401, Humana Press, New Jersey, 1980.

36. Holmes, E. H. and Hakomori, S., Enzymatic basis for changes in fucoganglioside during chemical carcinogenesis. *J. Biol. Chem.* **258**: 3706–3713, 1983.

37. Saito, M., Terui, Y. and Nojiri, H., An acidic glycosphingolipid, monosialoganglioside GM^3, is a potent physiological inducer for monocytic differentiation of human promyelocytic leukemia cell line HL-GO cells. *Biochem. Biophys. Res. Comm.* **132**: 223–231, 1985.

38. Ghazizadeh, M., Kagawa, S., Izumi, K. and Kurokawa, K., Immunochistochemical localization of T antigen-like substance in benign hyperplasia and adenocarcinoma of the prostate. *J. Urol.* **132**: 1127–1130, 1984.

39. Fukushi, Y., Orikasa, S., Shepard, T. and Hakomori, S., Changes of Le^x and dimeric Le^x haptens and their sialylated antigens during development of human kidney and kidney tumors. *J. Urol.* **135**: 1048–1056, 1986.

40. Solter, D. and Knowles, B. B., Monoclonal antibody defining a stage-specific embryonic antigen (SSEA-1). *P.N.A.S.* **75**: 5565–5568, 1978.

41. Gooi, H. C., Jones, N. J., Hounsell, E. F., Scudder, P., Hilkens, J., Hilgers, J. and Feizi, T., Novel antigenic specificity involving the blood group antigen, Le^a in combination with onco-developmental antigen, SSEA-1, recognized by two monoclonal antibodies to human milk-fat globule membranes. *Biochem. Biophys. Res. Comm.* **131**: 543–550, 1985.

42. Hakomori, S. I. and Kannagi, R., Glycosphingolipids as tumor-associated and differentiation markers. *J. Natl. Cancer Inst.* **71**: 231–241, 1983.
43. Brockhaus, M., Magnani, J. L., Herlyn, M., Blaszczyk, M., Steplewski, Z., Koprowski, H. and Ginsburg, V., Monoclonal antibodies directed against the sugar sequence of lacto-N-fucopentaose III are obtained from mice immunized with human tumors. *Arch. Biochem. Biophys.* **217**: 647–651, 1982.
44. Fukushi, Y., Hakomori, S., Nudelman, E. and Cochran, N., Novel fucolipids accumulating in human adenocarcinoma. II. Selective isolation of hybridoma antibodies that differentially recognize mono-, di-, and trifucosylated type 2 chain. *J. Biol. Chem.* **259**: 4681–4687, 1984.
45. Fukushi, Y., Hakomori, S. and Shepard, T., Localization and alteration of mono-, di-, and trifucosyl al → 3 type 2 chain structures during human embryogenesis and in human cancer. *J. Exp. Med.* **159**: 506–515, 1984.
46. Yogeeswaran, G. and Salk, P. L., Metastatic potential is positively correlated with cell surface sialylation of cultured murine tumor cell lines. *Science* **212**: 1514–1516, 1981.
47. Pearlstein, E., Salk, P. L., Yogeeswaran, G. and Karpatkin, S., Correlation between spontaneous metastatic potential, platelet-aggregating activity of cell surface extracts, and cell surface sialylation in 10 metastatic-variant derivatives of a rat renal sarcoma cell line. *Proc. Natl. Acad. Sci, USA* **77**: No. 7, 4336–4339, 1980.
48. Arends, J. W., Bosman, P. T. and Hilgers, J., Tissue antigens in large-bowel carcinoma. *Biochimica and Biophysica. Acta* **780**: 1–19, 1985.
49. Arends, J. W., Wiggers, T., Verstijnen, C., Hilgers, J. and Bosmann, F. T., Gastrointestinal cancer-associated antigen (GICA) immunoreactivity in colorectal carcinoma in relation to patient survival. *Int. J. Cancer* **34**: 193–196, 1984.
50. Gong, E., Hirohasi, S., Shimosato, Y., Watanabe, M., Ino, Y., Teshima, S. and Kodaira, S., Expression of carbohydrate antigen 19–9 and stage-specific embryonic antigen 1 in nontumorous and tumorous epithelia of the human colon and rectum. *J.N.C.I.* **75**: 447–454, 1985.
51. Haglund, C., Lindgren, J., Roberts, P. J. and Nordling, S., Gastrointestinal cancer-associated antigen CA 19–9 in histological specimens of pancreatic tumors and pancreatitis. *Br. J. Cancer* **53**: 189–195, 1986.
52. Haglund, C., Lindgren, J., Roberts, P. J. and Nordling, S., Tissue expression of the tumor marker CA 50 in benign and malignant pancreatic lesions. A comparison with CA 19–9. *Int. J. Cancer* (in press).
53. Berra, B., Gaini, S. M. and Riboni, L., Correlation between ganglioside distribution and histological grading of human astrocytomas. *Int. J. Cancer* **36**: 363–366, 1985.
54. Schengrund, C. L., Repman, M. A. and Shochat, S. J., Ganglioside composition of human neuroblastomas. *Cancer* **56**: 2640–2646, 1985.
55. Coon, J. S., Weinstein, R. S. and Summers, J. L., Blood group precursor T-antigen expression in human urinary bladder carcinoma. *Amer. J. Clin. Pathol.* **17**: 692–699, 1982.
56. Ohoka, H., Shinomiya, H., Yokoyama, M., Ochi, K., Takeuchi, M., and Utsumi, S., Thomsen-Freidenreich antigen in bladder tumors as detected by specific antibody: a possible marker of recurrence. *Urol. Res.* **13**: 47–50, 1985.
57. Springer, G. F., Desai, P. R., Robinson, M. K., Tegtmeyer, H. and Scanlon, E. F., The fundamental and diagnostic role of T and Th antigens in breast carcinoma at the earliest histologic stage and throughout. In *Tumor Markers and their Significance in the Management of Breast Cancer*, (T. Dao, Ed.), *Prog. Clin. Biol. Res.* Series, **204**: pp. 47–70. Alan R. Liss, Inc., 1986.

58. Howard, D. R. and Batsakis, J. G., Cytostructural localization of a tumor-associated antigen. *Science* **210**: 201–203, 1980.
59. Pihl, E., Nairn, R. C., Hughes, E. S. R., Cuthbertson, A. M. and Rollo, A. J., Mucinous colorectal carcinoma: immunopathology and prognosis. *Pathology* **12**: 439–447, 1980.
60. Yonezawa, S., Nakamura, T., Tanaka, S. and Sato, E., Glycoconjugate with Ulex europaeus agglutinin-I-binding sites in normal mucosa, adenoma, and carcinoma of the large bowel. *J. Natl. Cancer. Inst.* **69**: 777–781, 1982.
61. Boland, C. R., Montgomery, C. K. and Kim, Y. S., A cancer-associated mucin alteration in benign colonic polyps. *Gastroenterol.* **82**: 664–672, 1982.
62. Boland, C. R., Montgomery, C. K. and Kim, Y. S., Alterations in human colonic mucin occurring with cellular differentiation, and malignant transformation. *Proc. Natl. Acad. Sci. USA* **79**: 2051–2055, 1982.
63. Boland, C. R., Lance, P., Levin, B., Riddell, R. H., and Kim, Y. S., Abnormal goblet cell glycoconjugates in rectal biopsies associated with an increased risk of neoplasia in patients with ulcerative colitis: early results of a prospective study. *Gut* **25**: 1364–1371, 1984.
64. Listinsky, C. M. and Riddell, R. H., Patterns of mucin secretion in neoplastic and non-neoplastic disease of the colon. *Hum. Pathol.* **12**: 923–928, 1981.
65. Magani, J. L., Steplewski, Z., Koprowski, H. and Ginsburg, V., Identification of the gastrointestinal and pancreatic cancer-associated antigen detected by monoclonal, antibody 19–9 in the sera of patients as a mucin. *Cancer Res.* **43**: 5489–5492, 1983.
66. Herlyn, M., Blaszczyk, M., Bennicelli, J., Sears, H. F., Ernst, C., Ross, A. H. and Korprowski, H., Selection of monoclonal antibodies detecting serodiagnostic human tumor markers. *J. Immunol. Meth.* **80**: 107–116, 1985.
67. Herlyn, M., Sears, H. F., Verrilli, H. and Koprowski, H., Increased sensitivity in detecting tumor-associated antigens in sera of patients with colorectal carcinoma. *J. Immunol. Meth.* **75**: 15–21, 1984.
68. Summers, J. G., Coon, J. S., Ward, R. M., Falor, W. H., Miller, A. W. III, and Weinstein, R. S., Prognosis in carcinoma of the urinary bladder based upon tissue blood group ABH and Thomsen-Freidenreich antigen status and karyotype of the initial tumor. *Cancer Res.* **43**: 934–939, 1983.
69. Orntoft, T. F., Ole Mors, N. P., Eriksen, G., Jacobsen, N. O. and Skovgaard Poulsen, H., Comparative immunoperoxidase demonstration of T-antigens in human colorectal carcinomas and morphologically absnormal mucosa. *Cancer Res.* **45**: 447–452, 1986.
70. Cooper, H. S. and Reuter, V. E., Peanut lectin-binding sites in polyps of the colon and rectum. *Lab. Invest.* **49**: 655–661, 1983.
71. Levin, S., Russell, E. C., Blanchard, D., McWilliams, N. B., Maurer, H. M. and Mohanakuma, T., Receptors for peanut agglutinin (Arachus hyupogaea) in childhood acute lymphocytic leukemia: possible clinical significance. *Blood* **55**: 37–42, 1980.
72. Walker, R. A. and Day, S. J., Expression of the antigen detected by the monoclonal antibody CA 19.9 in human breast tissues. *Virchows Arch.* **409**: 375–383, 1986.
73. Nomoto, S., Muramatsu, H., Ozawa, M. and Muramatus, T., An anti-carbohydrate monoclonal antibody inhibits cell-substratum adhesion of F9 embryonal carcinoma cells. *Exp. Cell Res.* **164**: 49–62, 1986.
74. Blaszczyk-Thurin, M., Thurin, J., Hindsgaul, O., Karlsson, K., Steplewski, Z. and Koprowski, H., Y and blood group B type 2 glycolipid antigens accumulate in a human gastric carcinoma cell line as detected by monoclonal antibody. *J. Biol. Chem.* **262**: 372–379, 1987.

75. Hallgren, P. and Lundblad, A., Structural analysis of oligosaccharides isolated from the urine of a blood group A, secretor, woman during pregnancy and lactation. *J. Biol. Chem.* **252**: 1023–1033, 1977.
76. Lependu, J., Fredman, P., Richter, N., Magnani, J. L., Willingham, M. C., Pastan, I., Oriol, R. and Ginsburg, V., Monoclonal antibody 101 that precipitates the glycoprotein receptor for epidermal growth factor is directed against the Y antigen, not the H type 1 antigen. *Carbohydr. Res.* **141**: 347–349, 1985.
77. Brown, A., Ellis, I. O., Embleton, M. J., Baldwin, R. W., Turner, D. R. and Hardcastle, J. D., Immunohistochemical localization of Y hapten and the structurally related H type-2 blood group antigen on large-bowel tumors and normal adult tissues. *Int. J. Cancer* **33**: 727–736, 1984.
78. Siddiui, B., Buehler, J., Degregorio, M. W. and Macher, B. A., Differential expression of ganglioside GD_3 by human leukocytes and leukemia cells. *Cancer Res.* **44**: 5262–5265, 1984.

5

Commentary on Part I: Tumor Histology and Molecular Pathology

Robert F. Kallman, Ian F. Tannock, and Raymond S. Bush

Presentations throughout this monograph can be classified into two groups: (1) studies designed to predict response to a particular treatment and (2) studies of prognostic factors. Four of the proferred papers (A-2, A-3, A-7 and A-10) were designed to provide information about the effectiveness of a particular treatment—while most of the other presentations described more general prognostic factors.

HORMONE RESPONSIVENESS

Hug *et al.* (A-2) described an *in vitro* assay which might predict the response of human breast cancer to hormonal management. The assay involved cloning of cells in agar in the presence or absence of steroids (estradiol and hydrocortisone) and peptide hormones (epidermal growth factor and insulin). These investigators reported that, in a sample of 33 patients, *in vitro* hormone responsiveness was inversely related to cloning efficiency. They also found that an increase in cloning efficiency of 180% or more when hormones were added to the cultures appeared to identify those patients who would respond to hormonal manipulation. This assay might therefore augment or substitute for predictive information obtained from determination of estrogen and progestin receptors. One potential advantage of this assay, over the use of steroid receptors as a predictive test, is that colonies may grow from small amounts of tissue, as might be obtained using a needle biopsy. This advantage may decrease, however, since techniques are also being developed to measure steroid receptor levels in small volumes of tissue.

THE USE OF ANTIBODIES TO ADDUCTS OF DNA/PROTEINS

One promising approach to predicting whether cells will interact with a specific cytotoxic drug, a tumor marker, a sensitizer or the like, lies in the use of specific antibodies. Terheggen *et al.* (A-3) sought to utilize an assay that would be predictive of response to cis-diammine-dichloroplatinum (II) (c-DDP). The rationale was to use an antibody against DNA that had been coupled with c-DDP to detect whether this cytotoxic drug binds to cellular DNA in a given tissue or tumor; if it does, cytotoxic activity might be expected. Rabbits were immunized with calf thymus DNA that had been exposed *in vitro* to c-DDP and complexed with methylated BSA. Coupling of the resultant antiserum with cellular DNA was visualized by double peroxidase anti-peroxidase (PAP) staining. The polyclonal antibody assay predicted the rank order of drug sensitivity among four experimental tumor lines. The number of PAP-stained nuclei was dependent upon the dose of c-DDP administered i.p. to the tumor-bearing mice. *In vitro* experiments confirmed the results with tumors and demonstrated moreover, a good correlation between cell survival and c-DDP-DNA adduct formation. These data are encouraging, in that predictions of the cis-DDP sensitivity of human tumor cells to this chemotherapeutic drug could be made quite quickly and easily by the use of this relatively fast PAP assay for adduct detection.

In discussion of this work, the relative merits of the use of rabbit polyclonal antibodies in the manner described by Terheggen *et al.* (A-3) was contrasted with assays based upon the use of monoclonal antibodies against specific DNA adducts. Lohman and his colleagues [1,2] have produced several monoclonal antibodies by the customary method of deriving hybrid antibody-producing cells by fusing myeloma cells with spleen cells from an immunized mouse. Such antibodies, visualized by means of the recently developed laser-scanning miscroscope, made possible the detection of low numbers of specific adducts. It remains to be seen how the faster and relatively simpler polyclonal antibody method compares in efficiency and accuracy with such monoclonal methods. A related question deals with the specificity of the antibodies that have been raised. Would such antibodies be more specific and more likely to reveal antigenic adducts if the DNA moiety used in the antigenic adduct was homologous? That is to say, why use calf thymus DNA to produce antibodies that are to be detected in murine or, more importantly, in human cells? Indeed, there is precedent for the belief that homologous antigenic DNA adducts would be superior to heterologous molecules.

An analogous approach was taken by Miller *et al.* (A-4) who described the use of polyclonal antibodies to protein adducts of a hypoxic cell radiosensitizer, a derivative of misonidazole. A fluorescent antibody technique was used to detect the presence of hypoxic cells in EMT6 tumor cell spheroids and in a variety of solid tumors both *in vivo* and *in vitro*. Qualitatively, the distribution of fluorescence in such preparations is comparable with that of autoradiographic grains when similar tissues are incubated with radioactively labeled misonidazole. (The derivative used in these experiments, termed CC1-103F, is also capable of sensitization.)

This study is apparently the latest chapter in the development by the Edmonton group of quantitative means of visualizing hypoxic cells in tumors, a technique that has been shown to be quantitatively accurate and reproducible. (Several related facets of this same approach are described by Rasey *et al.* (E-1), Raleigh *et al.* (E-2), Urtasun *et al.* (E-3), and Kolar *et al.* (E-4) in Part V, Chapter 22 of this monograph.) As discussed in Part V, the development of non-invasive methods is the logical and desirable extension of the basic finding that hypoxic cells can be labeled in this manner either radioisotopically or with this kind of fluorescent antibody.

COLORIMETRIC MEASUREMENT OF CELL GROWTH *IN VITRO*

Twentyman *et al.* (A-7) reported their experience with the MTT color-imetric assay, which can be used to determine the number of viable cells in culture at a suitable interval after drug treatment. These investigators have selected cell lines that are resistant to doxorubicin and showed that the calcium channel blocker verapamil or the immunosuppressive drug cyclosporin A could modify drug resistance. They are currently extending these studies to cells taken directly from patients with leukemia. A disadvantage of the assay is that it seems necessary to modify the conditions for each drug and tumor type, but its use to study modifiers may give important clues about the nature of drug resistance in human malignancy.

MER ENZYME ASSAY

Yarosh *et al.* (A-10) measured the activity of the enzyme O-6-methyl-guanine-DNA methyltransferase (MER) in human tumor cells. They reported that cells deficient in this activity (the MER-phenotype) are very sensitive to alkylating agents and also to interferon. A simple biochemical assay of MER might therefore predict for tumor response to these agents. A question was asked about the relationship between this enzyme and glutathione (GSH) levels in the cell, since GSH may bind free radicals and hence protect cells from the toxicity of alkylating agents. Information does not appear to be available on the relationship, if any, between GSH and MER.

GLUTATHIONE

It is a principal theme of this monograph, documented thoroughly throughout this volume, that there is extensive heterogeneity in sensitivity to therapeutic agents within tumors. For the present discussion, it is largely irrelevant whether intratumor heterogeneity exists because of genetic or epigenetic factors. Heterogeneity in the state of oxygenation of individual cells within a tumor accounts for major differences in sensitivity to ionizing radiation, and protection against such O_2-dependent sensitivity may be afforded by sulfhydryl groups on various intracellular molecules. Glutathione (GSH) is the major SH-containing molecule that plays an important role in modulating cellular sensitivity, so it is important to determine its quantitative distribution throughout typical tumor cell populations. The methods for GSH measurement are, however, relatively few and are largely incapable of disclosing small differences in GSH content from cell to cell. Usually, one can make only average measurements of GSH concentration over many tumor cells.

When the fluorescent DNA stain, Hoechst 33342, is injected i.v. into tumor-bearing mice, it diffuses slowly away from blood vessels within a tumor, creating a gradient of fluorescence such that the intensity of staining decreases with increasing distance of cells from the blood supply.[3] Cell suspensions are prepared from solid tumors and, using fluorescence-activated cell sorting, the cells are separated into fractions that differ in dye content, where dye content depends upon the distance from blood capillaries. Instead of Hoechst 33342, one can also use a different diffusion-limited carbo-cyanine dye in order to sort cells according to their location, and can stain simultaneously with monobromobimane—which fluoresces at a different wavelength—to reveal intracellular GSH. By this means, one can investigate whether GSH content is uniform or is heterogenous within a given tumor. Significantly, cells that were situated farthest from vascular channels and were therefore likely to be more hypoxic, contained less GSH. Minchinton and Grulkey (A-6) were able to cause the depletion of intracellular GSH by using the enzyme inhibitor buthionine sulphoximine (BSO).

In doing so, one can narrow the width of the distribution of SH radicals, and therefore the cellular radiosensitivity, for the tumor as a whole. This should cause both an increase and a homogenization of radiosensitivity from cell to cell.

The importance of whether the cells of a given tumor have high or low average GSH concentrations is obvious, and the discrepancy in the findings of several authors takes on major significance. On the one hand, it has been reported that the cells of several human tumor lines, tested *in vitro*, contain more GSH than Chinese hamster V79 cells;[4,5] but Guichard et al.[6] determined GSH levels in five human tumor xenografts and found them to be comparable with V79 cells.

In their current study Guichard et al. (A-5) determined the GSH values of five human tumor cell lines both *in vitro* and *in vivo*. *In vitro*, cells in exponential growth were found to have at least double the mean GSH levels than they had when they were in plateau phase. The GSH content of xenografts fell between the values found for exponential and plateau phase cells, and they were comparable to the GSH levels of V79 hamster cells. However, the GSH content of the parenchymal cells of a human tumor growing as a xenograft in mice cannot be determined without interference from the stroma. Until it is possible to differentiate between these two major components of a tumor, it will be impossible to resolve the question of species-dependent GSH content. This is because in a human-mouse xenograft the parenchymal cells are of human donor origin, whereas the stromal cells are of murine host origin. Because GSH has not been measured histochemically in a manner which allows one to discriminate stroma from parenchyma, one cannot rule out the possibility that the cells of mice and of men contain rather different GSH levels. If this is so, measurements made on total xenografted tumors are incapable of providing the desired cell-specific GSH measurements. Once it is possible to discriminate tumor cells from stroma, pre-therapeutic measurements of GSH levels made in human tumor xenografts could contribute useful information relevant to optimizing therapeutic strategies.

Tumor regression

The studies of Moat et al. (A-1) were not designed to provide a predictive assay but described measurements made on primary human breast tumors treated with radiation or single agent chemotherapy. The rate of regression has been found to be highly variable and the results of others have suggested that rate of regression does not seem to be a useful indicator of ultimate response. Moat and his colleagues quantitated the initial proportions of parenchyma and collagen by using automated image analysis of drill biopsies and reported a significant correlation between the maximum rate of regression and the mean proportion of collagen in the tumor. The rate of tumor regression may therefore depend more on noncellular factors than on the number of clonogenic cells within the tumor, offering an explanation as to why rate of regression is not generally useful in prediction of response.

Oxygen regulated proteins (ORPs)

In studies on the regulation of metabolism of rodent and human tumor cells grown mainly in multicell spheroids *in vitro* under hypoxic and oxygenated conditions, Sutherland and his associates have identified a number (at least five) of specific proteins whose synthesis appears to be increased under conditions of either oxygen or glucose deprivation. Further details were provided by their contribution (A-8) to this session. One of these proteins (molecular weight, 260 kD) can be seen after one hour of hypoxia, and it reaches a maximum by four hours, while the others begin to increase at between two and four hours, but then show similar kinetics. The synthesis of all these proteins returns to the aerobic levels by between ten and twelve hours after reoxygenation, and they have been identified in at least 10 rodent and human tumor cell lines. Knowledge of the synthesis patterns of these oxygen-regulated proteins should be of considerable value in understanding the biology of diverse tumors, and may even potentiate the prediction of their response to treatment. In a related but entirely independent investigation, Rice, Hoy, and Schimke[7] have reported that Chinese hamster ovary AA8 cells, maintained under hypoxic conditions, show a marked enhancement in the frequency of methotrexate resistance and dihydrofolate reductase gene amplification. This kind of overreplication of nuclear DNA can be seen about four to 12 hours after the start of hypoxia and appears to reach a peak considerably later. Thus, the concentrations of these two major macromolecular classes appear to be increased under supposedly adverse conditions, and it remains to be determined whether and how they are interrelated. Overreplicated DNA certainly contributes to drug resistance, but the role of ORPs in cancer therapy remains to be elucidated. In order to improve our ability to predict tumor response, it is essential that there be a better understanding of 1) the controls over synthesis of these molecules, 2) the mechanism by which molecules enter into the physiology of the tumor cell and 3) the tumor's response to treatment.

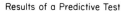

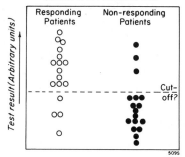

FIG. 5.1 Results of a hypothetical test conducted on tumor biopsies of patients who do or do not respond to treatment.

PREDICTIVE ASSAYS – DISCUSSION

Several points have been raised about methods that might be used to evaluate predictive tests or prognostic factors. For tests which attempt to predict response to a given treatment, test results are often presented as in Fig. 5.1. In this hypothetical example there is a significant difference between test results for responding and non-responding patients. However, as with almost all medical tests, there is overlap between the two sets of results. A cutoff must therefore be established which best discriminates responders from non-responders. Important determinants of the utility of the test include the sensitivity of the cutoff to: (i) the dose of the agent used in conducting the test, (ii) the type and stage of tumor on which the test is performed, and (iii) the definition of clinical response. Determination of the cutoff and its generalization to different tumors will be important in the development of the various predictive assays described in Part I of this monograph.

The most important question that can be asked of a predictive test is whether or not its results will be sufficiently reliable to base a course of treatment upon it. Since no test is perfect, the utility of a test depends on 1) the proportion of false negative and false positive results, 2) the "cost" of failing to treat a patient who would have responded (related to the benefit of treatment in responders) and 3) the "cost" of treating a patient who does not respond (related to the toxicity of treatment and the effectiveness of alternatives). If these factors can be quantitated, decision-making analysis, similar to that used in the field of economics, can estimate costs and benefits to similar groups of patients who are managed with or without using the results of a predictive assay for guidance. Few tests have as yet been evaluated in this way.

For the assays described in Part I of this monograph, it seems unlikely that prediction of hormone response in metastatic breast cancer will be particularly cost effective, since this desease cannot be cured, and there is little "cost" in prescribing the non-toxic drug tamoxifen as initial management for all patients. However, the assay may be more important if it can predict benefit from hormonal therapy in the adjuvant setting. In contrast, sparing patients treatment with toxic drugs such as cisplatin or interferon when they are unlikely to respond well would be useful if reliable tests were available. The "costs" of failing to treat even one patient with metastatic testicular cancer who might be cured by cisplatin-based chemotherapy would be high, however, so that a predictive test in this setting must have a very low proportion of false negative results.

It is easier to predict prognosis in general than to devise a useful test which predicts response to a particular treatment. The stage and grade of tumors and performance status of patients are familiar prognostic factors. The utility of a prognostic test which adds to these factors depends on the availability of therapy to alter that prognosis. If such therapy is not available, the test is only useful if the clinician has sufficient confidence in its result (a) to treat curable tumors aggressively and (b) to manage incurable tumors symptomatically. At present, few prognostic tests other than stage and grade of disease are used in determining treatment.

The above concepts were subjected to lively discussion, and it was pointed out that there are alternative treatments for some types of tumors. Examples include the use of either radiation or surgery to treat locoregional tumors of the head and neck, bladder, or prostate. Tests of radioresponsiveness might therefore aid in decision-making. It will probably require quite extensive clinical trials, however, before we can determine whether or not a given test can provide overall benefit to a substantial group of patients.

REFERENCES

1. Baan R. A., Zaalberg O. B., Fichtinger-Schepman, A. M. J., Muysken-Schoen, M. A., Lansbergen, M. J. and Lohman, P. H. M., Use of monoclonal and polyclonal antibodies against DNA adducts for the detection of DNA lesions in isolated DNA and in single cells. *Environ. Health Perspect.* **62**: 81–88, 1985.
2. Fichtinger-Schepman, A. M. J., van der Veer, J. L, Den Hartog, H. J. J., Lohman, P. H. M. and Reedijk, J., Adducts of the antitumor drug *cis*-diamminedichloroplatinum (II) with DNA: formation, identification and quantitation. *Biochem.* **24**: 707–713, 1984.
3. Chaplin, D. J., Durand, R. E. and Olive, P. L., Cell selection from a murine tumour using the fluorescent probe Hoechst 33342. *Br. J. Cancer* **51**: 569–572, 1985.
4. Mitchell, J. B., Phillips, T. L., De Graff, W., Carmichael, J., Rajpal, R. K., and Russo, A., The relationship of SR-2508 sensitizer enhancement ratio to cellular

glutathione levels in human tumor cell lines. *Int. J. Radiat. Oncol. Biol. Phys.* **12**: 1143–1146, 1986.

5. Biaglow, J. E., Varnes, M. E., Epp, E. R., Clark, E. P. and Aster, M., Factors involved in depletion of glutathione from A549 human lung carcinoma cells: implications for radiotherapy. *Int. J. Radiat. Oncol. Biol. Phys.* **10**: 1221–1227, 1984.
6. Guichard, M., Lespinasse, F. and Malaise, E. P., Influence of buthionine sulfoximine and misonidazole on glutathione level and radiosensitivity of human tumor xenografts. *Radiat. Res.* **105**: 115–125, 1986.
7. Rice, G. C., Hoy, C. and Schimke, R. T., Transient hypoxia enhances the frequency of dihydrofolate reductase gene amplification in Chinese hamster ovary cells. *Proc. Natl. Acad. Sci.* **83**: 5978–5982, 1986.

POSTERS

(A-1) The Prediction of Tumor Response from the Measurement of Tumor Regression: The Import of Computerized Quantitative Histology. N. E. Moat, A. E. Johnson, D. Cheung, and R. H. Thomlinson. Breast Study Centre, Mount Vernon Hospital, Northwood, Middlesex.

(A-2) A New Predictor for Response to Endocrine Treatment. V. Hug, H. Thames, D. Johnston, and G. Hortobagyi. U.T.M.D. Anderson Hospital and Tumor Institute, Houston, Texas 77030.

(A-3) Immunocytochemical Detection of cis-Diamminedichloroplatinum (II) (cDDP)-DNA Adducts in Tumor Cells. P.M.A.B. Terheggen, A. C. Begg, B. G. J. Floot, and L. den Engelse. The Netherlands Cancer Institute, Plesmanlaan 121, 1066 CX, Amsterdam.

(A-4) Quantitation of Tissue Hypoxia Using a Specific Fluorescent Probe. G. G. Miller, A. J. Franko, C. J. Koch, and J. A. Raleigh. Radiobiology, Cross Cancer Institute, 11560 University Avenue, Edmonton, Alberta, Canada T6G 1Z2.

(A-5) Glutathione Level in Human Tumor Cells (Biopsies, Xenografts and Cells *in vitro*). M. Guichard, F. Lespinasse, R. Estelin, A. Gerbaulet, C. Haie, E. Lartigau, E. P. Malaise, C. Micheau, M. Prade, J. M. Richard, P. Weeger, and G. Girinsky. Unite Inserm 247 and Institut Gustave-Roussy, 94805 Villejuif Cedex, France.

(A-6) Spatial Heterogeneity in the Concentration of Glutathione Within Solid Tumors. A. I. Minchinton, and B. Grulkey. British Columbia Cancer Research Centre, 601 West 10th Avenue, Vancouver, British Columbia, Canada V5Z 1L3.

(A-7) Use of Colorimetric (MTT) Assay to Study Modifiers of Cytotoxic Drug Resistance. P. R. Twentyman, J. G. Reeve, N. E. Fox, and J. Rees. MRC Clinical Oncology and Radiotherapeutics Unit and University Department of Haematological Medicine, Hills Road, Cambridge CB2 2QH, England.

(A-8) Relation to Therapeutic Responsiveness of Specific Proteins Induced by Oxygen and Glucose Deprivation. R. M. Sutherland, C. S. Heacock, T. T. Kwok, J. J. Sciandra, H. C. Smith, and R. E. Wilson. University of Rochester, Rochester, New York 14642.

(A-9) Tumor Necrosis as a Predictor of Treatment Response in Canine Osteosarcoma. B. E. Powers, S. J. Withrow, E. L. Gillette, S. M. LaRue, and D. E. Thrall. Colorado State University, Fort Collins, Colorado 80523 and North Carolina State University, Raleigh, North Carolina 27606.

(A-10) A Biochemical Marker in Tumor Cells for Hypersensitivity to Interferon. D. B. Yarosh, M. Goldstein, and N. Rosales. Applied Genetics Inc., Freeport, New York 11520.

PART II

TUMOR CELL KINETICS AND CYTOGENETICS

6

Flow Cytometric Analysis of Archival Tumor Specimens

Michael L. Friedlander

INTRODUCTION

The management of malignant disease on an individual patient basis could be made more rational if it were based on objective data reflecting inherent difference in biological behavior and likelihood of response to specific treatments within tumors of a similar type. In recent years, there has been a growing recognition that failure to appreciate the significance of prognostic factors contributed to the design of inefficient studies, inappropriate choice of treatment for many patients, erroneous interpretation of the results of therapy, and consequently the development of an inconsistent literature. By recognizing and incorporating multiple independent prognostic factors patients might be stratified according to risk of treatment failure, thus improving the ability of the medical community to make appropriate decisions. In the absence of any new and more effective cancer chemotherapeutic agents, there is now an aura of considerable interest being paid to enable individualization of therapies according to risk and probability of therapeutic gain. Basic biological research into the inherent properties of tumors, into their tendency to invade and metastasize, and into their subsequent variability in clinical course has been expanded enormously and has been facilitated by recent technological advances, many of which will be discussed in this monograph. One of these technological developments is *flow cytometry*, which permits high speed analysis of morphological, molecular, biophysical, and functional characteristics of individual cells within heterogeneous populations. The potential applications are many, but of particular interest to applied cancer research is the analysis of cellular DNA content and proliferating fraction (% S-phase), because previous studies using less sensitive techniques have suggested their potential value in predicting the biological behavior of human tumors.[1]

Although the flow cytometric measurement of cellular DNA content is straightforward enough, a major limitation (until recently) has been the absolute requirement for fresh unfixed tissue. In practice this has meant that the rate at which tumor specimens are accrued is restricted by the number of biopsies performed, the availability of suitable patients, and the cooperation of ancillary medical and laboratory personnel. Thus, it is difficult to study large numbers of tumors of the same histological type and stage from patients treated in a standard fashion. Added to this has been the problem of patient follow-up and the fact that in many tumor types treatment failure is delayed, requiring prolonged follow-up before the impact on survival can be assessed. These constraints prompted us to develop a method to obtain single cell suspensions from archival paraffin-embedded tumor tissue that would be satisfactory for flow cytometric analysis.[2] Most diagnostic histopathology laboratories retain paraffin-embedded blocks of fixed tissue indefinitely, providing a readily available source of tumor tissue from patients whose outcome is already known.

MATERIALS AND METHODS

The method to determine cellular DNA content of paraffin-embedded tumor tissue has been described by Hedley et al.[2,3] and will only be briefly outlined in this chapter, as will the potential advantages and disadvantages of the technique. Thick (30 μm) sections are cut from a paraffin-embedded block of tumor tissue using a microtome. Usually, a single section yields sufficient cells for analysis ($> 10^5$ cells), but for small samples, two, or occasionally three sections are required. The choice of 30 μm is somewhat arbitrary, but we found that the use of "thick" sections minimized the number of partly sectioned nuclei in the sample and improved the coefficient of variation (CV). This method has been subsequently corroborated by other researchers.[4] The sections are placed in 10ml glass centrifuge tubes and dewaxed using two changes of xylene (or Histoclear—National Diagnostics, Somerville, N.J.), followed by rehydration in a sequence of 100, 95, 70 and 50% ethanol for 10 minutes each at room temperature. The tissue is then washed in distilled water and resuspended in 0.5% pepsin (Sigma P7012, activity 2500–3200 units/mg protein) in 0.9% NaCl, adjusted to pH 1.5 in a 30°C water bath. Frequent vortex mixing improves the yield of nuclei. After a 30 minute incubation, examination under phase contrast microscopy

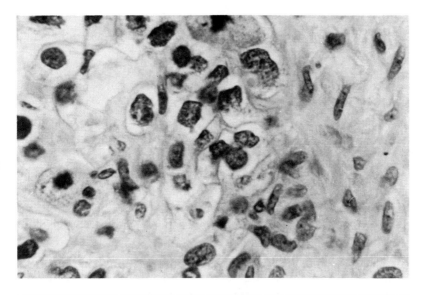

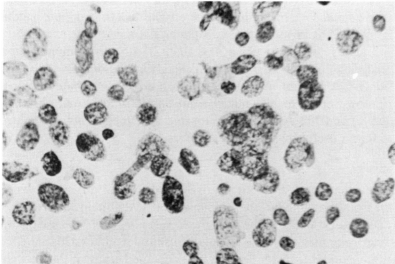

FIG. 6.1 (*a*) Comparison of nuclear morphology of a serous ovarian tumor *before* processing to isolate nuclei from paraffin-embedded tumor tissue.

6.1 (*b*) Comparison of nuclear morphology of a serous ovarian tumor *after* processing to isolate nuclei from paraffin-embedded tumor tissue.

usually reveals large numbers of cells or bare nuclei (Fig. 6.1) that closely resemble the original unfixed cell population. After washing and filtration, these nuclei can be analyzed using flow cytometry. Of the various DNA fluorochromes, 1 µg/ml 4′,6′-diaminido-2-phenylindole dichloride (DAPI) is the most satisfactory. Propidium iodide and ethidium bromide can also be used, but the CVs obtained tend to be greater.

METHODS AND MATERIALS

Internal Standards

The use of paraffin-embedded material precludes using an internal standard such as chicken red blood cells (CRBC) to determine absolute DNA content, as neither CRBC nor human peripheral blood lymphocytes elicit consistent ratios to a normal diploid G_1 peak. This is not, however, a problem in practice, as we and others have reported that a G_1 peak corresponding to a diploid population is a constant feature in DNA histograms obtained from human cancers, and can be used as an internal standard.[1,5,6] An excellent correlation is observed between the DNA indices obtained from the analysis of ploidy in fresh and paraffin-embedded tissue—confirming that the binding of DAPI to the pepsin digests is stochiometric[2,7] (Fig. 6.2). We have therefore taken the presence of a *single* G_1 peak to indicate a diploid tumor and *more than one* G_1 peak to indicate an aneuploid tumor. Thus, with the exception of hypodiploidy, which occurs in less than 2% of most human tumors, hyperdiploid tumors can be distinguished from diploid tumors by their greater DNA content. An alternative technique to estimate the ploidy level, however, is to mix nuclei from paraffin-embedded normal (if available) and tumor tissue of the same specimen. This method has been found useful by some investigators.[7]

Fixatives

An evaluation of different fixatives used to treat different portions taken from the same biopsy sample indicated that neutral formalin or formalin/acetic acid/acetone gave the lowest CV, while the use of Bouins fixative or mercury-based fixatives resulted in either a higher CV or an uninterpretable histogram.[3] A more detailed study of the effects of fixation on flow cytometric analysis of DNA in paraffin-embedded tissue has been reported by Quirke *et al.*[8] Human tonsil was fixed using a variety of agents prior to paraffin-embedding, and the effects of prolonged fixation (up to 28 days) in formalin or of prior immersion in saline before formalin fixation were also studied. Formalin, neutral buffered formalin, formal sublimate, periodate-lysine-paraformaldehyde (PLP), PLP-dichromate, Clarke's, Carnoy's, and formal saline acetic fixatives all allowed satisfactory retrospective DNA analysis. Tissues fixed in Bouin's, Susa's, Gendre's, Regaud's, and saturated picric

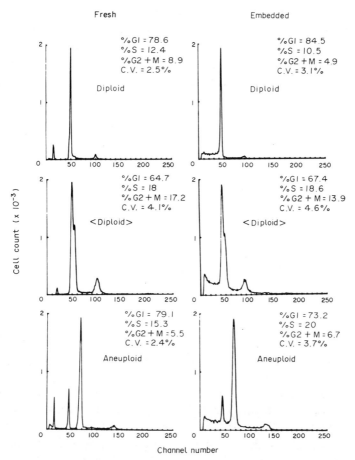

FIG. 6.2 Frequency distribution histograms of cellular DNA content obtained from three malignant tumors. Comparison of results using fresh or paraffin-embedded material from the same tissue sample.

acid with 3% mercuric chloride were unsatisfactory for DNA analysis. Apparently, delay in fixation of up to 48 hours and the length of time in formalin were not important factors in obtaining optimum CV's. We have, however, previously noted that formalin-fixed paraffin-embedded tissue of autopsy specimens are generally not satisfactory for DNA analysis, suggesting that autolysis can be an important adverse contributory factor.[3]

Resolution

Major problems encountered with early flow cytometric studies related to difficulties in cell monodispersion and quantitative cell staining, contributed to the relatively poor resolution of the technique.

These problems have now been largely overcome by technical improvements, and with optimum staining and instrument alignment, it should be possible to obtain CV's below 2% for most fresh tumor specimens. The CV's obtained from paraffin-embedded tumor tissues are, however, somewhat higher, and although the lowest CV's obtained by us using a standard ICP22 flow cytometer (Ortho Instruments, Westwood, MA) have been around 2%, they usually range between 3 and 5% (see Fig. 6.2). Some CV's, however, have been as high as 10% while still appearing diploid, and this is a concern since near-diploid aneuploid populations may be missed. In such cases, it is worth repeating the DNA analysis after cutting additional tissue sections from the same or different paraffin block (if available). Cutting thicker sections (i.e., 50–100 μm) may also improve the resolution.[4] These "wide CV" diploid histograms may still, however, not be improved by such maneuvers, and it is probable that they reflect problems with the fixation or with the embedding processes.

Sensitivity of Detection of Aneuploid Cells

Tumor tissue samples may contain only a small percentage of malignant cells which could be missed in flow cytometric analysis irrespective of whether fresh or paraffin-embedded tissue is being analyzed. By admixing experiments, we have shown that under ideal conditions a 1% population of aneuploid cells can be detected,[9] but for practical purposes, the limit of detection is between 5 and 10% of cells analyzed due to the possible masking effect of S-phase and $G_2 + M$ components of diploid cells commonly present in tumor cell suspensions. An advantage of using paraffin-embedded tumor tissue is that a section can be selected from a block of tissue on the basis that it contains a satisfactory number of tumor cells and thus ensures that the tumor population will not be overlooked. One group has recently stressed the importance of cutting thick sections (50 μm or greater) for analysis, as they noted that as the section thickness decreased, there was a progressive increase in baseline noise and a decrease in the relative peak height of the aneuploid DNA and thus the possibility of decreased sensitivity of detection of an aneuploid population.[3] Oud et al.[10] have recently described a technique of extracting nuclei from selected regions in paraffin-embedded tissue for flow cytometric analysis. This has potential value in analyzing tissues where only a small percentage of the cells present are malignant and could possibly be missed if the whole section was subjected to DNA analysis.

Diagnosis of Diploid Tumors

One drawback of flow cytometric analysis of either fresh or paraffin-embedded tissue is that one cannot discriminate between "normal" host cells and tumor cells that have a diploid DNA content. This underplays the importance of selecting tumor sections according to the proportion of morphologically identifiable tumor cells present. It is generally believed that in aneuploid tumors, the diploid component represents normal stromal cells, but there is also some evidence to suggest that diploid tumor cells may at times coexist with aneuploid tumor cells,[11] although the incidence of this phenomenon is not known. It would be, potentially extremely valuable if we could better identify diploid tumor cells. Despite numerous attempts, no good method is currently available.

Tumor Heterogeneity

Flow cytometric analysis of cellular DNA content and proliferative activity are being widely investigated with respect to their relationship to prognosis and to therapy response. The value of a single estimation of tumor ploidy would be very limited if tumors commonly exhibited a variability of ploidy within different regions. This prompted a study by us into the stability of DNA content in epithelial ovarian cancer.[9] With few notable exceptions, most tumors (87%) exhibited stability of ploidy both spatially and temporally. Similar findings have been noted in a number of other tumor types; including breast cancer, renal cancer, thyroid cancer, and malignant lymphomas.[1] However, regional variability has been documented to be relatively common in small cell lung cancer,[12] melanomas,[13] and colonic cancer.[14] This highlights the importance of determining the representative value of a single estimation of ploidy in the tumor type of interest before embarking on prospective studies.

The S-phase, as determined by flow cytometrically, has been reported to be of prognostic significance in a number of tumor types and may clearly be of clinical value. As with the case of ploidy, it is important to determine the representative value of a single estimation of S-phase. In a detailed study in epithelial ovarian cancer, we found that up to 50% of tumors showed a significant regional variation in S-phase (defined as a greater than 40% variation in different areas).[9] It is not clear to what extent this is true of other tumors and this trial requires evaluation. The reasons for this variability in ovarian cancer is not known, but could relate either to different proliferative states among cells in different nutritional environments, or to variable contamination of tumor cells by normal non-cycling cell populations.

Estimation of "S–" Phase

The S-phase, as determined by flow cytometry, generally correlates well with the degree of proliferative activity obtained using autoradiographic techniques and has the added advantage that it can be performed rapidly and with relative ease.[15,16] Although there is an excellent correlation between the DNA index of paraffin-embedded and unfixed tumor tissue,[1] the same cannot be said of proliferative activity in *all* tumor types. Baur *et al.*[17] found very similar proliferative activity in patients with diffuse lymphomas when single cell suspensions and paraffin-embedded tissue from the same biopsy were compared, while Schutte *et al.*[7] noted that in colonic tumors the relationship, while being statistically significant, was nevertheless quite variable in some tumors. The reasons for this may include tumor heterogeneity as well as the slightly lower resolution of the DNA histograms obtained from paraffin-embedded tissues.

There are a number of practical limitations associated with the determination of S-phase that apply equally to fresh and paraffin-embedded tumor tissue which should be considered here briefly. The S-phase can be determined in all diploid tumors, but overlapping of tumor populations precludes the accurate analysis of S-phase in up to 50% of aneuploid tumors[9,18] although some researchers claim to be able to approximate the S-phase in 90 to 95% of histograms.[19] Diploid tumors generally have a lower S-phase than do aneuploid tumors, but this may be artefactual—in some instances due to the admixture of normal non-cycling cells. In contrast, the estimation of the aneuploid S-phase population could be falsely elevated by the presence of overlapping populations, tetraploid normal cells, and cell debris.

APPLICATIONS

Ploidy as a Prognostic Variable

The potential application of flow cytometric DNA analysis has been greatly extended by using paraffin-embedded tissue, as retrospective studies can rapidly address the question of whether DNA content has any prognostic or therapeutic implications. There is now a large body of evidence to indicate that tumor ploidy reflects biological behaviour in a large number of patients, but importantly, not in all tumor types.[1,20,21] In those tumors in which ploidy has prognostic value, it is the diploid tumors that are usually associated with a better prognosis, while paradoxically, in some childhood tumors, notably neuroblastoma[22,23] and acute lymphoblastic leukemia,[24] patients with aneuploid tumors have a more favorable outcome. While numerous studies of tumor ploidy in a wide range of malignancies show generally good basic agreement regarding the prognostic value of ploidy in similar histological types, conflicting findings have been reported in melanomas,[13,25] myeloma,[26-28] small cell lung cancer,[29-31] and cervical cancer.[32,33] The reasons for this are not known, but may reflect technological differences, patient variability, and the effect of different forms of therapy. Unfortunately, many of the studies have been rather small or have included patients treated in one institution over many years, when many other factors such as time of diagnosis, staging procedures, tumor specific therapy, and supportive care may have changed and thus have had an important impact on outcome. This underlines the importance of applying the technique of flow cytometric analysis of paraffin-embedded tissue to specimens obtained from patients treated, preferably in large cooperative studies, over a similar time period and in a similar fashion. Only in this manner can the independent value of ploidy, as well as its relationship to other recognised prognostic variables and the type of treatment received, be properly assessed.

Rather than detailing the results of the many studies that have been published on the relationship between ploidy and prognosis, we have provided a summary of the different studies. The results are shown in Table 6.1, and I will only briefly review the updated results of three large retrospective studies in ovarian cancer, breast cancer, and adenocarcinoma of unknown primary that have been performed by our group. It should be noted that many of the studies referred to in Table 6.1 are rather small and may not have adequately assessed whether ploidy was an independent prognostic factor by using multivariate analysis.

Ovarian Cancer

In a recent flow cytometric study of paraffin-embedded tumor blocks from 128 patients with FIGO stage III and IV ovarian cancer who were entered onto a randomized clinical trial of combination versus sequential chemotherapy with chlorambucil and cisplatinum, it was found that 27% of tumors were diploid and the remainder were aneuploid.[34] Product limit survival analysis demonstrated a highly significant association between tumor ploidy and survival, with patients with diploid tumors having a median survival of 60 months and those

TABLE 6.1 *Tumors in Which Survival Advantage Demonstrated for Patients With Diploid Tumors*

Tumor Type
Ovarian
Breast
Thyroid
Prostate
Kidney
Bladder
Endometrium
Non Small Cell Lung
Bone
Acute Myeloid Leukemia
Mycosis Fungoides

Tumors in Which No Survival Advantage Demonstrated for Diploid Tumors or for Which Conflicting Data Exists

Tumor Type
ACUP
Lymphomas
Colon
Cervix
Melanoma
Small Cell Lung Cancer[a]

[a] Conflicting data regarding relationship between ploidy and survival.

with aneuploid tumors a median survival of 12 months (Fig. 6.3). When the effects of histological subtype, grade, clinical stage, amount of residual tumor and treatment were corrected for by multivariate analysis, only cellular DNA content and stage remained as significant prognostic factors for survival. Of the tumors analyzed, 97 were Stage III and 31 were Stage IV. The distribution of diploid and aneuploid tumor populations were similar in both stages. It was of considerable interest, therefore, to find that the relatively good prognosis associated with diploid tumors was limited to patients with Stage III disease, while patients with Stage IV disease had poor prognoses, irrespective of ploidy.[3] We have also found analysis of DNA content to be a useful adjunct to the histopathological diagnoses of ovarian tumors of border-line malignancy, as these tumors are, for the most part, diploid and therefore present an excellent prognoses.[35]

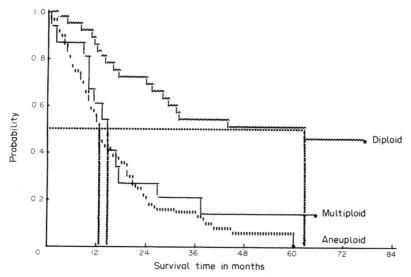

FIG. 6.3 Survival by ploidy in patients with advanced ovarian cancer.

The relationship of cellular DNA content to survival was also examined retrospectively in 61 patients with early stage (FIGO Stage I and II) invasive ovarian cancer who had prolonged follow-up. Forty-three per cent of early stage tumors were diploid, and 57% were aneuploid. As in the case of patients with FIGO Stage II ovarian cancer, patients with diploid tumors had a significantly longer survival rate than did those with aneuploid tumors (P < 0.006). Recently, similar findings have been reported by Erhardt et al.,[36] using Feulgen cytophotometry to analyze DNA content in patients with FIGO Stage I and II ovarian cancer, and by Volm et al.,[37] using flow cytometric analysis of fresh tumor specimens.

Breast Cancer

Aneuploidy has been reported to occur in 50 to 80% of breast tumors, and there is some evidence from static cytometric studies that cellular DNA content reflects the biology of breast cancer and therefore has prognostic value.[38] Several flow cytometric studies examining the cellular DNA content of fresh or frozen breast tumor specimens have been published but, because of the natural history of breast cancer, it is difficult to draw conclusions from any one of these studies. Hedley, Rugg, and Gelber[39] have recently analyzed the DNA content in 473 patients with Stage II breast cancer and have concluded that while aneuploidy correlated with the number of nodes involved, oestrogen

receptor status, tumor grade, and survival, ploidy did not have independent prognostic significance when allowance was made for its correlation with other prognostic features.

Adenocarcinoma of Unknown Primary Site

Adenocarcinomas of unknown primary site (ACUP) make up 7% of
all referrals to our unit, and it is well recognized that the vast majority of
such patients have a poor prognosis—with their tumors being generally
resistant to chemotherapy. However, a small percentage of patients
appear to have an indolent course, which cannot be predicted by clinical
or histological parameters. Hedley, Leary, and Kirsten, [40] have recently
investigated the prognostic value of cellular DNA content in 152
patients with ACUP for whom paraffin-embedded tumor blocks and
follow-up data was available. Thirty percent of the tumors were diploid, and the remainder were aneuploid. Median survival for patients
with diploid tumours was four to five months, similar to that of patients
with aneuploid tumors. It was not possible to predict the small percentage of long-term survivors on the basis of ploidy.[40]

Proliferative Fraction

The potential problems inherent in the estimation of S-phase or
proliferative fraction have been discussed earlier in this chapter, but
still there is good evidence that S-phase correlates well with clinical
outcome and has been demonstrated to have independent prognostic
significance in a number of tumor types. The correlation between flow
cytometric S-phase and thymidine labeling is generally good and is
probably best when one uses a simple method of histogram analysis
that will prevent any skew in the G_1 or G_2 profile from contributing
spurious S-phase cells.[15,16,19]

The S-phase has been studied in particular detail in breast cancer
and lymphomas where the results obtained by flow cytometric analysis
of fresh or paraffin-embedded tissue approximate the results of thymidine labeling studies. Hedley et al.[39] found S-phase to be of prognostic
value in a large retrospective flow cytometric study of patients with
Stage II breast cancer. The percentage of cells in S-phase could be
estimated in 287 patients and of these, 152 patients had an S-
phase $< 10\%$ and these patients had a significantly better prognosis
($P = 0.0008$) than did those with a high S-phase. S-phase $> 10\%$ was
strongly correlated with high tumor grade and abnormal DNA index,
but only weakly correlated with nodal status, hormone receptor status,
and menopausal status. However, multivariate analysis showed that

the prognostic significance of % S-phase was largely explained by its correlation with tumor grade. Similar results have been reported by Meyer,[41] who utilized thymidine labeling in a series of 278 patients in whom the labeling index was demonstrated to be a prognostic indicator independent of stage and estrogen receptor content.

It has been previously recognized that lymphoma cells with high proliferative activity are found in morphologic subgroups with grave prognoses, and that S-phase may have prognostic significance in patients with lymphomas.[15,16,42,43] There have been at least three reasonably extensive retrospective studies of S-phase on tumor blocks from patients with lymphomas—all of which demonstrated that percentage S-phase was a valuable prognostic parameter.[44,45] In one study by Bauer et al.,[17] high proliferative activity was found to be the single most important pre-treatment adverse prognostic factor in patients with diffuse large cell lymphoma (DLCL). Patients with DLCL with high proliferative activity had a median survival of seven months, compared to 39 months for those with low proliferative activity.

Similar results attesting to the prognostic value of proliferative fraction have also been reported for patients with cervical cancer.[46] This is an area that deserves further study.

Prediction of Tumor Response
Tumor Ploidy

Although there is good evidence in a variety of tumor types that ploidy and proliferative activity correlate well with patient outcome, the reasons for this are not clear. They may reflect the relative indolence of the particular tumor rather than the effect of treatment. There are limited data available that do suggest, however, that for certain tumor types, ploidy does predict or influence response to therapy. This appears to be the case particularly in childhood cancers, such as neuroblastoma and acute lymphoblastic leukemia (ALL). Look et al.[22] investigated the predictive value of cellular DNA content in determining the response to chemotherapy in infants under one year of age presenting with unresectable neuroblastoma. Of the 17 evaluable patients with hyperdiploid tumors, 15 had complete responses and two had partial responses to cyclophosphamide and doxorubicin, while six others with diploid tumors did not respond to therapy. From this study, it would seem that the prognostic information conveyed by the diploid stem line has therapeutic implications and argues that such patients should be treated with alternative chemotherapy. Similar results were also obtained by Gansler et al.,[23] in a retrospective study of paraffin-embedded blocks from 38 patients presenting with neuroblastoma. Look *et al.*[24] have reported on the relationship between ploidy and response to treatment in 205 children with ALL. Aneuploidy was present in 74 of the patients (36% to 70% hyperdiploid and 4 hypodiploid). It became apparent that patients with hyperdiploidy (DI > 1.16–n = 51) had significantly higher responses to treatment, longer durations of remission. Multivariate regression analysis indicated that ploidy was independent of the other known prognostic features. By combining prognostic factors, Look *et al.*[22] report that patients with a D1 ≥ 1.16 and white cell counts < +10^9/L have a very low probability of relapse when treated with current standard therapy. The MD Anderson experience of 194 patients with acute myeloid leukemia indicated a superior response rate and longer survival in patients with diploid blasts, while in adult ALL the reverse was true.[20] This data indicate that similar abnormalities in DNA content may have different prognostic implications in different tumor types.

My colleagues and I have correlated tumor ploidy with response to chemotherapy in 128 patients with Stage III and IV ovarian cancer treated in a prospective clinical trial and randomized to sequential therapy with chlorambucil followed by cisplatinum at relapse or a combination of both drugs *ab initio.*[47] The clinical response rate (CR + PR) was similar for all ploidy groups, but the results should be interpreted with caution, as 62% of patients with diploid tumors, 35% with aneuploid tumors, and 13% with multiploid tumors did not have measurable disease and were therefore not evaluable for our study. This may reflect inherent differences between the diploid and aneuploid group of tumors and suggests that the diploid types have a more complete resection-making evaluation of response difficulty. Similarly, the surgically documented response rates are difficult to interpret, as only 32% of patients had a second look laparotomy and therefore comprise a highly selected group. It is of interest that 68% of patients with diploid tumors, 18% with aneuploid tumors and 20% with multiploid tumors have been subjected to a second look laparotomy with the "true response rate" of diploid tumors appearing higher than that of the aneuploid group as a whole.

In view of the inherent problems in documenting response rates in ovarian cancer, an alternative method of comparing therapy results is determining the time that has elapsed to disease progression. In patients with diploid tumors, who were treated initially with combination chemotherapy, the median time to first treatment failure (58 weeks) was not significantly different (P = 0.5) from the time to the first treatment failure (134 weeks) of patients who received sequential therapy. By contrast, in patients with aneuploid tumors, combination therapy was superior to chlorambucil in prolonging the time to first treatment failure (36 weeks vs. 23 weeks, P = 0.05). However, when patients with aneuploid tumors relapsed on chlorambucil alone, the addition of cisplatinum resulted in further responses and the median time to overall treatment failure in these patients was not significantly different from time to disease progression in patients who initially received combination therapy.

There is not much information relating ploidy to chemo-responsiveness in other adult solid tumors, although Hedley (unpublished observation) has noted no relationship between ploidy and response to chemotherapy in 45 women with metastatic breast cancer who had been treated with a variety of treatment regimens.

There is limited evidence to suggest that ploidy correlates with hormonal responsiveness in prostrate cancer and possibly also breast cancer. Ploidy is a powerful prognostic indicator in patients with prostate cancer with diploid tumors having a relatively good prognosis.[48-50] Tavares et al.,[48] reported that ploidy predicted for estrogen response in patients with metastatic prostate cancer, and similar findings have also been reported by Zetterberg and Esposti.[49] There is a correlation between tumor ploidy and steroid receptor content in breast cancer, with diploid tumors tending to be receptor positive, but this relationship does not hold up in all studies.[18,39,51,52] Stuart-Harris et al. [53] could not demonstrate a relationship between ploidy and hormonal sensitivity in a retrospective study of tumor blocks from 42 patients with metastatic breast cancer treated with endocrine therapy.

Proliferative Activity

There is no good evidence to support the theory that cell kinetics predict the likelihood of curing a tumor by any particular therapeutic intervention, despite the interesting clinical observation that those adult cancers which are curable by cytotoxic therapy include those with the most rapid proliferative rates, such as germ cell tumors, choriocarcinoma, histiocytic lymphoma, and Burkitts lymphoma. Currently in clinically applied tumor cell kinetics, we only can measure phase distribution, which (as mentioned previously) may have prognostic significance, but there is a disappointing lack of correlation between the proportion of cells in S-phase and the achievement of complete remission in the small numbers of tumors in which this has been studied to date.

Other Applications

Bauer et al.[53] have recently described a technique of multiparameter flow cytometric analysis for the simultaneous quantitation of nuclear antigens and DNA content using paraffin-embedded tumor tissue. This approach appears to be useful for evaluating cellular heterogeneity within solid tumors and, by using monoclonal antibodies to proliferation, associated antigen opens the way for multiparameter studies of DNA content and "proliferative index" in human tumors. This technique has also been used to quantitate c-myc and DNA content in nuclei from paraffin-embedded tumor tissue.[54] The c-myc gene codes for a 62,000 molecular weight protein which binds within the nucleus and some evidence suggests that it may play a role in proliferation control. There may be considerable clinical value in quantitating oncogene products in biopsy material and the ability to do so on paraffin-embedded archival material will allow retrospective studies to be performed. Watson et al.[55] have reported the utility of the technique in analyzing c-myc oncoprotein in paraffin-embedded testicular and colonic tumors. This could be extended to measuring the protein products of c-fos and c-myb, which also have protein products localized to the cell nucleus and also appear to be proliferation and/or differentiation-associated. The use of paraffin-embedded material in the context of retrospective studies and FCM analysis should provide a useful approach for rapidly assessing the expression of tumor-associated oncoproteins within relevant tumor cell subpopulations, including aneuploid cells and proliferating cells in specific cancers.

CONCLUSIONS

The potential applications of flow cytometric DNA analysis are greatly extended by using paraffin-embedded tumor tissue. Although it is simpler and faster to analyze fresh tumor specimens, the ability to study archival material from patients for whom survival data and response to therapy are known has opened the way for detailed retrospective studies. The technique is particularly well suited for retrospective analyses to be performed on tumor specimens from patients who have been treated in large cooperative prospective clinical trials. Such patients should all have had similar staging investigations, treatment, methods of assessing response, pathological review, and a common computerized data base, allowing the question as to whether DNA content or proliferative activity has prognostic or therapeutic implications to be addressed rapidly.

ACKNOWLEDGMENTS

This work was conducted in and funded by the Ludwig Institute for Cancer Research (Sydney Branch).

I thank David Hedley for reading this chapter with a critical eye and I thank Judy Hood for her expert secretarial skills.

REFERENCES

1. Friedlander, M. L., Hedley, D. W. and Taylor, I. W., Clinical and biological significance of aneuploidy in human tumors. *J. Clin. Pathol.* **37**: 961–974, 1984.
2. Hedley, D. W., Friedlander, M. L., Taylor, I. W., Rugg, C. A. and Musgrove, E. A., Method for analysis of cellular DNA content of paraffin-embedded pathological material using flow cytometry. *J. Histochem. Cytochem.* **11**: 1333–1335, 1983.
3. Hedley, D. W., Friedlander, M. L. and Taylor, I. W., Application of DNA flow cytometry to paraffin-embedded archival material for the study of aneuploidy and its clinical significance. *Cytometry* **6**: 327–333, 1985.
4. Stephenson, R. A., Gay, H., Fair, W. R. and Melamed, M. R., Effect of section thickness on quality of flow cytometric DNA content determinations in paraffin-embedded tissues. *Cytometry* **7**: 41–44, 1986.
5. Barlogie, B., Drewinko, B., Schumann, J., Gohde, W., Dosik, G., Latreille, J., Johnston, D. A. and Freireich, E., Cellular DNA content as a marker of neoplasia in man. *Am. J. Med.* **69**: 195–203, 1980.
6. Friedlander, M. L., Taylor, I. W., Russell, P., Musgrove, E. A., Hedley, D. W. and Tattersall, M. H. M., Ploidy as a prognostic factor in ovarian cancer. *Int. J. Gynecol. Pathol.* **2**: 55–63, 1983.
7. Schutte, B., Reynders, M. M. J., Bosman, F. T. and Blijham, G. H., Flow cytometric determination of DNA ploidy level in nuclei isolated from paraffin-embedded tissue. *Cytometry* **6**: 26–30, 1985.
8. Quirke, P., North, C. L., Roberts, A. M. *et al.*, Effects of fixation on flow cytometric analysis of DNA in paraffin-embedded tissue. *Pathology* **146**: 278 (Abstract), 1985.
9. Friedlander, M. L., Taylor, I. W., Russell, P., Tattersall, M. H. N., Cellular DNA content—A stable marker in epithelial overian cancer. *Brit. J. Cancer* **49**: 173–179, 1984.
10. Oud, P. S., Hanselaar, T., Reubsaet-Veldhuizen, J. *et al.*, Extraction of nuclei from selected regions in paraffin-embedded tissue. *Cytometry* **7**: 595–600, 1986.
11. Perez, D. J., Taylor, I. W., Milthorpe, B. K., McGovern, V. J. and Tattersall, M. H. N., Identification and quantitation of tumour cells in cell suspensions: A comparison of cytology and flow cytometry. *Br. J. Cancer* **43**: 526–531, 1981.
12. Vindelov, L. L., Hansen, H. H., Christensen, I. J., Spang-Thomsen, M., Hirsh, F. R., Hansen, M. and Nissen, N. I., Clonal heterogeneity of small cell anaplastic carcinoma of the lung demonstrated by flow cytometric DNA analysis. *Cancer Res.* **40**: 4295–4300, 1980.
13. Sondergaard, K., Larsen, J. K., Moller, U., Christensen, I. J. and Jensen, K. H., DNA ploidy-characteristics of human malignant melanoma analysed by flow cytometry and compared with histology and clinical course. *Virchows Arch (Cell Pathol.)* **42**: 43–52, 1983.
14. Peterson, S. E., Lorentzen, H. and Bichel, P. A., A mosaic subpopulation structure of human colorectal carcinomas demonstrated by flow cytometry. In *Flow*

cytometry IV, Laerum, O. D., Lidmo, T., Thorud, E., eds. Oslo, Bergen and Trondheim: Universitetsforlaget, 412–416, 1980.

15. Braylan, R. C., Diamond, L. W., Pavell, M. L. and Harly-Golder, B., Percentage of cells in S-phase of the cell cycle in human lymphoma determined by flow cytometry. Correlation with labeling index and patient survival. *Cytometry* 1: 171–174, 1980.

16. Costa, A., Nazzini, G., Del Bino, G. and Silvestrini, R., DNA content and kinetic characteristics of non-Hodgkin's lymphoma: Determined by flow cytometry and autoradiography. *Cytometry* 2: 185–188, 1981.

17. Bauer, K. D., Merkel, D. E., Winter, J. N. *et al.*, Prognostic implications of ploidy and proliferative activity in diffuse large cell lymphomas. *Cancer Res.* 46: 3173–3178, 1986.

18. Taylor, I. W., Musgrove, E. A., Friedlander, M. L., Foo, M. S. and Hedley, D. W., The influence of age on the DNA ploidy levels of breast tumors. *Eur. J. Cancer. Clin. Oncol.* 19: 623–628, 1983.

19. McGuire, W. L., Meyer, J. S., Barlogie, B. and Kute, T. E. Impact of flow cytometry on predicting recurrence and survival in breast cancer patients. *Breast Cancer Res. and Treat.* 5: 117–128, 1985.

20. Barlogie, B., Raber, M. N., Schumann, J. *et al.*, Flow cytometry in clinical cancer research. *Cancer Res.* 43: 3982–3997, 1983.

21. Laerum, O. D. and Farsund, T., Clinical application of flow cytometry: A review. *Cytometry* 2: 1–13, 1981.

22. Look, A. T., Hayes, M. D., Nitschke, R., McWilliams, N. B. and Green, A. A., Cellular DNA content as a predictor of response to chemotherapy in infants with unresectable neuroblastoma, *N. Engl. J. Med.* 311: 231–235, 1984.

23. Gansler, T., Chatten, J., Varello, M., Bunn, G. and Atkinson, B., Flow cytometric DNA analysis of neuroblastoma correlation with histology and clinical outcome. *Cancer* 58: 2453–2458, 1986.

24. Look, A. T., Roberson, P. K., Williams, D. L., *et al.*, Prognostic importance of blast cell DNA content in childhood acute lymphoblastic leukemia. *Blood* 5: 1079–1086, 1985.

25. von Roenn, J., Kheir, S. M., Wolter, J. N. and Coon, J. S., Significance of DNA abnormalities in primary malignant melanoma and nevi, a retrospective flow cytometric study. *Cancer Res.* 46: 3192–3195, 1986.

26. Lavensohn, R., Tribukait, B. and Hansson, J., DNA content of human myeloma cells. *Eur. J. Clin. Oncol.* 19: 59–63, 1983.

27. Bunn, P. A., Krasnow, S., Makuch, R. W., Schlam, M. L., Schechter, G. P., Flow cytometric analysis of DNA content of bone marrow cells in patients with plasma cell myeloma: Clinical Implications. *Blood* 59: 528–535, 1982.

28. Barlogie, B., Alexanian, R., Gehan, E. A., *et al.*, Marrow cytometry and prognosis in myeloma. *J. Clin. Invest.* 72: 853–861, 1983.

29. Bunn, P. A., Carney, D. N., Gazdar, A. F., *et al.*, Diagnostic and biological implications of flow cytometric DNA content analysis in lung cancer. *Cancer Res.* 43: 5026–5032, 1983.

30. Johnson, T. S., Valdivieso, M., Barlogie, B., Jefferies, D., Williamson, K. and Keating, M., Flow cytometric ploidy and proliferative activity in human small cell lung carcinomas: Potential diagnostic and prognostic features. *Proc. Am. Assoc. Cancer. Res.* 488: 124, 1983.

31. Blondal, T. and Pontsen, J., DNA ploidy in small cell carcinoma of the lung. *Anticancer Res.* 3: 47–51, 1983.

32. Jacobsen, A., Prognostic impact of ploidy level in carcinoma of cervix. *Am. J. Clin. Oncol.* 7: 475–480, 1984.

33. Atkin, N. B. and Kay, R., Prognostic significance of modal DNA value and other factors in malignant tumours based on 1465 cases. *Br. J. Cancer* **10**: 210–221, 1979.
34. Friedlander, M. L., Hedley, D. W., Taylor, I. W., *et al.*, Influence of cellular DNA content on survival in advanced ovarian cancer. *Cancer Res.* **44**: 397–400, 1984.
35. Friedlander, M. L., Russell, P., Taylor, I. W., Hedley, D. W. and Tattersall, M. H. M., Flow cytometric analysis of cellular DNA content as an adjunct to the diagnosis of ovarian tumors of borderline malignancy. *Pathology* **16**: 301–306, 1984.
36. Erhardt, K., Aver, G., Bjorkolm, E., *et al.*, Prognostic significance of DNA content in serous ovarian tumors. *Cancer Res.* **44**: 2198–2202, 1984.
37. Volm, M., Bruggemann, A., Gunter, M. *et al.*, Prognostic relevance of ploidy and proliferation in ovarian carcinoma. *Cancer Res.* **45**: 5280–5185, 1985.
38. Auer, G. U., Caspersson, T. O. and Wallgren, A. S., DNA content and survival in mammary carcinoma, *Anal. Quant. Cytol.* **2**: 161–165, 1980.
39. Hedley, D. W., Rugg, C. A. and Gelber, R. D., Effects of DNA index and S-phase fraction on prognosis in Stage II breast cancer. *Cancer Res.* (in press), 1987.
40. Hedley, D. W., Leary, J. A. and Kirsten, F., Metastatic adenocarcinomas of unknown primary site. Abnormalities of cellular DNA content and survival. *Eur. J. Cancer Clin. Oncol.* **21**: 185–189, 1985.
41. Meyer, J. S., Cell kinetics in selection and stratification of patients for adjuvant therapy of breast cancer. *NCI Monograph* **1**: 1–167, 1986.
42. Shackney, S. E., Levin, A. M., Fisher, R. I., *et al.*, The biology of tumor growth in non-Hodgkin's lymphomas: A dual parameter flow cytometric study of 220 cases. *J. Clin. Invest.* **73**: 1201–1214, 1984.
43. Diamond, L. W. and Braylan, R. C., Flow analysis of DNA content and cell size in non-Hodgkin's lymphoma. *Cancer Res.* **40**: 703–712, 1980.
44. Roos, G., Dige, U., Lenner, P., *et al.*, Prognostic significance of DNA analysis by flow cytometry in non-Hodgkin's lymphoma. *Haematol. Oncol.* **3**: 233–242, 1985.
45. Young, G., Hedley, D., Rugg, C. and Iland, H., The prognostic significance of proliferative activity in poor histology non-Hodgkin's lymphoma—A flow cytometry study using archival material. *COSA Proceedings* #144, 1986.
46. Volm, M., Mattern, J., Sonka, J., *et al.*, DNA distribution in non small cell lung carcinomas and its relationship to clinical behaviour. *Cytometry* **6**: 348–356, 1985.
47. Gynaecological Group, Clinical Oncology Society of Australia, Chemotherapy of advanced ovarian adenocarcinoma: A randomised comparison of combination versus sequential therapy using chlorambucil and cisplatin. *Gynecol. Oncol.* **15**: 261–277, 1986.
48. Tavares, A. S., Costa, J., De Carvalho, A. and Reis, M., Tumor ploidy and prognosis in carcinomas of the bladder and prostrate. *Br. J. Cancer* **20**: 438–441, 1966.
49. Zetterberg, A. and Esposti, P. L., Prognostic significance of nuclear DNA levels in prostatic carcinoma. *Scand. J. Urol. Nephrol. Suppl.* **55**: 53–59, 1980.
50. Fordham, M. V. P., Burdge, A. H., Matthews, J., Williams, G. and Cook, T., Prostatic carcinoma cell DNA content measured by flow cytometry and its relation to clinical outcome. *Br. J. Surg.* **73**: 400–403, 1986.
51. Kute, T. E., Moss, H. B., Anderson, D., Crumb, K., Miller, B., Burns, D. and Dube, L. A., Relationship of steroid receptor, cell kinetics and clinical status in patients with breast cancer. *Cancer Res.* **41**: 3524–3529, 1981.

52. Raber, M. N., Barlogie, B., Latreille, J., Bedrossian, C., Fritsche, H., and Blumenschein, G., Ploidy, proliferative activity and estrogen receptor content in human breast cancer. *Cytometry* **3**: 36–41, 1982.
53. Bauer, K. D., Clevenger, C., Endow, R. K., *et al.*, Simultaneous nuclear antigen and DNA content quantitation using paraffin-embedded clonic tissue and multiparameter flow cytometry. *Cancer Res.* **46**: 2428–2434, 1986.
54. Watson, J. V., Sikora, K. and Evan, G. I., A simultaneous flow cytometric assay for C-myc oncoprotein and DNA in nuclei from paraffin-embedded material. *J. Immunol. Methods* **83**: 179–192, 1985.
55. Watson, J. V., Oncogenes, cancer and analytical cytology. *Cytometry* **7**: 400–410, 1986.

7

Human Tumor Cell Cycle Parameters

Rosella Silvestrini

The past treatment of human tumors has been executed according to biologic and therapeutic information collected on experimental tumors. However, subsequent evidence has led physicians to realize the large inadequacy of experimental information for planning highly effective clinical treatments.

The primary transplantable animal tumors used in biologic and therapeutic studies have highly reproducible patterns of growth but are not representative of potentially metastatic human disease or the variety of human tumor types with biologic heterogeneity. As a result, some of the basic assumptions claimed for experimental tumors have lost their relevance to the treatment of human tumors. For example, very few pathologic instances fit an exponential growth, and the more likely gompertzian growth model cannot be considered an absolute, general law of growth for solid tumors, since it poorly fits much of the human tumor measurements.

Similarly, a relation between the growth rate or tumor aggressiveness as defined according to morphologic, clinical, or pathologic criteria and sensitivity to drugs is not a general finding in clinical practice. The Goldie and Coldman hypothesis of resistant clones as an age-dependent phenomenon and pleiotropic resistance could explain the chemo-resistance of some tumors and the treatment failures with alternating courses of different drugs.

Since the seventies, a major interest of scientists has thus been to investigate individual human tumors to obtain information about biology and sensitivity to chemical and physical therapeutic agents. Much data worthy of analysis and preliminary conclusions have been gathered. Obviously, experimental approaches quite different from those used in animal models were required and set up due to logistic and ethical limitations.

In the specific field of tumor growth control, the possibility to predict clinical response has been investigated with groups of patients with similar disease resulting in population probabilities or with individual patients with the hope of determining yes or no response. Preclinical *in vitro* chemosensitivity tests, whose potentials and limits have been extensively studied,[1] mainly fulfilled the first purpose. Conversely, the availability of an indicator of biologic aggressiveness implies a larger number of applications for both purposes.

TABLE 7.1. *Potential and perspectives of a prognostic marker to optimize treatment and improve clinical success*

Potentials	Perspectives
For large groups	
Prognostic indications	Modulation of treatment
Indications for treatment response	Treatment of subsets which can benefit from specific therapies
For individual tumors	
Monitoring of cytokinetic perturbations induced by few treatment courses	Early assessment of clinical response
Indications of the effect of cell cycle manipulation	Increased therapeutic effect on synchronized cell populations

The potential and perspectives of a prognostic marker to optimize treatment and improve clinical success are shown in Table 7.1. These potentials have been more or less extensively investigated, not only in relation to their clinical importance, but also as regards their practical realization.

CELL KINETICS AS A PROGNOSTIC INDICATOR

In addition to the clinical and pathologic risk factors introduced in clinical practice for their high reproducibility and consolidated prognostic relevance (tumor size, stage), other morphologic and biologic features have been proposed. Among these, one which has drawn increased attention in the last 10 years is the potential proliferative activity of cell populations.

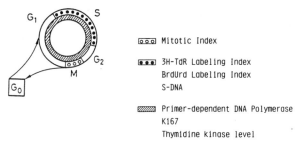

FIG. 7.1. A schematic representation of the mammalian cell cycle which indicates which phases can be measured by various procedures. M = mitosis, G_1 = gap between cytokinesis and onset of DNA synthesis, S = DNA synthetic phase, G_2 = gap between termination of DNA synthenise and prophase, and G_0 = resting or quiescent phase.

Many approaches have been set up and can be grouped according to their target in the cell cycle (Fig. 7.1). These different methods of determining cell kinetics are characterized by different degrees of accuracy, simplicity, cost and rapidity, and for some of them the prognostic relevance still requires definitive verification on large series of cases and for different tumor types.

Determination of the number of proliferating cells, evaluated on biopsies as the ^{3}H-thymidine labeling index,[2,3] has the main advantages of being feasible on consecutive series of patients and performable on solid samples, so as to avoid any cell disaggregation procedure and to preserve histologic architecture.

Cell kinetic information obtained in the last 10 years has shown different median labeling index values for different tumor types.[4-15] However, the wide ranges are indicative of a high cell kinetic heterogeneity among tumors of the same type (Fig. 7.2). For an accurate evaluation of the prognostic potential of cell kinetics it is important to exclude patients in which the natural history of the tumor might have been modified by systemic treatments. The possible prognostic potential has thus been primarily analyzed in relation to probability of relapse in patients submitted to only locoregional control, radiotherapy, and/or surgery. In patients with breast[16-18] or head and neck cancers,[19] the pretreatment labeling index determined on the primary lesion is able to discriminate between two subgroups with significantly different relapse-free survival and also overall survival regardless of multiple treatments after first relapse (Table 7.2). Similarly, cell kinetics determined on nodal metastases from melanoma is related to probability of overall survival.[8]

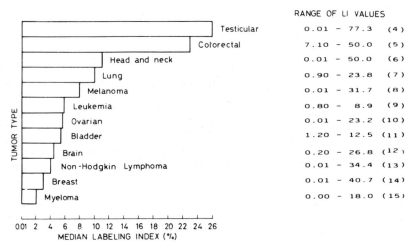

FIG. 7.2. The median labeling index (%) and range of labeling index values measured for various human tumors. The numbers in parentheses refer to the reference from which each specific value was taken.

The potential of cell kinetics in predicting overall survival has also been observed in patients with advanced breast[20] and colorectal cancers or with systemic diseases, such as myeloma[21] and non-Hodgkin lymphoma (NHL),[22] treated with combined modalities or different drug combinations as the first-line of therapy (Table 7.3). Only for operable node-positive breast cancers has a similar probability of overall survival been observed for the two kinetic subsets,[23] probably due to an actual impact of adjuvant treatment on fast-proliferating tumors. Therefore, in spite of the benefit from treatment which has been clinically demonstrated in many cases, pretreatment cell kinetics eventually emerges as an important long-term prognostic factor in subsets of tumors defined homogeneous according to morphologic, clinical, or pathologic criteria. It also has a high score in multivariate analyses performed to evaluate the relative importance of different prognostic variables.[17,18,21,24]

In conclusion, pretreatment cell kinetics is an indicator of risk common to all tumor types considered and deserves special consideration as a stratification parameter for the planning of adequately intensive therapy.

TABLE 7.2. *Clinical outcome as a function of cell kinetics in patients submitted to locoregional treatment*

Tumor type	First-line treatment	Follow-up (yrs.)	Relapse-free survival (%)			Overall survival (%)		
			Low LI	High LI	p value	Low LI	High LI	p value
Breast[a]								
operable N- (16) (258 cases)	Radical surgery	6	81	60	< 0.01	91	75	< 0.01
operable N- (17) (117 cases)	Radical surgery	4	86	52	< 0.01	—	—	—
operable Mo (18) (125 cases)	Surgery + RT	10	74	45–30	0.02	77	50	0.02
Head and Neck[a]								
operable N+ (19) (39 cases)	Radical surgery + RT	3	62	24	0.05	87	48	0.04
Melanoma[b]								
stage II (8)	Radical surgery	2	46	41	n.s.	87	40	0.054

[a] Primary lesion
[b] Nodal lesion

TABLE 7.3. *Overall survival as a function of cell kinetics in patients treated with systemic therapy*

Tumor type	Lesion	First-line treatment	Follow-up (yrs.)	Overall survival (%)		
				Low LI	High LI	p value
Breast						
operable N+ (23) (197 cases)	Primary	Surgery + CMF	6	73	63	n.s.
locally advanced (20) (52 cases)	Primary	AV→RT or S→AV	4	68	37	0.02
Colorectal						
advanced[a] (30 cases)	Liver	5FU or FUDR	0.5	92	51	0.03
Myeloma (21)						
stages I, II, II (79 cases)	Bone marrow	C or LPam and P ± BCNU, A, V	4	40	25	0.02
NHL (22)						
stage II, III, IV (151 cases)	Lymph node	CVP ~ ABP or miscellanea	6	67	22	< 0.01

[a] Metastatic to liver

TABLE 7.4. Objective clinical response as a function of tumor cell kinetics

Tumor type	Lesion	Treatment	Response rate (%)		
			Low LI	High LI	p value
NHL (22) stages II, III, IV (151 cases)	Lymph node	CVP ~ ABP or miscellanea	74	44	< 0.01
Leukemia (25)					
(a) myeloblastic (51 cases)	Bone marrow	Ara-C ± C, V, P	17	71	< 0.01
(b) lymphoblastic (20 cases)	Bone marrow	Ara-C ± C, V, P	60	67	n.s.
Myeloma (21) stages I, II, III (79 cases)	Bone marrow	C or LPam and P ± BCNU, A, V	40	45	n.s.
Melanoma[a] advanced (24 cases)	Node	DTIC	27	33	n.s.
Breast					
(a) locally advanced (20) (52 cases)	Primary	AV	50	50	n.s.
(b) advanced (26) (25 cases)	Effusion	FAC ± V	18	82	< 0.01
Head and Neck (27) advanced (35 cases)	Primary	RT	56	74	n.s.
Miscellanea (28) advanced (16 cases)	Node	RT	90	83	n.s.

[a] A. Costa, unpublished results

CELL KINETICS AS AN INDICATOR OF TREATMENT RESPONSE

Clinical evidence does not support a general direct relationship between actual tumor volume growth and response to therapy, as derived from experimental tumors—not only for metastic lesions but also for primary tumors. Such evidence is substantiated by analysis of the relationship between the known clinical sensitivity of the various tumor types to different therapeutic approaches and the median potential proliferative rate of the same tumor types defined from experimental determinations on individual tumors (Fig. 7.2). In fact, although it is true that germ cell testicular tumors (which exhibit the highest proliferative activity) are the most drug-sensitive tumors, it is also true that gastrointestinal tumors (which show a similarly high proliferative activity) are extremely resistant to chemotherapy, including S-phase-specific drugs. Similarly, the high and moderate resistance of melanomas and ovarian cancers, and the relatively high sensitivity of NHL to different clinical treatments do not reflect their cell kinetic allocation.

The definition of the role of cell kinetics on response to treatment on the basis of available information is hampered by two main factors. The first is the heterogeneity of drug combinations and treatment schedules and of tumor types and stages involved. The second critical point is the confusion about which clinical end point to use. In fact, the relevance of short-term treatment response on the long-term clinical outcome still needs to be precisely defined for many tumors. However, this perplexity should not exclude the importance of knowing the relationship between cell kinetics and objective clinical response.

Available data refer to systemic diseaseas at different stages, to advanced solid tumors treated with drug combinations, and to advanced head and neck cancers and miscellaneous tumors treated with radiotherapy (Table 7.4). All the different types of patterns between cell kinetics and objective clinical response were observed after chemotherapy, but they mainly consisted of a lack of any relationship. An inverse correlation, i.e., a higher response rate in slow-proliferating rather than in fast-proliferating tumors, was observed on a large series of NHL. Most were treated with CVP and ABP and the rest were treated with BACOP or other drug combinations.[22] A direct relationship has been reported only for myeoblastic leukemias[25] and for a small series of effusions from breast cancer.[26] Neither does pretreatment labeling index seem to be, at least significantly, related in response to radiotherapy.[27,28]

Also, in consideration of the rough determination of tumor volume and the potential bias in producing false positives due to inflammatory component reduction or false negatives due to residual necrotic mass, it is reasonable to conclude that response to chemical or physical agents is largely independent of cell kinetic status. The presence of drug-resistant clones or of repair mechanisms of treatment-induced damage could explain the different situation observed with experimental tumors.

TABLE 7.5. *Cell kinetics and treatment response as a function of pathologic stage in operable breast cancer*

Pathologic stage	First-line treatment	Follow-up (yrs)	Relapse-free survival (%)		
			Low LI	High LI	p value
N⁻ (175 cases)	Surgery	6	76	57	< 0.01
N⁻/ER⁻ (60 cases)	Surgery	4	80	30	
	Surgery + CMF	4	87	80	
N⁺ 1–3 nodes[a] (86 cases)	Surgery + CMF	6	69	69	n.s.
N⁺ > 3 nodes[a] (70 cases)	Surgery + CMF	6	54	32	0.03

[a] R. Silvestrini, unpublished results

Whether resistance phenomena is a primary characteristic or only an acquired age-dependent feature is difficult to determine, since the length of the undetectable preclinical phase is not known for different tumor types. Moreover, clinical protocols on adequate series of patients have never been planned on a cell kinetic basis or directed to verify cell kinetic hypotheses. Some information derived from different clinical protocols on operable breast cancers can be tentatively considered to analyze the role of the kinetic variable as a predictor of response to treatment in relation to pathologic stage. An analysis was performed in premenopausal patients (Table 7.5) for whom a benefit from adjuvant therapy has since been reported.[29] Cell kinetics is an indicator of natural aggressiveness, as is consistently shown by the worst prognosis observed for patients with operable, fast-proliferating tumors as compared to those with slow proliferating tumors treated with surgery alone.[16] However, at this stage a recent randomized trial of surgery alone versus surgery plus CMF performed on a series of estrogen receptor negative (ER⁻) tumors[30] has indicated considerable benefit from adjuvant treatment for fast-proliferating tumors which show a probability of relapse-free survival at four years similar to that observed for indolent tumors. Probably due to the effect of adjuvant therapy, a similar probability of relapse-free survival at six years has been observed for patients with slow or fast-proliferating node-positive tumors, but only when metastatic spread was limited to three or less axillary nodes. Conversely, a worse prognosis has been observed for patients with fast-proliferating tumors than those with indolent tumors when associated with nodal involvement of more than three nodes.

By limiting the comments to the prediction of cell kinetics on treatment response, we can conclude that in operable breast cancers, a high labeling index is indicative of response to therapy, at least up to an invasion of three nodes, and classical CMF seems to reduce the poor potential of fast-proliferating tumors to that of the indolent ones. The failure of adjuvant treatment in patients with fast-proliferating tumors and more than three positive nodes could be explained by a tumor cell proliferating compartment greater than the therapeutic potential of adjuvant treatment, or to the extensive presence of resistant clones in more advanced and faster-growing older tumors. The reliability of one or both of these hypotheses will be verified by using suitable methodologic approaches and study designs to acquire information in order to plan even more effective protocols. The consistency of this finding for breast cancer makes investigation for other human tumor types, a feasible possiblity.

CELL KINETIC CHANGES FOR AN EARLY MONITORING

Cell kinetics is an important short and long-term clinical predictor, but a poor indicator of response to treatment. The concept of utilizing changes in proliferative activity induced by a few treatment courses as a predictor of treatment response has been devised. Cell kinetic changes have been determined mainly on tumor biopsies obtained before and after the first radiation or drug courses or on pretreatment samples incubated for different lengths of time with serum taken from the same patient after drug administration.[31] The reliability of these monitoring systems has been analyzed on systemic and solid tumors. A study performed on a series of 48 miscellaneous tumors[32] demonstrated the response predictivity of early cell kinetic changes. A two-fold or greater inhibition of the pretreatment LI value has always been associated with an objective clinical response.

TABLE 7.6. *Clinical response to radiotherapy in relation to early cell kinetics in patients with oral cavity carcinoma*

Change in LI (%)[a]	No. of cases	Clinical Response (%)		
		Objective response	Freedom from progression[b]	Overall survival[b]
≤ − 70%	19	53	10	16
> − 70%	16	81	71	56
p value		0.07	0.01	< 0.01

[a] Variation after 10 Gy/5 fractions
[b] Follow-up: 3 years

Controversial results have been obtained about the reliability of these systems in monitoring response to chemotherapy in acute leukemia,[31] probably due to the different agents included in clinical protocols. Results from the studies directed to monitor response to radiotherapy have been more concordant. In a study performed on a series of 20 cases, including solid and systemic diseases,[28] a decrease by at least two-thirds of the pretreatment LI by radiation therapy was always associated with an objective clinical response. In a more recent study on patients with oral cavity carcinoma (Table 7.6), a reduction of more than 70% of pretreatment LI after 10 Gy was more frequently associated with an objective clinical response and was highly indicative of freedom from progression and of overall survival.[27] There are reasons to believe that these monitoring systems will find extensive applications in the future treatment of cancer.

TUMOR CELL SYNCHRONIZATION

Manipulation to synchronize cell populations has been thought to make most of the cells susceptible to the effect of specific drugs in order to reach maximum cell kill during a relatively short drug exposure. These attempts, which have been successful in cell lines, have led to more deluding results in *in vivo* experimental models and have shown failures in human tumors. The main limiting factors are incomplete drug penetration to all tumor areas and severe toxicity produced by drugs on normal proliferating cells. Moreover, successive tumor sampling mainly for solid tumors is ethically limiting and psychologically refused, so that it may be possible and justified on only a small number of patients to define the effect of new synchronization systems but not for long-term monitoring on individual patients. On the other hand, considering intratumor and intertumor cell kinetic heterogeneity, some doubts remain about the representativeness of each sample and the possibility of extrapolating the results obtained on a small group of tumors to all the tumors of the same type.

Some problems can be overcome when the success of synchronization can be expected on the basis of a defined biologic marker—for example hormone receptors for hormonal manipulation.[33] In such a way, the eligibility of tumors is defined by a single determination. However, once cell proliferating recruitment has been reached, the lack of effective drugs may prove to be dramatic.

Cell synchronization of human tumors is a major problem which has not been extensively investigated to date. Intrinsic drug resistance and natural cell kinetic status, which range widely from tumor to tumor, even within those with similar cytohistopathologic features, need to be known and considered in utilizing synchronization manipulations and in interpreting the results. An attempt to synchronize indolent tumors with low growth fractions is a big problem and could lead to unwarranted results, and tumors with high growth fractions might already be adequately affected by conventional drug combinations and treatment schedules. The main prospectives for cell synchronization and the most important results could be expected for intermediate proliferating tumors.

ACKNOWLEDGMENTS

The author thanks Drs. A. Costa and M. G. Daidone for collaboration and data analyses.

Supported by Grant no. 8602609.44, special project "Oncology" from CNR Rome, Italy.

REFERENCES

1. Dendy, P. P., Hill, B. T., eds., Human Tumor Drug Sensitivity Testing *In Vitro*. In: *Techniques and Clinical Applications*, Academic Press, London, 1983.
2. Silvestrini, R., Sanfilippo, O. and Tedesco, G., Kinetics of human mammary carcinomas and their correlation with the cancer and the host characteristics. *Cancer* **34**: 1252–1258, 1974.
3. Silvestrini, R., Piazza, R., Riccardi, A. and Rilke, F., Correlation of cell kinetic findings with morphology of non-Hodgkin's malignant lymphomas. *J. Natl. Cancer Inst.* **58**: 499–504, 1977.
4. Silvestrini, R., Costa, A., Pilotti, S. and Pizzocaro, G., Cell kinetics in human germ cell tumors of the testis. In *Testicular cancer and other tumors of the genitourinary tract* (M. Pavone-Macaluso, P. H. Smith, M. A. Bagshaw, eds.) pp. 55–62. Plenum Publishing Corporation, New York, 1985.
5. Kanemitsu, T., Koike, A. and Yamamoto, S., Study of the cell proliferation kinetics in ulcerative colitis, adenomatous polyps, and cancer. *Cancer* **56**: 1094–1098, 1985.

6. Molinari, R., Costa, A., Silvestrini, R., Mattavelli, F., Cantu, G., Chiesa, F. and Volterrani, F., Cell kinetics in the study and treatment of head and neck cancer. In *Head and Neck Oncology* (G. T. Wolf, ed.) pp. 229–248. Martinus Nihoff Publishers, Boston, 1984.
7. Muggia, F. M., Cell kinetic studies in patients with lung cancer. *Oncology* **30**: 353–361, 1974.
8. Costa, A., Silvestrini, R., Cascinelli, N., Attili, A. and Testori, A., Cell kinetics of human malignant melanoma: Basic studies and potential clinical prospectives. Proceedings of First International Conference on Skin Melanoma 68, 1985.
9. Yosheida, T., Hattori, K. I., Nakamura, S., Mitamura, T., Kobayashi, S., Ohtake, S. and Tanimoto, K., A simple rapid autoradiography for 3H-thymidine labeling index and its application to therapy of adult acute leukemia. *Cancer* **46**: 2298–2307, 1980.
10. Paradiso, A., Silvestrini, R., Daidone, M. G., Coltro Campi, C. and Grignolio, E., Cell kinetics of human epithelial ovarian cancers. *Bas. Appl. Histochem.* **30**: 215–220, 1986.
11. Awwad, H., Ezzat, S., Hegazy, M., Dahaba, N., El Bolkaini, N., Abd El Baki, H., Abd El Moneim, H., Mansour, M., Aboul Ela, M., Abd El Meguid, H. and Ismail, S., Cell proliferation in carcinoma in bilharzial bladder: Influence of pre-operative irradiation and clinical implications. *Int. J. Radiation Oncology Biol. Phys.* **10**: 2265–2272, 1984.
12. Hoshino, T. and Wilson, C. B., Cell kinetic analyses of human malignant brain tumors (gliomas). *Cancer* **44**: 956–962, 1979.
13. Costa, A., Bonadonna, G., Villa, E., Valagussa, P. and Silvestrini, R., Labeling index as a prognostic marker in non-Hodgkin's lymphomas. *J. Natl. Cancer Inst.* **66**: 1–5, 1981.
14. Gentili, C., Sanfilippo, O. and Silvestrini, R., Cell proliferation and its relationship to clinical features and relapse in breast cancers. *Cancer* **48**: 974–979, 1981.
15. Durie, G. M., Young, L. A. and Salmon, S. E., Human myeloma *in vitro* colony growth: interrelationships between drug sensitivity, cell kinetics, and patients survival duration. *Blood* **5**: 929–934, 1983.
16. Silvestrini, R., Daidone, M. G. and Gasparini, G., Cell kinetics as a prognostic marker in node-negative breast cancer. *Cancer* **56**: 1982–1987, 1985.
17. Meyer, J. S., Friedman, E., McCrate, M. M. and Bauer, W. C., Prediction of early course of breast carcinoma by thymidine labeling. *Cancer* **51**: 1879–1886, 1983.
18. Tubiana, M., Pejovic, M. H., Chavaudra, G., Contesso, G. and Malaise, E. P., The long-term prognostic significance of the thymidine labeling index in breast cancer. *Int. J. Cancer* **33**: 441–445, 1984.
19. Costa, A., Silvestrini, R., Molinari, R., Salvatori, P., Veneroni, S. and Motta, R., Cell kinetics to predict biologic aggressivity and radioresponsivity in head and neck cancers. *Proceedings of the Cell Kinetics Society and the International Cell Cycle Society.* Denver, 1985.
20. Silvestrini, R., Daidone, M. G., Valagussa, P., Salvadori, B., Rovini, D. and Bonadonna, G., Cell kinetics and prognosis in locally advanced breast cancer. *Cancer Treat. Rep.* **71**: 375–379, 1987.
21. Durie, B. G. M., Salmon, S. E. and Moon, T. E., Pretreatment tumor mass, cell kinetics and prognosis in multiple myeloma. *Blood* **55**: 3364–3372, 1980.
22. Del Bino, G., Silvestrini, R., Costa, A., Veneroni, S. and Giardini, R., Morphological and clinical significance of cell kinetics in non-Hodgkin's lymphomas. *Bas. Appl. Histochem.* **30**: 197–202, 1986.
23. Silvestrini, R. and Daidone, M. G., Clinical relevance of proliferative activity of human breast cancer in comparison to other prognostic variables. In: *Endocrin-*

ology and Malignancies: Basic and Clinical Issues (E. E. Bealieu, S. Iacobelli, W. L. McGuire, eds.) Parthenon Publishing, 1986.

24. Silvestrini, R., Daidone, M. G., Di Fronzo, G., Morabito, A., Valagussa, P. and Bonadonna, G., Prognostic implication of labeling index versus estrogen receptors and tumor size in node-negative breast cancer. *Breast Cancer Res. Treat.* **7**: 161–169, 1986.

25. Hart, J. S., George, S. L., Frei III, E., Bodey, G. P., Nickerson, R. C. and Freireich, E. J., Prognostic significance of pretreatment proliferative activity in adult acute leukemia. *Cancer* **39**: 1603–1617, 1977.

26. Sulkes, A., Livingston, R. B. and Murphy, W. K., Tritiated thymidine labeling index and response in human breast cancer. *J. Natl. Cancer Inst.* **62**: 513–515, 1979.

27. Costa, A., Salvatori, P., Molinari, R., Motta, R., Cerutti, A. and Silvestrini, R., Cell kinetics to monitor radioresponsivity in human epidermoid carcinoma. *Bas. Appl. Histochem.* **30**: 209–213, 1986.

28. Elequin, F. T., Muggia, F. M., Ghossein, N. A., Ager, P. J. and Krishnaswamy, V., Correlation between *in vitro* labeling indices (LIs) and tumor regression following radiotherapy. *Int. J. Radiation Oncology Biol. Phys.* **4**: 207–213, 1978.

29. Bonadonna, G. and Valagussa, P., Adjuvant systemic therapy for resectable breast cancer. *J. Clin. Oncol.* **3**: 259–275, 1985.

30. Bonadonna, G., Valagussa, P., Tancini, G., Rossi, A., Brambilla, C., Zambetti, M., Bignami, P., Di Fronzo, G. and Silvestrini, R., Current status of Milan adjuvant chemotherapy trials for node-positive and node-negative breast cancer. *NCI Monogr 1*, 45–49, 1986.

31. Livingston, R. B., Titus, G. A. and Heilbrun, L. K., *In vitro* effects on DNA synthesis as a predictor of biological effect from chemotherapy. *Cancer. Res.* **40**: 2209–2213, 1980.

32. Murphy, W. K., Livingston, R. B., Ruiz, V. G., Gercovich, F. G., George, S. L., Hart, J. S. and Freireich, E. J., Serial labeling index determination as a predictor of response in human solid tumors. *Cancer Res.* **35**: 1438–1444, 1975.

33. Conte, P. F., Alama, A., Di Marco, E., Rosso, R. and Nicolin, A., *In vivo* cytokinetic effects of oestrogens and anti-oestrogens in human breast cancer. In *Anti-oestrogens in oncology: past, present and prospects* (F. Pannuti, ed.) pp. 71–78. Excerpta Medica, Amsterdam, 1985.

8

Analytical Cytology Applied to Detection of Prognostically Important Cytogenetic Aberrations: Current Status and Future Directions

J. W. Gray, D. Pinkel, B. Trask, G. van den Engh, M. Pallavicini,
J. Fuscoe, J. Mullikin and H. van Dekken

INTRODUCTION

The development of techniques for chromosome banding has lead to the discovery of specific cytogenetic abnormalities that are diagnostically and prognostically useful in the treatment of a variety of human cancers.[1-3] Identification of these aberrations has focused on the search for the molecular genetic events associated with tumor development or progression. For example, the strong correlation between chronic myelogeneous leukemia (CML) and the Philadelphia chromosome, eventually identified as t(9;22),[3,4] motivated molecular analyses of the breakpoints on chromosomes 9 and 22 that has demonstrated the consistent translocation of the c-abl oncogene (normally on chromosome 9) into the break point cluster region (bcr) on chromosome 22.[5] The oncogenic role of the atypical c-abl protein that results from this translocation[6] is being investigated and may ultimately lead to an understanding of the oncogenic event(s) responsible for CML. Numerous other prognostically or diagnostically useful chromosome aberrations have been discovered since the Philadelphia chromosome. Some seem to involve the loss or gain of one or a few specific chromosome types or portions thereof. Trisomy 7, for example, has been associated with clear cell carcinoma of the kidney,[7] malignant glioma,[8,9] and renal adenocarcinoma.[10,11] Monosomy 18 and the loss of 17p are associated with colo rectal cancers.[12,13] A deletion of all or part of chromosome 11 is associated with Wilm's tumor,[14] while a duplication of 3p and loss of 11p indicates a poor prognosis in transitional cell carcinoma of the bladder.[15] These studies suggest that: (1) Specific chromosomal abnormalities are associated with one or more tumor types, (2) chromosomal abnormalities may be diagnostically, prognostically, and therapeutically important, and (3) identification of disease-linked chromosomal aberrations opens the way for investigation of the molecular basis of the disease.

THE DNA INDEX

Cytogenetic studies of human tumors are not simple, especially solid tumors. In many cases it is not possible to produce sufficient high quality metaphase spreads for analysis. Even when metaphase spreads can be produced and banded, the culture procedures required to produce the mitotic cells may select for tumor subpopulations that are not representative of the malignant stem line. As a result, one has had to be content with approaches that yield less complete information than would ideally be desired. One such approach has been measurement of tumor cell DNA content as a general indication of the cytogenetic status of the tumor.[16] Tumor cell DNA content measurements are desirable because they can be accomplished quickly using flow cytometry and without cell culture. In fact, developments in recent years have allowed measurement of the DNA contents of cells isolated from paraffin blocks, so that extensive retrospective studies have become possible using archival material.[17]

DNA distribution analysis

Quantitative analysis of tumor cell DNA content is conceptually straightforward. Individual cells are isolated from fresh, frozen, or paraffin-embedded tumors; treated with RNAse, stained with a nucleic acid-specific fluorescent dye, and processed through a flow cytometer. Total fluorescence is measured as an estimate of cellular DNA content. Standard cells are often mixed with the tumor population to provide a DNA content reference against which the tumor population can be compared. Alternatively, the normal diploid cells in the tumor itself may be used as an internal reference. The DNA index (DI) for the tumor is defined as the ratio of the mean of the G1/G0 tumor peak to the mean of the G1/G0 peak for the normal diploid cells. Estimation of the DI is straightforward when the separation between the normal and tumor peaks is considerably larger than the widths of the peaks. However, the calculation of the DI becomes difficult as the means of the two peaks move together or as the relative frequency of one population becomes smaller. The width of the normal and tumor peaks is usually expressed as a coefficient of variation (CV = standard deviation/mean). It is difficult to recognize the presence of an abnormal population if the fractional difference in the means of the normal and abnormal populations is less than about 2.5 times the CV, even when the normal and abnormal populations are of equal frequency. Thus, measurements with a CV of 0.05 would allow detection of aneuploidy in tumors with DI>1.125, while measurements with a CV of 0.01 would allow detection of aneuploid tumors with DI>1.025. In practice, CVs ranging from 0.07 down to 0.01 are achieved for various human tumors, depending on experimental technique, instrument rational adjustment, and tumor type. The CVs achieved for leukemias are generally smaller than the CVs for solid tumors.

Correlation between the DI and tumor characteristics

The simplicity, broad applicability, and speed of DNA distribution analysis has allowed numerous studies in which abnormalities in tumor cell DNA content have been correlated with karyotype, tumor stage, and prognosis.

Comparison with karyotype

Several studies have examined the correlation between the DI determined by flow cytometric DNA distribution analysis and the DI expected from cytogenetic analysis of tumor metaphase spreads.[16,18-20] In general, the correlation between the DIs measured by the two methods has been strong for solid tumors[19] and for leukemias.[16,20] However, a few discrepancies were noted in which samples found to be diploid by conventional karyotyping were found to have DIs greater than 1 by flow cytometry. It seems reasonable to conclude from these studies that a DI>1 or DI<1 measured by flow cytometry indicates the addition at loss of chromosomes or chromosomal fragments. However, this approach yields no information about which chromosomes are involved or about chromosome rearrangements.

Prognostic utility of the DI

DIs have been measured for a broad spectrum of human tumors. In general, DI>1 seems to be associated with an unfavorable prognosis in solid tumors. The DIs for solid tumors tend to fall anywhere in the range of 1.0 to >2.0.[21] DIs for acute leukemias, on the other hand, are in the range of 1.0 to 1.1.[22] Interestingly, DI<1 is associated with an unfavorable prognosis in myelodysplasia.[20] Table 8.1 shows DIs and information about the correlation between DI and prognosis for several human tumors. Table 8.1 also shows commonly occurring chromosomal changes that have been found by banding analysis for these tumor types.

TABLE 8.1. *Comparison of tumor cytogenetic endpoints*

Tumor Type	% aneuploid	Model DI	Prognostic ?	Common Karyotypic Findings	Reference No.
Bladder	50	1.7	Yes	+7, −9, +3p, −5p, −11p	15,16,21
Breast	65	1.7	Yes	Rearranged 1	13,16,17,24–28
Colorectal	65	1.7	Yes/No[a]	+7, −17p, −18	12,16,19,21–29
Ovarian	65	1.4	Yes	i(6p), i(12p)	16,23
Renal	70	1.6	Yes	+7	10,11,16,28
AML	40	1.1	No		16.22
All	24–40	1.1–1.2	Possible[b]	+8	3,13,16,20,22

[a] Indicates conflicting reports
[b] Childhood ALL

In spite of the correlations that have been established between the DI and prognosis in some tumors, the utlimate utility of the DI remains unclear. One limiting feature of the assay is its poor cytogenetic specificity. That is, a number of different cytogenetic events may lead to the same DI. In addition, the assay depends critically on the precision achieved during DNA distribution analysis. These points are illustrated in Figure 8.1, which shows the minimum detectable level of chromosome aneuploidy as a function of the measurement CV achieved during DNA distribution analysis. Thus, establishment of direct correlations between tumor phenotypes and genetic events linked to specific chromosomes will probably be impossible based on the DI alone.

FLOW KARYOTYPING

Flow karyotyping is a flow cytometric approach to chromosome classification that does allow detection of specific chromosome aberrations. In this approach, mitotic cells are collected from the population of interest, swollen and then ruptured to release the chromosomes into an aqueous buffer designed to maintain the structural integrity of the isolated chromosomes. In our laboratory, the chromosomes are then stained with the DNA specific dyes Hoechst 333258 (Ho; binds preferentially to AT rich DNA) and chromomycin A3 (CA3: binds preferen-

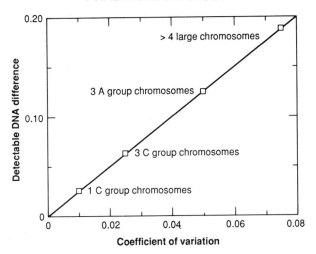

FIG. 8.1 Illustration of the minimum detectable DNA content difference as a function of DNA measurement CV. DNA content difference is related to chromosomal loss or gain at several points.

tially to GC rich DNA) and analyzed using dual beam flow cytometry.[30–32] The Ho and CA3 contents of each chromosome are measured as the chromosomes pass one by one through two laser beams, one emitting 351+363nm and the other emitting 458nm. The measurements of about 10^5 chromosomes are accumulated in a few minutes to form a bivariate Ho vs CA3 distribution (called a flow karyotype) like those shown in Figure 8.2 for human cells. These distributions show numerous peaks, each produced by one or a few chromosome types. The mean position of a peak is characteristic of the chromosomal DNA content and DNA base composition, while the peak volume is proportional to the frequency of that chromosome or chromosome group in the population. Figure 8.2a shows that a distinct peak is produced by each human chromosome type except for chromosomes 9 through 12 in a normal diploid cell population. Chromosomes 9 through 12 have nearly identical DNA contents and DNA base composition and thus cannot be distinguished. Measurement of a sample containing an aneuploidy would yield an abnormal value for the relative volume of the peak corresponding to the aneuploid chromosome. For example, the peak for chromosome 7 in the flow karyotype for a population trisomic for that chromosome would be 50% larger than in a normal flow karyotype. Structural aberrations resulting in derivative chromosome with altered DNA contents or DNA base composition result in the formation of new peaks in the flow karyotype. For example, Figure 8.2b shows the flow karyotype measured for chromo-

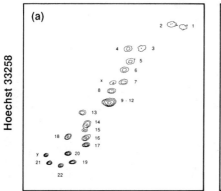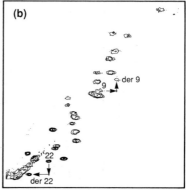

Chromomycin A3

FIG. 8.2 Bivariate flow karyotypes measured for chromosomes isolated from human cells: (a) Flow karyotype measured for normal diploid cells. The numbers indicate the chromosome types responsible for each peak. (b) Flow karyotype measured for leukemic cells from a patient with chronic myelogenous leukemia. The peaks for the derivative chromosomes resulting from t(9;22) are indicated.

somes isolated from leukemic cells from a patient with chronic myelogenous leukemia. The leukemic cells from this patient had the characteristic t(9;22) associated with this disease. The derivative chromosomes have formed two new, distinct peaks in the flow karyotype.[56]

Flow karyotyping thus appears especially useful for characterization of chromosomal changes in human tumors that can be grown sufficiently well in culture to permit chromosome isolation. This has been demonstrated to be routinely possible for chronic myelogenous leukemia (Fig. 8.2b) and it seems likely that the technique can be extended to other leukemias and possibly even to solid tumors. The technique is less well suited to detection of chromosome-specific aneuploidy; especially for cell populations containing multiple aneuploidies. In this case, it is difficult to determine the relative frequency of a chromosome type, since the total number of chromosomes per cell in the population may be variable or unknown. In addition, flow karyotyping is limited to tumors which can be cultured, and the culturing may lead to selective growth of cells that are not representative of the tumor cell stem line.

FLUORESCENCE HYBRIDIZATION

Some of the limitations in the DI assay and in flow karyotyping may be reduced by application of new techniques that allow quantitative analysis of the number of chromosomes of a specific type or the amount of particular DNA sequences present in individual interphase nuclei. These techniques are based on the use of fluorescence *in situ* hybridiz-

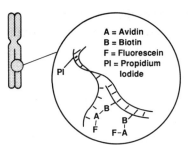

FIG. 8.3 Cytochemical principles of fluorescence hybridization. The DNA in the target nucleus or chromosome is partially denatured to expose single-stranded DNA. Denatured, chemically modified probe DNA (biotin labeled, in this example) is added and the probe and target DNA are allowed to reanneal under conditions where the probe binds only to target DNA sequences to which it has high homology. The bound probe DNA is detected by treating with a fluorescent reagent that binds with high specificity to the chemically modified probe (fluorescein labeled avidin in this example). The double-stranded DNA is counterstained with a reagent (PI in this example) that fluoresces in a wavelength region different from the probe-linked fluorescent reagent.

ation (called fluorescence hybridization hereafter) to specifically and intensely stain selected chromosomes or portions thereof so that they can be readily identified and enumerated in metaphase and interphase nuclei. The remainder of this chapter describes the concept of fluorescence hybridization and illustrates how it may be applied to detect chromosome-specific aneuploidy and to study the chromosomal organization of the interphase nucleus.

Chromosome staining by fluorescence hybridization

The cytochemical principles of fluorescence hybridization are illustrated in Figure 8.3. In this approach,[33-36] the DNA in the target cell population is denatured to form single-stranded DNA. The denatured cells are then incubated with chemically-modified (e.g., biotin or 2-acetylaminofluorene (AAF))[37,38] single-stranded "probe" DNA under conditions where the probe binds only to DNA sequences in the target cells to which it is homologous. The bound probe is rendered fluorescent using fluorescently labeled affinity reagents specific for the chemical modification in the probe. The binding of several different probes, each carrying a unique chemical modification, can be distinguished by detection with reagents labeled with different fluorophores. For example, biotin-labeled probes may be detected using fluorescein-labeled avidin and AAF-labeled probes may be detected using rhodamine-labeled antibody against the AAF-DNA adducts. The cells or chromosomes may be counterstained with a DNA specific dye (e.g., propidium iodide or DAPI) that fluoresces in a different wavelength region than from the detection reagent(s). Figure 8.4 shows photomicrographs for the same metaphase chromosomes from a human × hamster cell line carrying a few human chromosomes. Hybridization was carried out using AAF-labeled human genomic DNA and biotin-labeled hamster genomic DNA as probes. The AAF-labeled probe was detected using red fluorescing rhodamine-labeled goat anti-AAF antibody and the biotin-labeled probe was detected using green fluorescing, fluorescein-labeled avidin. The chromosomes were counterstained with the blue fluorescing dye, DAPI. These fluorochromes can be independently excited.

Human chromosome—specific probes

We are pursuing two strategies for specifically staining individual human chromosomes. The first involves use of probes for DNA sequences that occur repetitively on a single chromosome type. These are typically concentrated on one region of a chromosome, usually near the centromere. Frequently, they are members of a family of related sequences whose members are distributed on many chromosomes. Thus, careful control of the hybridization stringency is required to optimize the chromosome-specificity of probe binding. Repetitive probes with useful specificity for both sex chromosomes and a large number of the autosomes have been discovered. We are currently using or evaluating probes for chromosomes 1[39,40], 6[41], 7[42], 9[43], 11[44], 13/21[45], 15[46], 17[47], 18[45], 20[48], 22[49], X[41,50], and Y[51]. The rapid discovery of new repetitive probes suggests that such probes will be available for most of the human chromosomes in the near future. Repetitive probes are particularly useful for cytogenetic analysis involving aneuploidy. However, this approach is sensitive only to aneuploidy involving the labeled portion of the chromosome. For example, duplication or loss of a chromosome arm may not be detectable using a centromeric probe. The utility of repetitive probes for translocation detection is limited because there is only a small probability that the rearrangement will split the fluorescent label between the derivative chromosomes.

Translocation detection becomes more effecient as the portion of a chromosome that is spanned by the probe is enlarged. Thus the second approach to chromosome staining involves the use of combinations of repetitive or unique sequence probes that bind to different places on the same chromosome.[57] The combined probes may be repetitive probes such as those that bind to the telomeric[40] and centromeric regions[39] of chromosome 1. Alternately, the combined probes may

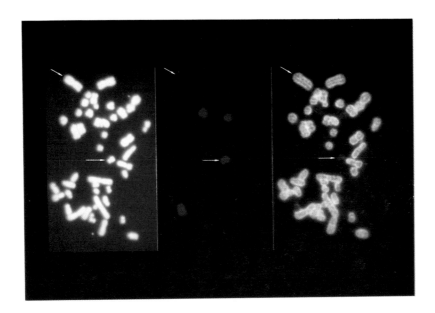

FIG. 8.4. Fluorescence photomicrograph of human and hamster metaphase chromosomes following hybridization with AAF-labeled human genomic DNA and biotin-labeled genomic DNA. Fluorescence detection and staining was accomplished as described in the text: (a) DAPI fluorescence image; (b) Rhodamine (AAF-linked) fluorescence from human chromosomes; and (c) Fluorescein (biotin-linked) fluorescence from hamster chromosomes. The upper arrow in each figure indicates a hamster chromosome and the lower arrow indicates a human chromosome.

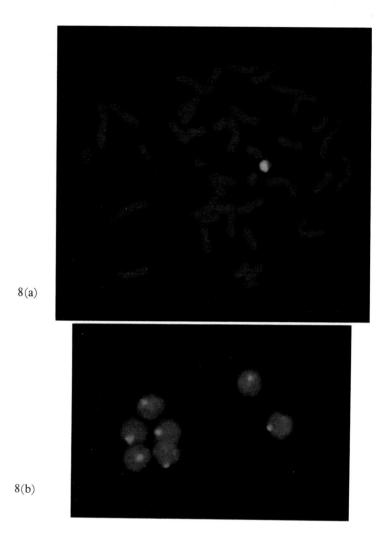

8(a)

8(b)

FIG. 8.5. Hybridization to human nuclei and metaphase spreads with chromosome specific probes: (a) Hybridization with a Y specific probe to a metaphase spread from a normal male; (b) Y chromosomes in nuclei from a normal 47XY male; (c) Y chromosomes in nuclei from a 47XYY male; (d) Hybridization with a probe for the telomeric region of the short arm of the number 1 human chromosome to a metaphase spread; and (e) Chromosome 1p telomeric regions in interphase nuclei. Probes were labeled with biotin and detected with fluorescein-avidin. The DNA was counterstained with Pl. Thus, regions of probe hybridization appear yellow and the remaining DNA appears red.

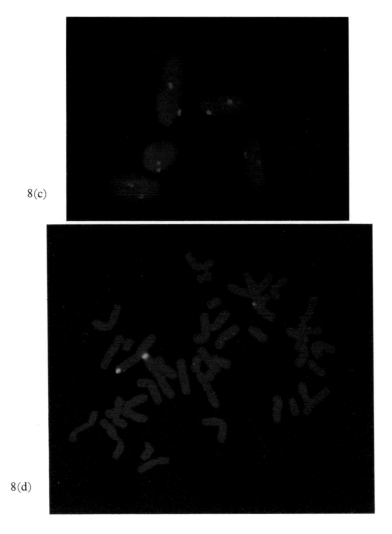

8(c)

8(d)

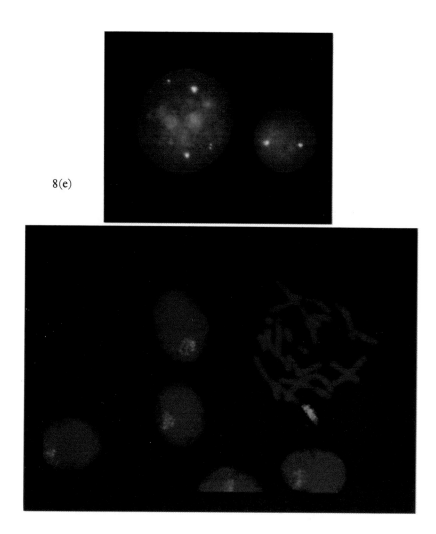

8(e)

FIG. 8.6. Hybridization with a probe for the c-myc gene to a metaphase spread of a hamster cell line carrying approximately 2,000 copies of the c-myc gene. Hybridization detection and counterstaining were accomplished as described in Figure 8.5.

be collections of chromosome-specific unique sequences isolated from chromosome-specific libraries to stain continuously along any desired portion of a chromosome.

FLUORESCENCE HYBRIDIZATION APPLIED TO CYTOGENETIC ANALYSIS

We demonstrate in the following sections several cytogenetic applications of fluorescence hybridization with repetitive probes. The results can be analyzed using fluorescence microscopy, quantitative image processing, or flow cytometry. This approach should allow improved analysis of tumor aneuploidy, may allow for quantitative analysis of specific gene amplification, and may provide information about changes in the chromosomal positions in interphase nuclei that result from or lead to oncogenesis.

Fluorescence microscopy applied to aneuploidy detection

The hybridization of chromosome-specific repetitive probes is easily seen both in metaphase spreads and interphase nuclei using standard microscopy.[33,53-55] Figure 8.5a, for example, illustrates hybridization of a Y-specific probe to a human metaphase spread. The single Y-chromosome is distinctively labeled and can be recognized immediately. Figures 8.5b and 8.5c shown fluorescence hybridization with a Y-specific probe to 46XY and 47XYY interphase nuclei, respectively. The single compact fluorescent domains in 46XY nuclei and the two domains in the 47XYY nuclei are clearly visible. Figures 8.5d and 8.5e illustrate hybridization with a probe specific to the telomere of the short arm of human chromosome #1 to a metaphase spread and to an interphase nucleus. Figures 8.5b, 8.5c and 8.5d show that the probe-binding in nuclei is concentrated in compact regions (domains), one for each copy of the chromosome that is present. Results to date indicate that the homologues of a given chromosome tend to be well separated in interphase nuclei. Thus, a cell population containing a specific aneuploidy can be detected simply by counting the fluorescent domains in the nuclei.[33,36,52-55] These examples suggest that aneuploidy involving specific chromosomes should be detectable using this approach as long as suitable repetitive probes are available. Perhaps the main limitations of the "domain counting" approach to analysis of two dimensional nuclear images is the inevitability that two spots will appear overlapped due to a chance orientation of the nucleus. This would cause an erroneous count. Quantitative intensity measurements of probe binding may alleviate this problem to some extent.

Fluorescence hybridization may also be used to detect specific DNA content changes resulting from amplification of specific gene sequences when the level of amplification is high. Figure 8.6, for example, shows fluorescence hybridization of a biotin labeled 2.2kb probe for c-myc to a metaphase spread of a hamster cell line (Pallavicini *et al*; manuscript in preparation) that was constructed by co-transfecting with plasmids carrying genes for dihydrofolate reductase and c-myc. The transfected c-myc sequence in this cell line was amplified approximately 2000-fold by growth in successively higher concentrations of methotrexate.[34] The site of incorporation of the c-myc sequence is clearly visible on one chromosome in the metaphase spread and in the interphase nucleus as well.

Flow cytometric analysis of chromosome-specific aneuploidy

Flow cytometry can be used to measure the amount of target sequence for a probe that is present in a nucleus. This requires the fluorescence hybridization to be carried out for the nuclei in liquid suspension.[35,36] Flow cytometric measurements have been taken of a series of human $\times$ hamster hybrid cell lines containing different amounts of human DNA made after fluorescence hybridization with human genomic DNA. This probe bound only to the human chromosomes under the hybridization conditions used. The probe-linked fluorescence was shown to be proportional to the amount of human DNA present.[36] This result suggests the use of flow cytometry for analysis of the number of copies of a specific amplified or repeated sequence present in nuclei. The method is currently limited to analysis of sequences in which the amount of target is above 10^6 bases. This sensitivity is adequate for use with many chromosome-specific repetitive probes.

Figure 8.7 illustrates a flow cytometric measurement of the intensity of probe-linked fluorescence following hybridization with a Y-specific probe to a mixed cell population containing roughly equal numbers of 46XX, 46XY, and 47XYY nuclei. Three distinct peaks are visible in the distribution, as expected. Of course, this method of aneuploidy detection will be accurate only if the amount of target sequence to which the probe binds is not highly polymorphic. Currently, the CV of the flow measurements of probe-linked fluorescence intensities is in the range of 15 to 20%. If the precision can be improved, the high processing speed of flow cytometry may allow large numbers of cells to be scanned in search of low frequency aneuploid populations.

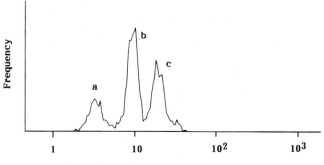

FITC (probe) fluorescence intensity

FIG. 8.7 Probe-linked fluorescence intensity distribution measured flow cytometrically for 46XX(a), 46XY(b), and 47XYY(c) nuclei. The nuclei were hybridized to a Y-specific probe in suspension.

Quantitative image analysis of the chromosomal positions in interphase nuclei

Quantitative image processing, coupled with fluorescence hybridization of chromosome-specific probes to nuclei in suspension, promises a further improvement in our ability to characterize the cytogenetic status of tumor cells. Hybridization in suspension appears to preserve the three-dimensional structure of the nucleus. This allows analysis of the interphase chromosome domains in three dimensions (van Dekken *et al.*, manuscript in preparation).[36,52] With this approach, digitized fluorescence microscope images are acquired at several focal planes through a hybridized nucleus. These images are then computer-processed and assembled to show the three-dimensional distribution of the fluorescing domains resulting from the hybridization process. Use of a DNA counterstain allows reconstruction of the nuclear shape in the same manner. Figure 8.8 shows three-dimensional views of human × hamster hybrid nuclei containing two human chromosomes. Human genomic DNA was used as the probe to specifically label the human chromosomes. The nuclear boundary, estimated from images acquired while exciting DAPI fluorescence are illustrated as well. These techniques, when applied to human nuclei, should allow improved detection of aneuploidy, since the chance overlap of chromosomal domains that will occur in two-dimensional nuclear images will be resolved in three-dimensional images. More importantly, this technology should allow general analysis of the relative positions of different chromosomes in interphase nuclei. Important questions that might be addressed include: (1) Is the organization constant for cells of the same type and stage of differentiation? (2) Does the organization change with

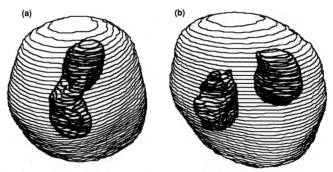

FIG. 8.8 Reconstruction showing the three-dimensional locations of two human chromosomes in human × hamster hybrid nuclei. The heavy lines show the locations of the two human chromosomes obtained from a fluorescein image (blue excitation, green fluorescence). The light lines show the location of the nuclear boundary obtained from a DAPI image (UV excitation, blue fluorescence).

differentiation or oncogenesis? and (3) Does the organization of the interphase nucleus play a role in aberration formation and/or oncogenesis?

DISCUSSION

Conventional cytogenetic analyses and flow cytometry of human tumors have provided valuable clues to cytogenetic events that may have diagnostic and/or prognostic use. Abnormal DIs are so strongly correlated with poor prognosis in some tumors that staging according to DI seems appropriate. However, specific information about which chromosomes are involved is not available from flow measurements at this point in time.

Conventional cytogenetic analyses have revealed specific chromosome additions or deletions (e.g., trisomy 7) that occur with such high frequency in human solid tumors that the dosage of one or more genes on this chromosome appears to play a role in the malignant process.[8] The recent report that the tumorigenicity of Wilm's tumor can be altered by addition of an intact number 11 chromosome tends support to the hypothesis that changes in gene dosage associated with tumor aneuploidy may play an important role in the formation of progression of selected tumors.[14] However, these techniques are difficult to apply to large numbers of human tumors, especially solid tumors.

Flourescence hybridization with chromosome-specific probes now promises substantially improved analysis of tumor aneuploidy. The assay is already sufficiently sensitive to allow detection of the gain or loss of the labeled subregion of a specific chromosome following hybridization with a repetitive probe. The specificity of this approach may be further increased by hybridizing with collections of chromosome-specific unique sequence probes tailored to optimize detection of loss or gain in a particular chromosomal region. Fluorescence hybridization also has the potential to allow analysis of gene amplification. This new capability will dramatically increase the rate at which the importance of chromosome-specific aneuploidy and gene amplification in human malignancy can be evaluated. If, as seems likely, important correlations are found, diagnosis, prognosis, and eventually therapy should be improved. Quantitative analysis of the relative chromosome positions in the interphase nucleus should allow study of the role of their organization in translocation formation and should provide useful information about the response of the interphase organization during oncogenesis.

ACKNOWLEDGMENTS

This work was performed under the auspices of the US Department of Energy by the Lawrence Livermore National Laboratory under contract number W–4705–ENG–48 with support from USPHS grants HD 17655 and CA45919. H.vD. was supported by FUNGO, the Netherlands. The authors are grateful for probes generously provided by Drs. F. Wurm (c–myc), K. Smith (Y), and M. Litt (#1 telomere).

REFERENCES

1. Mitelman, F., Restricted number of chromosomal abnormalities implications in the aetiology of human cancer and leukemia. *Nature* **310**: 325–327, 1984.
2. Rowley, J. and Ultmann, J. eds. In: *Chromosomes and Cancer, from Molecules to Man.* Academic Press, NY, 1982.
3. Mitelman, F. In: Catalog of Chromosome Aberrations in Cancer, 2nd ed. Academic Press, New York, 1985.
4. Nowell, P. and Hungerford, D., A minute chromosome in human chronic granulocytric leukemia. *Science* **132**: 1497, 1960.
5. Bartram, C., Kleihauer, E., de Klein, A., Grosveld, G., Teyssier, J., Heisterkamp, N. and Groffen, J., c-abl and bcr are rearranged in a Ph-negative CML patient. *The EMBO Journal* **4**: 683–686, 1985.
6. Varmus, H., The molecular genetics of cellular oncogenes. *Ann. Rev. Genet.* **18**: 55–612, 1984.
7. Wolman, S., Golimbu, M., Morales, P. and Schinella, R., Characterization of human clear cell carcinoma. *Proceedings of AACR* **27**: 38, 1986.
8. Bell, C., Rosenblum, M., Harsh, G., Korc, M., Meltzer, P. and Trent, J., Correlation of chromosome 7 alterations with expression of epidermal growth factor receptor (EGF) in human glial and pancreatic carcinomas. *Proceedings—Second International Conference on Chromosomes in Solid Tumors*, January 18–21, 1987.
9. Bigner, S., Wong, A., Mark, J., Kinzler, K., Vogelstein, B. and Bigner, D., Chromosomes and gene amplication in malignant human gliomas (MHG). *Pro-*

ceedings—Second International Conference on Chromosomes in Solid Tumors, January 18–21, 1987.

10. de Jong, B., Idenburg, V., Dam, A. and Wolter, J., Cytogenetics of renal adeno-carcinoma in 13 patients. *Proceedings—Second International Conference on Chromosomes in Solid Tumors.* January 18–21, 1987.

11. Nordenson, I., Ljungberg, B. and Roos, G., Chromosomal heterogeneity in renal cancer. *Proceedings—Second International Conference on Chromosomes in Solid Tumors*, January 18–21, 1987.

12. Muleris, M., Salmon, R., Zafrani, B., Girodet, J. and Dutrillaux, B., Involvement of chromosomes 17 and 18 in sixteen human colo-rectal cancers. *Proceedings of AACR 27*, 38, 1986.

13. Sandberg, A., Cytogenetic definition of cancer subtypes. *Proceedings—Second International Conference on Chromosomes in Solid Tumors*, January 18–21, 1987.

14. Weissman, B., Saxon, P., Pasquale, S., Jones, G., Geiser, A. and Stanbridge, E., Introduction of a normal human chromosome 11 into Wilms' tumor cell line controls its tumorigenic expression. *Science* **236**: 175–180, 1987.

15. Falor, W. and Ward-Skinner, R., Chromosomal analysis of 37 noninvasive and 13 sub-mucosal invasive transitional cell carcinomas of the bladder following up to seventeen years. *Proceedings—Second International Conference on Chromosomes in Solid Tumors*, January 18–21, 1987.

16. Barlogie, B., Raber, M., Schumann, J., Johnson, T., Drewinko, B., Swartzen-druber, D., Godhe, W., Andreeff, M. and Freireich, E., Flow cytometry in clinical cancer research. *Cancer Res.* **43**: 3982–3997, 1983.

17. Hedley, D., Friedlander, M. and Taylor, I., Application of DNA flow cytometry to paraffin-embedded archival material for the study of aneuploidy and its clinical significance. *Cytometry* **6**: 327–333, 1985.

18. Tribukait, B., Granberg-Ohman, I. and Wilkstrom, H., Flow cytometric DNA and cytogenetic studies in human tumors: A comparison and discussion of differences in modal values obtained by the two methods. *Cytometry* **7**: 194–199, 1986.

19. Petersen, S. and Friedrich, U., A comparison between flow cytometric ploidy investigation and chromosome analysis of 32 human colorectal tumors. *Cytometry* **7**: 307–312, 1986.

20. Look, A. T., Melvin, S., Williams, D., Brodeur, G., Dahi, G., Kalwinsky, D., Murphy, S. and Mauer, A., Aneuploidy and percentage of S-phase cells determined by flow cytometry correlate with cell phenotype in childhood acute leukemia. *Blood* **60**: 959–967, 1982.

21. Frankfurt, O., Arbuck, S., Chin, J., Greco, W., Pavelic, Z., Slocum, H., Mittelman, A., Piver, S., Pontes, E. and Rustum, Y., Prognostic applications of DNA flow cytometry for human solid tumors. In: *Clinical Cytometry* (M. Andreeff, Ed.) pp. 276–290. *Ann. NY Acad. Sci.*, New York, 1986.

22. Hiddemann, W., Wormann, B., Ritter, J., Thiel, E., Gohde, W., Lahme, B., Henze, G., Schellong, G., Riehm, H. and Buchner, T., Frequency and clinical significance of DNA aneuploidy in acute leukemia. In *Clinical Cytometry* (M. Andreeff, Ed.) pp. 227–240. *Ann. NY Acad. Sci.*, New York, 1986.

23. Friedlander, M., Hedley, D., Taylor, I., Russell, P., Coates, A. and Tattersall, M., Influence of cellular DNA content on survival in advanced ovarian cancer. *Cancer Res.* **44**: 397–400, 1984.

24. Ewers, S. B., Langstron, E., Baldetorp, B. and Killander, D., Flow-cytometric DNA analysis in primary breast carcinomas and clinicopathological correlations. *Cytometry* **5**: 408–419, 1984.

25. Boon, M., Auer, G., van Kaam, H. and Schwinghammer, H., Classifying breast carcinomas with DNA measurements and morphometry. *Cytometry* **5**: 469–472, 1984.

26. Auer, G., Fallenius, A., Erhardt, K. and Sundelin, B., Progression of mammary adenocarcinomas as reflected by nuclear DNA content. *Cytometry* 5: 420–425, 1984.

27. Frankfurt, O., Slocum, H., Rustum, Y., Arbuck, S., Pavelic, Z., Petrelli, N., Huben, R., Pontes, E. and Greco, W., Flow cytometric analysis of DNA aneuploidy in primary and metastatic human solid tumors. *Cytometry* 5: 71–80, 1984.

28. Baisch, H., Otto, U. and Kloppel, K., Malignancy index based on flow cytometry and histology for renal cell carcinomas and its correlation to prognosis. *Cytometry* 7: 200–204, 1986.

29. Kokal, W., Shelban, K., Terz, J. and Haroda, J. R., Tumor DNA content in the prognosis of colo-rectal carcinoma. *J. Am. Medical Assn.* 255: 3123–3127, 1986.

30. Gray, J., Langlois, R., Carrano, A., Burkhart-Schultz, K. and Van Dilla, M., High resolution chromosome analysis. One and two parameter flow cytometry. *Chromosoma.* 63: 9–27, 1979.

31. van den Engh, G., Trask, B., Gray, J., Langlois, R. and Yu, L. C., Preparation and bivariate analysis of suspension of human chromosomes. *Cytometry* 6: 92–100, 1985.

32. Gray, J. and Langlois, R., Chromosome classification and purification using flow cytometry and sorting. *Ann. Rev. Biophys. Biophys. Chem.* 15: 195–235, 1986.

33. Pinkel, D., Straume, T. and Gray, J., Cytogenetic analysis using quantitative, high sensitivity, fluorescence hybridization *Proc. Natl. Acad. Sci.* USA 83: 2934–2939, 1986.

34. Wurm, F. M., Gwinn, K. A. and Kingston, R. E., Inducible overproduction of the mouse c-myc protein in mammalian cells. *Proc. Natl. Acad. Sci.* USA 83: 5414–5418, 1986.

35. Trask, B., van den Engh, G., Landegent, J., Jansen, in de Wal N. and van der Ploeg, M., Detection of DNA sequences in nuclei in suspension by *in situ* hybridization and dual beam flow cytometry. *Science* 230: 1401–1403, 1985.

36. Trask, B., van den Engh, G., Pinkel, D., Mullikin, J., van Dekken, H. and Gray, J., Fluorescence *in situ* hybridization to interphase cell nuclei in suspension allows flow cytometric analysis of chromosome content and microscopic analysis of nuclear organization. *Human Genetics* 42: 49–59, 1988.

37. Langer, P., Waldrop, A. and Ward, D., Enzymatic synthesis of biotin—labeled polynucleotides: Novel nucleic acid affinity probes. *Proc. Natl. Acad. Sci.* USA 78: 6633–6637, 1981.

38. Landegent, J., Jansen, in de Wal, N. Baan, R., Hoeijmakers, J. and van der Ploeg, M., 2-Acetylaminofluorene-modified probes for indirect hybridochemical detection of specific nucleic acid sequences. *Exp. Cell Res.* 153: 61–72, 1984.

39. Waye, J. S., Durfy, S. J., Pinkel, D., Kenwrick, S., Patterson, M., Davies, K. E. and Willard, H. F., Chromosome-specific alpha satellite DNA from human chromosome 1: Hierarchical structure and genomic organization of a polymorphic domain spanning several hundred kilobase pairs of centromeric DNA. *Genomics* 1: 43–51, 1987.

40. Buroker, N., Bestwick, R., Haight, G., Magenix, R. E. and Litt, M., A hypervariable region of human chromosome 1p36.3. *Human Genetics* (in press).

41. Jabs, E. W., Wolf, S. F. and Migeon, B. R., Characterization of a cloned DNA sequence that is present at centromeres of all human autosomes and the X chromosome and shows polymorphic variation. *Proc. Natl. Acad. Sci.* USA, 81: 4884–4888, 1984.

42. Waye, J. S., England, S. B. and Willard, H. F., Genomic organization of alpha satellite DNA on human chromosome 7: Evidence for two distinct alphoid domains on a single chromosome. *Molecular and Cellular Biol.* 7: 349–356, 1987.

43. Moyzis, R., Albright, K., Bartholdi, M., Cram, S., Deaven, L., Hildebrand, E., Joste, N., Longmire, J., Meyne, J. and Schwarzacher-Robinson, T., Human chromosome specific repetitive DNA sequences: Novel markers for genetic analysis. *Chromosoma* (in press).

44. Waye, J. S., Creeper, L. A. and Willard, H. F., Organization and evolution of alpha satellite DNA from human chromosome 11. *Chromosoma* (in press).

45. Devilee, P., Cremer, T., Slagboom, P., Bakker, E., Scholl, H., Hager, H., Stevenson, A., Cornelisse, C. and Pearson, P., Two subsets of human alphoid repetitive DNA show distinct preferential localization in the pericentric regions of chromosomes 13, 18 and 21. *Cytogenet. Cell Genet.* **412**: 193–201, 1986.

46. Higgins, M. J., Wang, H., Shtromas, I., Haliotis, T., Roder, J. C., Holden, J. J. A. and White, B. N., Organization of a repetitive human 1.8 kb Kpnl sequence localized in the heterochromatin of chromosome 15. *Chromosoma* **93**: 77–86, 1985.

47. Waye, J. S. and Willard, H. F., Structure, organization, and sequence of alpha Satellite DNA from human chromosome 17: Evidence for evolution by unequal crossing-over and an ancestral pentamer repeat shared with the human X chromosome. *Molecular and Cellular Biol.* **6**: 3156–3165, 1986.

48. Waye, J. S. and Willard, H. F., (private communication).

49. McDermid, H. E., Duncan, A. M. V., Higgins, M. J., Hamerton, J. L., Rector, E., Brasch, K. R. and White, B. N., Isolation and characterization of an α-satellite repeated sequence from human chromosome 22. *Chromosoma* **94**: 228–234, 1986.

50. Waye, J. S. and Willard, H. F., Chromosome-specific alpha satellite DNA: Nucleotide sequence analysis of the 2.0 kilobasepair repeat from human X chromosome. *Nuc. Acid. Res.* **13**: 2731–2743, 1985.

51. Burk, R., Szabo, P., O'Brian, O., Nash, W., Yu, Y. and Smith, K., Organization and chromosome specificity of autosomal homologs of human Y chromosome repeated DNA. *Chromosoma* **92**: 225–233, 1985.

52. Pinkel, D., Gray, J., Trask, B., van den Engh, G., Fuscoe, J. and van Dekken, H., Cytogenetic analysis by *in situ* hybridization with fluorescently labeled nucleic acid probes. *Cold Spring Harbor Symposia on Quantitative Biology*, LI: 151–157, 1986.

53. Manuelidis, L., Individual interphase chromosome domains revealed by *in situ* hybridization. *Hum. Genet.* **71**: 288–293, 1985.

54. Cremer, T., Landegent, J., Bruckner, A., Scholl, H., Schardin, M., Hager, H., Devilee, P., Pearson, P. and van der Ploeg, M., Detection of chromosome aberrations in the human interphase nucleus by visualization of specific target DNAs with radioactive and non-radioactive *in situ* hybridization techniques: Diagnosis of trisomy 18 with probe L1.84. *Hum. Genet.* **74**: 346–352, 1986.

55. Rappold, G., Cremer, T., Hager, H., Davies, K., Muller, C. and Yang, T., Sex chromosome positions in human interphase nuclei as studied by *in situ* hybridization with chromosome specific DNA probes. *Hum. Genet.* **67**: 317–325, 1984.

56. Van den Engh, G., Trask, B., Lansdorp, and Gray, J. W., Improved resolution of flow cytometric measurements of Hoechst/Chromomycin-stained human chromosomes after addition of citrate and sulfite. Cytometry **9**: 266–270, 1988.

57. Pinkel, D., Landegent, J., Collins, C., Fuscoe, J., Segraves, R., Lucas, J., and Gray, J. W., Fluorescence in situ hybridization with human chromosome specific libraries: Deletion of trisomy 21 and translocations of chromosome 4. Proc. Natl. Acad. Sci (US) (in press).

9

Commentary on Part II
Tumor Cell Kinetics and
Cytogenetics

R. P. Hill, W. P. Vaughan, and N. McNally

The earliest "cell kinetic" observations on the natural history of human malignancy showed that tumors grew uncontrollably and had a higher mitotic rate than did the surrounding normal tissue. Some variability in growth rates over time and between tumors was noted. Early treatment experience demonstrated that, in general, rapidly growing tumors responded more rapidly than did slowly growing tumors. This seemed logical, since experimental studies indicated that early response to radiation and drug therapy was relatively cell cycle specific. These observations suggested that a component of cancer treatment might be the design of therapies which would expose the viable malignant cells to cytotoxic agents during a sensitive phase of the cell cycle. Results of early attempts at such "recruitment" and "synchronization" of malignant cells were unconvincing.

The reasons for this failure were unclear and empiric approaches to improving drugs and radiation treatment have become the standard for clinical trials. Most often, treatment schedules and doses are chosen on the basis of avoiding toxicity and for patient and physician convenience without regard for whether therapeutic index becomes improved. Fortunately, these empiric approaches and the development of drugs with improved therapeutic indices have resulted in cures for a significant number of malignant neoplasms. The observation that rapidly growing neoplasms were more often curable than slowly growing neoplasms again suggested that cell kinetic measurements might predict response and that cell-kinetic-based treatments might improve the chances of survival.

In the meantime, a number of advances in technology have made it possible to study the kinetic behavior of malignant cell populations more efficiently. Mitotic index has been joined by thymidine labeling index, percent labeled mitosis curves, proliferation-dependent polymerase assays, other cell cycle specific proteins, premature chromosome condensation, DNA content analysis, and BrdUrd incorporation as measurable parameters. Flow cytometry, monoclonal antibodies, molecular biology, along with improvements in specimen sampling, preparation, and preservation have tremendously increased the efficacy of these methods and have also spawned a new interest in the application of cell kinetic and cytogenetic measurements for the accurate prediction of tumor treatment response.

In the previous chapters the ploidy (or DNA content) of tumor cells, and the percent of tumor cells in S-phase as predictors of tumor response have been discussed. Gray et al. describe elegant new approaches for refining the gross measurement of DNA content of cells to allow identification of increases (or decreases) in specific chromosomes or (potentially) specific genes. Friedlander describes the application of flow cytometry to measure the DNA content and the S-phase proportion of tumor cells from paraffin blocks of fixed tissue. He demonstrates the power of such an approach, which can utilize retrospective analysis of results of previously conducted clinical trials, thus circumventing the often long delay inherent in assessing the outcome of prospective trials. Silvestrini addresses the question of whether measurements of the thymidine labeling index in tumors can be used either as an indicator of treatment response or as a prognostic indicator, drawing on results of her own studies to illustrate her discussion.

The posters presented in Part II could, in general, be split into two groups: (1) those which dealt with the application of existing techniques for the prediction of treatment outcome or response and (2) those which described new experimental approaches. In the former group, two posters (B-5 and B-6) described the use of an assay involving in vitro uptake of tritiated thymidine by tumor cells from biopsies as a predictor of treatment response for five different types of tumors (ovarian, breast, testicular, melanoma, and non-Hodgkin's lymphomas). The authors concluded from the study of nearly 200 cases that the assay predicted clinical response to conventional drugs for the tumor types considered, but they noted a higher accuracy for predicting resistance rather than for predicting sensitivity—a finding which is similar to results reported by others using the tumor stem cell assay (Selby et al., 1983).[2] An interesting aspect of the study described in Poster B-6 was the finding that the *in vitro* drug sensitivity of primary and metastatic lesions from the same patient were remarkably different.

Three posters (B-7, B-8, and B-11) discussed various aspects of measurements of ploidy (or DNA-index). The first (B-7) used the technique described by Friedlander to examine tissue from 40 patients with epithelial malignancies of the ovary. The authors concluded that DNA-index provided an independent indicator of poor prognosis for five-year survival with aneuploid tumors. Poster B-8 discussed three variables (fresh or frozen specimen, enzymatic or mechanical tissue dispersal, and method of analysis of the DNA histogram) affecting measurements of ploidy and percent S-phase cells using flow cytometry. Ploidy measurements were reasonably consistent but percent of S-phase cells could vary substantially, depending on the method of analysis and the quality of the histogram obtained from the flow cytometer. Flow cytometric analysis of 36 dog osteosarcomas was described in Poster B-11 and indicated that when multiple biopsies were taken, there were significant differences in the measurement of DNA-index between the biopsies for 25% of the tumors.

A further three posters (B-9, B-13, B-14) dealt with various aspects of measuring the percent of S-phase cells in tumors. The first of these posters (B-9) described measurements on samples of cells taken at various times from the abdominal cavity of patients with advanced gynecological and gastrointestinal cancers. The authors found that in 28 of 31 patients, there was a diurnal rhythm in the fraction of cells in S-phase with a range of less than 1% to more than 30%. The rhythm was different for tumor cells and for normal diploid cells. The other two posters related measurements of thymidine labeling index in locally advanced (B-13) or node negative breast cancer and head and neck cancer (B-14) to outcome of treatment with drugs and radiation respectively. High labeling index prior to treatment was found to correlate with response to drug treatment for 36 patients, but the results were not statistically significant. For radiotherapy, low labeling index was a prognostic indicator of good patient outcome for 76 node-negative breast cancers and 87 head and neck cancers.

The final two posters in this group (B-12 and B-15) discussed the use of the BrdUrd labeling technique for estimating the percent of cells in S-phase (labeling index) and the length of S-phase in cells within tumors (hence allowing an estimate of the potential doubling time) as described initially by Begg *et al.*, 1985[1]. The rationale for such measurements is that they may allow identification of tumors for which treatment outcome would be improved if overall treatment time was reduced. Poster B-12 addressed some of the theoretical difficulties in the required analysis and applied three different methods to analyze data from a model system. The authors concluded that all three methods elicited similar results in their system, but had different limitations with the most theoretically rigorous model requiring very high quality data. Poster B-14 described application of the method to 18 solid and 21 hematological malignancies of various types. The potential doubling time of the solid tumors ranged from 2.2 to 12 days and that of the hematological malignancies from 1.9 to 21.5 days. A major limitation of the technique is the need to prepare a suspension containing a large number of intact single tumor cells.

There were five posters which discussed new experimental approaches. Poster B-1 described the use of fluorescent probes to assess cell viability after cytotoxic treatment of an *in vitro* tumor model (V79 cell spheroids). Two probes, dichlorofluoresin diacetate and orthophthaldialdehyde were found to be indicative of toxicity from diverse anti-neoplastic agents but, based on studies with X-rays and BCNU, the author concluded that multiparameter measurements showed more promise than did single probes. Poster B-2 described measurements of DNA strand breaks and DNA-protein cross-links in CHO cells following irradiation under conditions of different oxygenation. The yield of strand breaks (measured using the alkaline elution technique) was reduced at low oxygen concentrations, with the K-value (O_2 concentration for half-maximum effect) similar to that for cell survival. DNA-protein cross-links increased at low oxygen concentrations, but again, the K-value was similar to that for cell survival. Analysis of cells from tumors irradiated *in vivo* demonstrated significant levels of DNA-protein cross-links, suggesting the possibility that this lesion might be used as a marker for hypoxic cells *in vivo*. Poster B-3 also described measurements of DNA damage using the alkaline elution technique, following treatment of tumor cells *in vitro* with cisplatin and/or hyperthermia. Combination treatment was found to induce more DNA strand breaks than cisplatin alone, and this correlated with increased cytotoxicity as assessed by a 72-hour growth inhibition assay.

The formation of hybrid spheroids from cells of different types was described in poster B-4. This technique potentially allows determination, in this model, of the radiation sensitivity of cells which do not form spheroids themselves. The authors hope to be able to apply the technique to biopsies from human tumors. Poster B-10 also addressed measurement of radiation sensitivity of cells, but the emphasis was on variations associated with the position in the division cycle. As a first step in developing an approach to measuring such variations in cells from human tumor biopsies, the authors described the use of a cell analyzer, which is capable of automatic recognition of live unstained cells grown in culture, to measure the specific stage in the cycle of individual cells. The radiation survival curves obtained for CHO cells of different cell cycle age using the cell analyzer were similar to those for cells separated by centrifugal elutriation.

The discussion which followed the viewing of the posters addressed four overlapping themes. The first related to the question of assessment of treatment response and the importance of defining this in a careful and consistent manner when predictive assays were being examined. Problems in correlating treatment response with pretreatment variables result from the heterogeneity of tumor biology and host tolerance in the clinical setting. Within even the most carefully selected groups of patients in clinical trials, there will be multiple endpoints which require careful sub-set analysis. Thus, median survival may be the most useful end point for evaluating correlations of cell kinetic measurements with the natural history of untreated disease. Median survival of patients who do not respond to treatment because of absolute resistance of the malignant cell population might demonstrate the same correlations. For responding patients, however, who may be cured or whose tumors may recur, median survival is too simplistic an end point. Time to recurrence/progression and survival of responders who are not cured are very different end points from cure or survival of non-responders. Finally, when therapy is continued until relapse, time to development of resistance is a confounding variable.

Several illustrations of apparently conflicting data, probably created by not being able to sort out the multiple end points, can be found in the chapters by Silvestrini and Friedlander, and the poster presentations. However, the consistency between investigators is improving dramatically. The results are sufficiently convincing within a growing number of tumors and clinical settings that we are now convinced that when cell kinetic data do not correlate as expected with natural history or treatment outcome, there is a technical fault or an uncontrolled missing variable. The emerging general hypothesis is that tumors with high fractions of S-phase cells or labeling index will have a short natural history but, if sensitive to therapy, will have a higher probability of cure. Failing cure, however, they will demonstrate a shorter relapse time after treatment is stopped or resistance develops. For example, apparently conflicting data for malignant lymphomas has tended to resolve itself, as the end point has been properly handled. The traditional "good" prognosis lymphomas have a long natural history, but are not curable with chemotherapy. These tend to have a lower S-phase fraction than do the "bad" prognosis lymphomas. However, many "bad" prognosis high S-phase fraction lymphomas will respond dramatically to chemotherapy and some patients will be cured. Since the cure rate is less than 50%, it is not surprising that within these "bad" prognosis lymphomas, overall survival remains better with low S-phase fraction. Unexplained is Silvestrini's apparently inconsistent observation that within these "bad" prognosis subtypes, the probability of obtaining complete remission is significantly *greater* when DNA content analysis reveals *low* S-phase fraction. Friedlander's group has obtained similar results. It may be that the fastest of these fast growth rate tumors would do better with therapy which did not await normal bone marrow recovery between courses and that resistance develops more rapidly in high S-phase fraction lymphomas. It may be that within the responders, curability will be higher with high S-phase fraction. These are testable hypotheses.

The second theme concerned the wide variation in measured values of cell kinetic and cytogenetic parameters, particularly of percent of S-phase cells (or labeling index), found between different human tumors—even those of similar histopathological type. This variation was documented in several of the posters and in Dr. Silvestrini's chapter. It was highlighted by data for colorectal tumors, which indicated a relatively high value of labeling index (range 7–50%) for such tumors, whereas other authors have reported much lower values (2–4%). The question was raised as to whether this variation was real or artifactual and therefore associated with measurement techniques. Silvestrini and Streffer argued that most of the variations were real, since even when a consistent measurement was adopted, considerable variation was still observed. It was noted, however, that most of the measurements were made on single biopsies. Streffer also made the point that measurements of labeling index usually demonstrate lower values than are obtained by estimating percent of S-phase cells from flow cytometric analysis, but that this or other systematic errors could not explain the observed variability.

Streffer stated that it would be useful to measure other parameters as well as labeling index and that it may be necessary to use multiple parameters for the purpose of prediction. McNally also espoused this viewpoint, arguing that, despite the general correlation observed between labeling index and potential doubling time in his BrdUrd labeling studies (B-15), determining the extra parameter was potentially useful, since the two parameters did not correlate in all tumors. Steel was not convinced that measuring cell kinetic parameters other than labeling index would be helpful. He suggested that creating problems of interpretation by trying to do too sophisticated an analysis of "fuzzy" clinical trials was a real possibility.

Heterogeneity within tumors was the third theme. The problems associated with single biopsies and their potential lack of representativeness was noted in relation to the wide variation observed in cell kinetic and cytogenetic parameters of tumors. The importance of sub-populations of cells within tumors was also raised. The proportion of stem cells in tumors had already been discussed in Dr. Suit's introductory chapter. An important unresolved question is whether cell kinetic measurements on the total tumor population reflect the kinetic parameters of the tumor stem cells. The role of micro-environmental heterogeneity in creating sub-populations of hypoxic cells and drug-resistant cells also needs to be considered. Do cell kinetic measurements reflect the parameters of these treatment resistant cells? It was pointed out by Dr. Lange that, if clonogenicity of cells from tumors is being assessed following treatment, sub-populations of resistant cells can potentially be identified by extending the analysis to low levels of survival.

The final theme arising out of these studies was the question of biological rationale for the approach or assay being proposed. The rationale for why a parameter such as DNA-index (or ploidy) can be used as a predictive measure needs to be clarified, but even more importantly proposed new assays need to have a clear rationale. Out of this issue arose some discussion concerning whether or not new experimental approaches need to be related to some "gold standard". Ultimately, such a standard would be the results of a clinical trial to test the assay method, but during development some standard such as a clonogenic assay is required. Lange suggested using loss of clonogenicity as a standard for comparing new assay procedure but, Buick pointed out that measurement of the clonogenicity of human tumor cells is fraught with problems and could not, at this time, be regarded as a suitable standard.

Denekamp raised the question of the rationale for making measurements of the potential doubling time of tumors. She suggested that tumors with short potential doubling times might be expected to undergo significant proliferation during the five to seven week course of standard fractionated radiation treatment and that such tumors might be better treated by shortening the overall treatment time, so-called "accelerated fractionation". She indicated that clinical trials at Mt. Vernon Hospital in London would address the validity of this rationale. Withers questioned this rationale, suggesting that there is little evidence for signicant growth in human tumors up to four weeks after the start of fractionated radiotherapy.

Overall, the discussion demonstrated that interest in the use of cell kinetic and cytogenetic parameters as predictors of tumor response has enjoyed a renewed interest in recent years, largely as a result of advances in technology which have allowed measurments to be made in times short enough that they could influence the choice of therapy. Trials are planned or are in progress to investigate the predictive value of measurements made using these newer techniques. Despite these advances, it was also clear from the discussion that a number of fundamental objections to the likely predictive value of such measurements remain unresolved. Particularly important are the problems of heterogeneity and sub-populations of cells in tumors. Further advances in technology will probably be required to identify and study these subpopulations.

REFERENCES

1. Begg, A. C., McNally, N. J., Shrieve, D. C., and Karcher, H., A method to measure the duration of DNA synthesis and the potential doubling time from a single sample. *Cytometry* **6**: 620–626, 1985.
2. Selby, P., Buick, R. N. and Tannock, I., A critical appraisal of the "Human Tumor Stem-Cell Assay". *New Eng. J. Med.* **308**: 129–134, 1983.

POSTERS

(B-1) Fluorescent Probes as Indicators of Cell Viability. R. E. Durand. B.C. Cancer Research Centre, Vancouver, British Columbia, Canada V5Z 1L3.

(B-2) Radiation-Induced DNA Lesions as an Indicator of Tumor Cell Hypoxia. S. C. vanAnkeren, D. Murray, and R. E. Meyn. M.D. Anderson Hospital and Tumor Institute, Houston, Texas 77030.

(B-3) The Effects of Hyperthermia and Cisplatin on Tumor DNA Integrity. T. C. K. Chan, G. Fennimore, and R. C. Richardson. Department of Physiology and Pharmacology and the Small Animal Clinic School of Veterinary Medicine, Purdue University, West Lafayette, Indiana 47907.

(B-4) Long- and Short-Term Approaches to the *In Vitro* Assay of Tumor Radiosensitivity. C. S. Lange and B. Djordjevic. SUNY Health Science Center at Brooklyn, Brooklyn, New York 11203.

(B-5) Predictivity of a Short-Term Assay on Clinical Response: A Ten-Year Experience. O. Sanfilippo, R. Silvestrini, N. Zaffaroni, M. Grazia Daidone, and E. Grignolio. Istituto Nazionale Tumori, Milan, Italy.

(B-6) Interlesion Variability in Drug Sensitivity of Human Tumors as a Determinant for Clinical Predictivity of *In Vitro* Assays. N. Zaffaroni, R. Silvestrini, O. Sanfilippo and M. Grazia Daidone. Istituto Nazionale Tumori, Milan, Italy.

(B-7) Cytofluorometric Analysis of the DNA Content in Ovarian Carcinoma and its Relationship to Patient Survival. K. J. Murray, L. E. Hopwood, and J. F. Wilson. Department of Radiation Oncology, Medical College of Wisconsin, Milwaukee, Wisconsin 53226.

(B-8) Variables Affecting DNA Ploidy Data Obtained from Breast Tumors. P. K. Horan, P. Wallace, K. Muirhead, W. Kashatus, and V. P. Perna. Smith Kline and French Laboratories, Philadelphia, Pennsylvania 19101 and Smith Kline Bio-Science Laboratories, King of Prussia, Pennsylvania 19406.

(B-9) Cell Kinetic Measurements in *In Vivo* Human Cancers—The Effect of Surgical Debulking and Chemotherapy. P. S. Braly, and R. R. Klevecz. Department of Gynecologic Oncology, City of Hope National Medical Center, Duarte, California and Department of Obstetrics and Gynecology, University of California at Irvine, Irvine, California and Cell Biology, Beckman Research Institute at the City of Hope National Medical Center, Duarte, California.

(B-10) Characterization of Tumor Cell Age Response and Subpopulations Using Various Analytical Cytology Techniques. P. C. Keng, R. L. Howell, and R. M. Sutherland. University of Rochester Cancer Center, Rochester, New York 14642.

(B-11) Flow Cytometric Analysis of Dog Osteosarcoma Aneuploidy. M. H. Fox, S. J. Withrow, B. D. Powers, and E. L. Gillette. Colorado State University, Fort Collins, Colorado 80523.

(B-12) Cell Kinetic Measurement from a Single Sample. M. L. Meistrich, R. A. White, D. P. Calkins, and W. Beisker. M.D. Anderson Hospital and Tumor Institute, Houston, Texas 77030.

(B-13) Tumor Cell Kinetics of Human Breast Cancer During Treatment with Diethylstilbestrol and Chemotherapy: A Predictor of Response? P. F. Conte, A. Alama, E. Di Marco, G. Gardin, A. Nicolin, P. Pronzato, and R. Rosso. Istituto Nazionale Ricerca Cancro, V. le Benedetto XV n. 10, 16132 Genova, Italy.

(B-14) The Labeling Index: A Predictor of Patient Outcome in Breast Cancer and in Head and Neck Cancer. A. Courdi, J. Gioanni, P. Chauvel, M. Hery, and F. Demard. Centre A. Lacassagne, 36 Voie Romaine, 06054. Nice, France.

(B-15) Human Tumour Potential Doubling Times Measured by *In Vivo* Labeling with Bromodeoxyuridine. N. J. McNally, G. D. Wilson, S. Dische, M. Bennett, and M. Danova. Cancer Research Campaign, Gray Laboratory and Departments of Radiotherapy and Pathology, Mount Vernon Hospital, Northwood, Middlesex, United Kingdom and Institute of Clinical Medicine II, University of Pavia, Italy.

PART III

TUMOR CELL RESPONSE *IN VITRO*

10

Tumor Cell Sensitivities to Drugs and Radiation

W. A. Brock, F. L. Baker, and P. J. Tofilon

INTRODUCTION

For the past 20 years, researchers have been developing and testing *in vitro* methods aimed at appraising the effectiveness of cytotoxic agents (chemotherapeutic drugs and radiation) on human tumor cells for the purpose of predicting response to therapy. Most of these assays have been based upon the clonogenic human tumor stem cell assay first introduced by Hamburger and Salmon,[1] although more recently, several non-clonogenic assays have been developed. The rationale behind these efforts is that: (1) significant differences in intrinsic cellular sensitivity exist between tumors to account for differences in tumor response to therapy, and (2) stem cells removed from the tumor environment and grown in culture continue to express the same relative sensitivities to cytotoxic treatment as they do in the tumor. These assumptions tend to minimize the roles of cell contacts in tumors, host factors, metabolic stringencies imposed by the tumor environment, oxygenation, and cellular heterogeneity. They also suggest that the most significant tumor parameter and, therefore, the best predictor of radiation treatment outcome is intrinsic cellular radiosensitivity. The purpose of this chapter is a review of some of the current methods for estimating drug and radiation sensitivity in human tumor cells and to determine what light the test results have shed upon the question: How important is intrinsic cellular sensitivity as an independent determinate of tumor response to therapy? Especially in the case of radiotherapy, we have yet to determine if cellular sensitivity differences are significant in tumor response.

THE RESPONSE OF TUMOR CELLS TO DRUGS AND RADIATION

It is clear from the composite of published chemotherapy drug survival curves that cell lines differ enormously in their sensitivity to essentially all agents. Such large differences, if expressed in tumors, could account for the entire range of clinical responses, from growth during treatment to complete remission. It is, therefore, reasonable to expect that in the case of chemotherapy, cell sensitivity is often the predominate critical determinate of tumor response. On the other hand, in the case of radiation, the common opinion has been that there are no significant differences in radiosensitivities among tumor cells; that is, when the terminal slopes (D_o) of radiation survival curves are compared. However, Fertil and Malaise[2,3] suggested an alternative method of describing radiation sensitivity, by comparing parameters that describe the initial portion of the curve such as survival at 2.0 Gy, mean inactivation dose ($\bar{D}$) or the alpha coefficient of the linear quadratic model. After comparing these parameters from a great number of published survival curves, they found that significant differences in sensitivity exist between cell strains derived from different histological tumor types. This suggested to them that cell sensitivity could account for the clinical response. This hypothesis was further supported by the additional observation that cell lines derived from tumors that are considered difficult to cure by radiotherapy, are, on the average, more resistant *in vitro*. Their work has been extended to over 200 different tumor cell lines and has also been confirmed by others.[4] Therefore, a rationale does exist for making *in vitro* measurements of both drug and radiation sensitivity and for comparing the results to the clinical outcome.

ASSAYS FOR MEASURING INTRINSIC CELLULAR SENSITIVITY
Clonogenic Assays

The advantage of a clonogenic assay is that it is an accepted measure of cell survival. The human tumor stem cell assay has been used extensively for drug and radiation testing and has the advantage that cloning of cells in soft agar is indicative of malignant cell growth. This system has been extensively characterized and applied to studies of cytogenetics,[5] tumor growth factors,[6] immunology,[7] cell-cell interactions, measuring the cytotoxicity of chemotherapeutic drugs,[8] radiation,[9] biological response modifiers,[7] and screening new drugs for their potential anticancer activity.[10] The main features of this assay include a one-hour drug exposure to the cell suspension, drug concentrations corresponding to one-tenth of the peak plasma concentration obtainable in humans, and plating of cells as a dispersion in 0.3% agar. The cloning efficiency in control and treated cultures is determined by colony counting and a tumor culture is defined as sensitive if the drug causes at least a 50% inhibition of colony formation.

The stringent requirements of clonogenic assays, however, cannot usually be met in primary cultures from human tumors. The biggest problem is setting up an assay such that all colonies arise from single cells; a significant number of colonies arising from a clump of more than one cell results in an artifactually high estimate of cell survival.[11] The consequences of this problem were first realized when the primary human tumor stem cell assay produced radioresistant survival curves that were biologically unlikely.[9,12] Radiation is an excellent cytotoxic agent to test a colony assay, since it is not possible to have a plateau on the survival curve due to truly radioresistant cells. Modifications of the stem cell assay have been made to minimize the problem, but many modifications tend to make the assay non-clonogenic. Other problems with soft agar assays that must be considered include the potential dependence of plating efficiency on cell seeding density, a non-linear relationship between cell number and colony formation,[13] and the problem of abortive colonies large enough that they are counted as survivors.[11]

A recently published modification of the Courtenay soft agar assay has yielded realistic radiation survival curves for human tumor cells.[14] Rofstad et al. [14] presented radiation survival curves with exponential terminal slopes. The curves were based upon complete dose-response data whose range of Do and survival at 2.0 Gy values were within the range of those published for cell lines.[3] Figure 10.1 shows several of these survival curves from bladder and head and neck cancers which exhibit a wide range of sensitivities with shouldered as well as exponential survival curves. The problems of multiplicity due to small clumps was avoided by not performing assays if the cell suspensions contained doublets and, in addition, all cultures were screened after the first day for any clumps that might later be scored as colonies. The results of this method may be useful for drugs and radiation in clinical studies, although the success rate is not clear and the number of cells required makes it impractical to perform with biopsies.

Non-Clonogenic Assays

A number of non-clonogenic assays have been described and tested. Non-clonogenic assays have common problems: (1) they are indirect measures of cell survival; (2) they must be validated against clonogenic

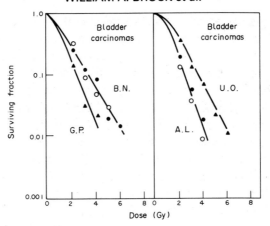

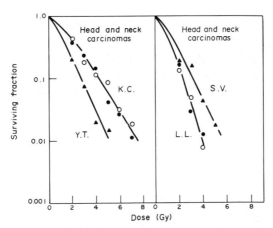

FIG. 10.1. X-ray survival curves from head and neck carcinomas (top) and bladder carcinomas (bottom) obtained by Rofstad *et al.*[14] Their method was a modification of the Courtenay soft agar colony assay. (From Reference 4, with permission of the publisher.)

assays using cell lines, and (3) they are usually accurate only under a defined range of conditions. Those conditions which yield an accurate measure of cell survival are not always the same from one cell line to another and from one primary culture to another. For example, most non-clonogenic assays are highly dependent upon both the number of cells inoculated and the growth rate of the cells and these parameters are not usually known for individual tumors. Nevertheless, non-clonogenic assays are important because they are designed to overcome the problems that often make clonogenic assays impossible.

An interesting example of a non-clonogenic assay has been recently described by Carmichael et al.[15] It is based upon the ability of living cells to reduce a tetrazolium salt (MTT) to an insoluble blue formazan product. This endpoint is based upon the assumption that only surviving cells are able to produce the reducing equivalents necessary to convert MTT to its crystalline form. Cell killing is then estimated by measuring the amount of blue material produced in treated cultures and comparing that value to controls. The presence in the starting population of cell clumps, dead cells, or abortive colonies will not influence the survival measurement. These researchers' results[15] showed that under defined conditions, this assay gives comparable results to control and parallel clonogenic assays. The MTT assay has been standardized against a number of established human tumor cell lines and has great potential as a method for screening investigational drugs.

The MTT assay has not yet been applied to primary cultures for two main reasons: (1) normal host cell contamination and growth must be controlled since those cells will also produce a positive reaction with MTT and (2) controls are needed to deal with the unpredictable cell growth, because the validity of the assay relative to clonogenic survival depends upon a fairly narrow range of cell densities. This problem stems from the limited space available for cell growth in a multiwell plate; the control cultures will reach a crowded state and slow their growth before treated cultures, which have more growth area per surviving cell due to cell killing. As a consequence, overplated or fast growing control and treated cultures have different rates of cell growth, producing fewer than expected total cells in control and low dose cultures which results in a more "resistant" survival curve. A solution to this problem is to run multiple survival curves using many different initial cell concentrations.

Another non-clonogenic assay has been developed and is currently undergoing extensive testing with both drugs and radiation. The culture system, developed by Baker et al.,[16] makes use of 24-well culture plates that have had their growing surfaces coated with Cell Adhesion Matrix (CAM; LifeTrac, Irvine, CA.). This coating efficiently promotes the attachment of cells and supports their growth. A highly enriched growth medium stimulates the growth of over 80% of cultures so far tested. Furthermore, cytogenetics, tumor induction in nude mice, and flow cytometry have demonstrated that this culture system predominately supports the growth of malignant cells.[16,17] Survival curves for chemotherapy drugs and radiation are established at different initial cell concentrations and produce useable data if they show a linear relationship between the number of cells inoculated and total growth. Drug and radiation treatments take place 24 hours after cultures are established, and the assay is terminated after a total of two weeks. At that time, each culture well contains the total number of cells produced by all survivors after treatment. The endpoint of the assay is the relative amount of crystal violet staining density in each culture, and experiments have shown that this value is directly related to the total cell number in each well. Therefore, this assay is based upon the relative two-week growth potential of cells that survive cytotoxic treatment.

Figure 10.2 shows a stained culture from a radiosensitivity test[18] in which the cells were inoculated at different seeding densities and treated with graded doses of radiation. The decreased cell density after increasing doses of radiation is apparent and the relative amounts of growth are determined by integrating the optical density of each well using a video image analyzer. Because a complete survival curve is generated for every cell inoculum, only data that is linear with respect to cell number inoculated and staining density is used. This eliminates artifacts due to a slowing of growth in unirradiated controls as the cells begin to become confluent. Control culture wells are also shown in Figure 10.2 in which a suicide level of tritiated thymidine was added during the culture period to kill all proliferating cells; the staining density in this well then represents the background staining due to non-dividing and killed cells. The difference between the background and total growth in controls is the maximum growth of the controls and is the target "density" for cytotoxic treatment.

Figure 10.3a shows a plot of the staining density of a human tumor cell primary culture.[19] The unirradiated control shows a non-linear relationship between cell number and staining density as the initial cell densities become large. At higher doses of radiation, the relationship becomes linear because enough cell killing takes place so that crowding of growing cells does not occur during culture. Figure 10.3b shows the radiation survival curve calculated from the linear portion of each curve in Figure 10.3a.

Figure 10.4 illustrates survival curves for several chemotherapy drugs that were obtained using this assay.[16] The endpoint used for clinical correlations is the IC-90 value, the concentration of drugs that results in 90% cell killing. These curves and others derived by the same method show sensitivities and shapes within the ranges expected for human tumor cells *in vitro*. Currently, clinical trials are underway in

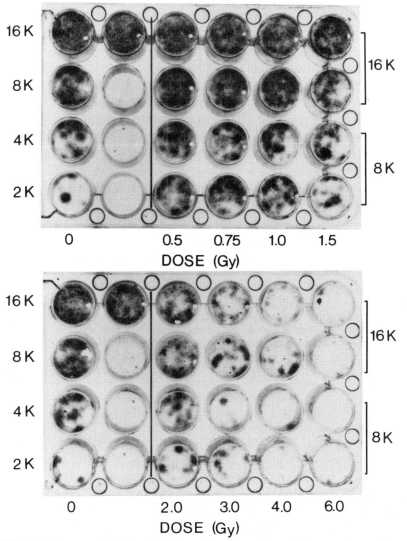

FIG. 10.2. Photograph of 24 well culture plates of a radiosensitivity test from a human melanoma primary culture in the adhesive tumor cell culture system.[19] The cultures were stained with crystal violet following two weeks of growth after irradiation. Survival curves were obtained from optical density measurements using a video system.

which the IC-90 values are being routinely determined for 8 drugs and are being compared to the tumor response to therapy.[20] Another use of this assay that is especially valuable is the initial *in vitro* screening of new chemotherapy agents. In this application, up to 100 different compounds can be tested against cells from the same tumor.[21]

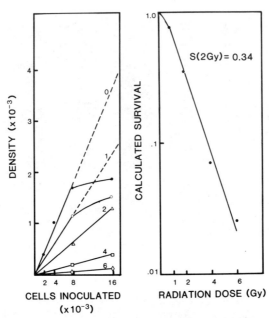

FIG. 10.3. Plot of the crystal violet staining density versus the number of cells inoculated (left) in the adhesive tumor cell culture system.[16] A non-linear relationship is observed above 8,000 cells due to crowded growth in the wells. Note that at the higher doses of radiation, linearity is regained due to cell killing. The right side of the figure shows the survival curve calculated as a ratio of the slopes of the linear portions of the curves on the left. Survival at 2.0 Gy is calculated from a fit of the data to the linear quadratic model.

Similar to the MTT assay described above, this assay is subject to several problems that, unless properly controlled, will lead to spurious results. Using a relationship between staining density and cell survival assumes that all surviving cells produce the same total number of progeny during the culture period. This assumption cannot be true under all conditions for several reasons, including radiation-induced division delay which is dose dependent, abortive colony formation, and differential growth rates of cells due to the effects of different surviving cell densities. In addition, there is not always linearity of total growth versus the number of cells inoculated, since some tumor cell specimens produce factors that influence cell growth (both stimulatory and inhibitory). For example, with most cytotoxic agents, especially radiation, surviving and killed cells are indistinguishable from each other for up to a few days after treatment. As a result, it is necessary to allow enough time for doomed cells to express their lethal damage and for surviving cells to grow enough to become the dominant population. This problem is typical of non-clonogenic assays because they rely on the accuracy of

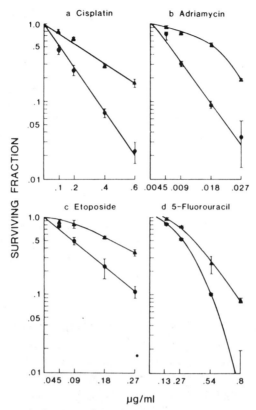

FIG. 10.4. Drug survival curves of a melanoma (▲) and a squamous cell carcinoma of the lung (●) primary culture in the adhesive tumor cell culture system. (From Reference 16, with permission of the publisher.)

several assumptions: (1) that doomed cells will die within a given time period and will not contribute to the measured endpoint, (2) that surviving cells will equally express the characteristic measured, and (3) that surviving cells from all treatment doses and untreated controls continue to grow and divide with similar kinetics. If all of these assumptions are true, then the results will correspond with clonogenic survival and, since these factors are dose-dependent, non-clonogenic assays often provide an accurate estimate of clonogenic survival.

THE RELATIONSHIP BETWEEN *IN VITRO* SENSITIVITY AND THE CLINICAL RESPONSE TO THERAPY

In vitro sensitivity measurements for both drugs and radiation in human tumor primary cultures have resulted in broad ranges of survival levels. These differences, if expressed in tumors during treatment, could account for the entire range of clinical responses. However, it is clear that several other factors could also account for differences in the clinical response of tumors to therapy, and it is not known whether or not those factors are so influential in determining tumor response that knowledge of intrinsic sensitivity would be of any value. For example, it is well known that tumor oxygenation, cell-cell contacts, host immune status, and clonogenic cell number all influence the response of tumors to therapy. The relative importance of these factors on individual treatment response cannot be predicted, and it is therefore likely that several factors will be required to accurately predict the response to therapy of individual tumors.

The reports of correlations between *in vitro* chemosensitivity testing and the clinical response of cancer patients suggest that there is a relationship between these measurements. Two types of information have led to this conclusion. The first is that significant differences in *in vitro* sensitivities have been found when tumors of different histologic types are compared,[19,22] and the relative sensitivity of each histologic group tends to generally rank with the clinical responsiveness of these tumors. Secondly, there has been an excellent correlation between *in vitro* response and patient response.[23,24] In general, researchers of clinical correlations often report greater than 90% success at predicting resistance and up to 70% success at predicting sensitivity. These observations suggest that intrinsic tumor cell sensitivity to drugs is an important determinant of tumor response and that even after tumors have been dispersed into single cells and grown in short-term culture, they retain and express the same relative sensitivity to cytotoxic agents. This means that other factors in tumor response, such as tumor blood flow or oxygenation, are probably of secondary importance. These results provide a rationale for continuing to develop and test new methods of measuring the sensitivity of tumor cells. However, at this time there is still considerable controversy as to the value of performing present generation tests for the purposes of individualizing cancer therapy. It is one thing to show that the cellular sensitivity is a determinant of tumor responsiveness by comparing large numbers of cases in which a relatively high error rate could be overcome, and it is another thing to perform the test for an individual patient when the probability is low that the culture will grow, that the proper drugs are tested, or that other factors controlling tumor response are not dominant in this particular case. In a prospective clinical trial by VonHoff,[24] it was reported that a higher patient response was observed when patients were treated with drugs that tested sensitive in an *in vitro* clonogenic assay. The final result of this controversy must await more prospective clinical trials and possibly for more trials that involve single agent therapy. Such studies are very difficult to organize, to carry out, and to analyze. It also seems likely that the ability to direct improved therapy for an individual from an *in vitro* test of intrinsic cellular sensitivity will be limited by many other factors controlling tumor response, but this likelihood should not discourage endeavors to optimize such measurements, because other tests will also be limited in the same way.

The radiation sensitivity of human tumor cells in primary culture has been determined in some systems, but clinical correlations have not yet been reported. The rationale for comparing parameters of the initial slope of the survival curve with clinical response has been provided by the work of Malaise[3] and others.[4] Their data suggests that survival at 2.0 Gy differentiates between cell lines derived from different tumor histologic types and their values line up on a similar rank order as the clinical sensitivities of these types. The wide and overlapping ranges of survival at 2.0 Gy observed for each histology may represent differences in clinical sensitivities of individual tumors.

The clonogenic assay results reported by Rofstad *et al.*[14] included survival measurements at 2.0 Gy for 66 primary cultures derived from seven tumor histologic types. Of those, the melanoma cultures were the most radioresistant, although a significant difference between the groups was not apparent and the parameters Do, Dq, and n did not distinguish the different histologic types. It is possible that with more case study results, significant differences will emerge.

The survival at 2.0 Gy values determined by a non-clonogenic assay[19] are summarized in Figure 10.5. This cumulative frequency histogram shows melanomas to be the most resistant histologic type, with a broad range of values and the most sensitive melanoma as one of the most sensitive cultures reported. Like the data reported by Fertil and Malaise for cell lines,[3] the values from the different histologic types agree, in general, with the clinical radiocurability of each type. This correlation suggests a possible value of this assay as a predictor of tumor response. The results of a clinical study are needed to test this hypothesis.

TUMOR CELL HETEROGENEITY IN SENSITIVITY TO DRUGS AND RADIATION

It has long been known that many tumors contain mixed populations of stem cells with different sensitivities to antineoplastic agents and that therapy can actually select for resistant populations or even induce

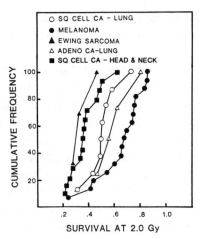

FIG. 10.5. Cumulative frequency histograms of survival at 2.0 Gy for primary cultures derived from different tumor histologies. The melanoma cultures were significantly more resistant than any other type. Considerable overlap in the sensitivities of the groups is apparent. (From Reference 19, with permission of the publisher.)

resistance. This is clear from studies that show greater *in vitro* resistance to specific drugs in recurrent tumors.[25] If these resistant cells are the majority population, an *in vitro* test result would most likely reflect this resistance. But if the resistant cells are not the majority population, then the *in vitro* test result would reflect the most sensitive cells present or at least the average of the population. As a result, prediction of sensitivity to a particular drug always carries with it the possibility that there are resistant cells within the tumor. In terms of clinical correlations for chemotherapy, an initial tumor response might correlate with a drug sensitivity, but a recurrent tumor may result from the resistant stem cells. In the case of radiotherapy, the chance to treat with an alternate protocol or modality might be lost if the resistant subpopulation is not identified before treatment. Therefore, along with the development of assays to measure intrinsic sensitivity—methods also need to be developed to identify the occurrence of heterogeneity.

While tumor cell heterogeneity to drug sensitivity has long been recognized, it has not been so clearly accepted with radiation. The analysis of Malaise and his co-workers[2,3,26] and Deacon *et al.*[4] illustrate that the initial slope of survival curves shows considerable variation even within lines derived from similar histologic types, and the suggestion is that similar variations might exist within a tumor. More direct evidence comes from the work of Weichselbaum,[27] who isolated multiple clones from a single squamous cell carcinoma of the head and neck that have very large differences in radiation sensitivity. These clones, in early passage, presumably reflect heterogeneity within the original tumor. The real problem for drugs and radiation sensitivity testing is how to determine if heterogeneity exists in individual tumors so that the results of *in vitro* sensitivity assays can be interpreted.

A new method for investigating heterogeneity in primary human tumor cultures, introduced by Tofilon *et al.*,[28,29] has the promise of usefulness for any cytotoxic agent, including radiation. Their technique is based upon the sister chromatid exchange (SCE) assay. Sister chromatid exchanges are induced by several chemotherapy drugs and reflect damage to the DNA. The levels of induced damage correlate with cell killing.[30] The specific attribute that this chromosome level assay provides is an individual sensitivity measurement for each cell. Therefore, a frequency histogram of induced levels in a group of treated metaphases represents the ranges of individual sensitivities existing within a given treated population. Figure 10.6 illustrates the results of this type of analysis in six human tumor primary cultures that were treated with cis-platinum (cPt) and then analyzed for sister chromatid exchanges. In most cases, a wide range of induced values was observed, suggesting that some heterogeneity is present in most cultures. Homogeneous cell lines analyzed in this manner exhibit histograms with relatively narrow ranges. Most interesting are the bottom three cases, which all show a similar wide range of responses but also a significant number of cells with SCE's not induced above untreated controls (the dark shaded area represents the overlap of treated and controls). These cells are, therefore, considered to be resistant to cPt as compared to the other more sensitive cells in the same culture.

Tofilon *et al.*[29] have extended this study to identify heterogeneity of response to virtually any other cytotoxic agent, even if that agent does not induce SCE's on its own, including radiation. In this protocol, an SCE-inducing agent is used to display a range of SCE responses in a cell population and a separate culture is treated with a test dose of radiation before cPt is used to display the range of sensitivities. Histograms of responses are compiled and analyzed to determine whether or not the test dose of radiation changes the distribution. If the test dose of radiation altered the histogram from cPt alone, then radiation non-randomly killed cells in the starting population, thus demonstrating heterogeneity in radiation sensitivity. In initial studies, four out of eight cases examined displayed heterogeneity in radiation sensitivity.

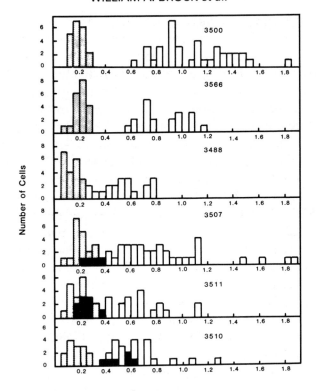

SCE's/Chromosome

FIG. 10.6. SCE frequency histograms from primary cultures derived from six different patients. Hatched areas, untreated cells; open areas, cells treated with 5 μM cPt; blackened areas, regions occupied by both untreated and treated cells (i.e. overlap). (From Reference 28, with permission of the publisher.)

CONCLUSIONS

In vitro testing of human tumor cells for their sensitivity to cytotoxic agents is still in a developmental stage. The culture methods are not optimal, the tumor sampling problems are not clearly understood, the relationship between tumor stem cells and the cells that grow in culture is not known, the dose of each cytotoxic agent used in culture is controversial, the cellular heterogeneity issue needs to be solved, and endpoints of clinical response are very difficult to quantitate objectively. Nevertheless, the results of clinical correlations to date have proven that intrinsic cellular sensitivity does play a significant role in the response of tumors to therapy. The differences in sensitivities reported between histology groups, the positive clinical correlations, and the fact that prospective clinical trials have been positive, clearly justify further development of these methodologies. The range of drug responses is very large, making it likely that this type of testing will be a useful aid for planning chemotherapy. The range of radiation sensitivities is less, although simple calculations show that even small differences in survival at 2.0 Gy would translate into very large differences in total cell killing after 30 fractions of radiotherapy.[4]

The problem of heterogeneous populations with respect to cell sensitivity now appears to be real for both chemotherapeutic agents and for radiation. As illustrated earlier, the presence of resistant subpopulations will tend to mask the accuracy of predictions from *in vitro* survival curves. Therefore, estimates of the presence and degree of heterogeneity must become an essential part of any *in vitro* test. It appears that a chromosome level assay is one approach that has potential for fulfilling this requirement. Finally, the fact that *in vitro* assays have not been accepted very widely because they have not been proven useful for more than a minority of patients, should not lead to the conclusion that they cannot be very important prognostic tools. Their value has been diluted by the many other confusing factors that influence the response of a tumor to therapy. It is likely that intrinsic sensitivity measurements will, eventually, be an important prognostic indicator, and will be supplemented by measurements of other important prognostic tumor parameters.

ACKNOWLEDGMENTS

This investigation was supported by National Institutes of Health research grant CA-06294, Contract CM57775, and the Katherine Unsworth Memorial Fund. The assistance of Sheri Lee Chase in preparation of this manuscript is appreciated.

REFERENCES

1. Hamburger, A. W. and Salmon, S. E., Primary bioassay of human tumor stem cells. *Science* **197**: 461–463, 1977.
2. Fertil, B. and Malaise, E. P., Inherent cellular radiosensitivity as a basic concept for human tumor radiotherapy. *Int. J. Radiation Oncology Biol. Phys.* **7**: 621–629, 1981.
3. Fertil, B. and Malaise, E. P., Intrinsic radiosensitivity of human cell lines is correlated with radioresponsiveness of human tumors: analysis of 101 published survival curves. *Int. J. Radiation Oncology Biol. Phys.* **11**: 1699–1707, 1985.
4. Deacon, J., Peckham, M. J. and Steel, G. G., The radioresponsiveness of human tumours and the initial slope of the cell survival curve. *Radiotherapy and Oncology* **2**: 317–323, 1984.
5. Trent, J. M. and Salmon, S. E., Human tumor karyology: marked analytic improvement by short-term agar culture. *Br. J. Cancer* **41**: 867–874, 1980.

154   WILLIAM A. BROCK et al.

6. Hamburger, A. W., White, C. P., Dunn, F. E., Citron, M. L. and Hummel, S., Modulation of human tumor colony growth in soft agar by serum. *Int. J. Cell Cloning* **1**: 216–229, 1983.

7. Bradley, E. C., Catino, J. J and Issell, B. F., Cell-mediated inhibition of tumor-colony formation in agarose by resting and inter-leukin 2-stimulated human lymphocytes. *Cancer Res.* **45**: 1464–1468, 1985.

8. Salmon, S. E., Developmental applications of a human tumor colony assay for chemosensitivity testing. *Recent Result Cancer Res.* **94**: 1–16, 1984.

9. Meyskens, F. L., Radiation sensitivity of clonogenic human melanoma cells by FSH. *Lancet* **2**: 219, 1983.

10. Shoemaker, R. H., Wolpert-DeFilippes, M. K. and Kern, D. H., Application of a human tumor colony-forming assay to new drug screening. *Cancer Res.* **45**: 2145–2153, 1985.

11. Rockwell, S., Effects of clumps and clusters on survival measurements with clonogenic assays. *Cancer Res.* **45**: 1601–1607, 1985.

12. Meyskens, F. L., Human melanoma colony formation in soft agar. In: *Cloning of Human Tumor Stem Cells*. Salmon, S. E., ed., New York, Alan R. Liss, pp. 85–99, 1980.

13. Eliason, J. F., Aapro, M. S., Decrey, D. and Brink-Petersen, M., Non-linearity of colony formation by human tumour cells from biopsy samples. *Br. J. Cancer* **52**: 311–318, 1985.

14. Rofstad, E. K., Wahl, A., and Brustad, T., Radiation sensitivity *in vitro* of cells isolated from human surgical specimens. *Cancer Res.* **47**: 106–110, 1987.

15. Carmichael, J., DeGraff, W. G., Gazdar, A. F., Minna, J. D. and Mitchell, J. B., Evaluation of a tetrazolium-based semi-automated colorimetric assay: assessment of chemo-sensitivity testing. *Cancer Res.* **47**: 936–942, 1987.

16. Baker, F., Spitzer, G., Ajani, J., Brock, W. A., Lukeman, J., Pathak, S., Tomasovic, B., Thielvoldt, D., Williams, M., Vines, C. and Tofilon, P., Drug and radiation sensitivity measurements of successful primary monolayer culturing of human tumor cells using cell-adhesive matrix and supplemented medium. *Cancer Res.* **46**: 1263–1274, 1986.

17. Baker, F. L., Spitzer, G., Ajani, J. A. and Brock, W. A., Assay of primary human tumor cells for drug sensitivity using the adhesive-tumor-cell culture system. Conference on: Prediction of Tumor Treatment Response, Banff, Alberta, Canada, April 21–24, 1987 (Abstract).

18. Brock, W. A., Maor, M. H. and Peters, L. J., Cellular radiosensitivity as a predictor of tumor radiocurability. *Radiation Research* **104**: 290–296, 1985.

19. Brock, W. A., Baker, F., Spitzer, G., Peters, L. J., Bock, S. and Williams, M., Radiosensitivity testing of human tumor cells in primary culture. (In press, 1987.)

20. Ajani, J. A., Baker, F. L., Kelly, A., Spitzer, G., Brock, W. A., Tomasovic, B., Singletary, S. E., Fan, D., McMurtrey, M. and Plager, C., Comparison of the clinical response with *in vitro* drug sensitivity profiles of the primary human tumors in the adhesive tumor cell culture system. (In press, 1987.)

21. Spitzer, G., Anjani, J. A., Baker, F. L., Brock, W. A., Tomasovic, B., Thielvoldt, D., and Dicke, K., Comparison of antitumor activity of standard and investigational drugs at equivalent granulocyte-macrophage colony-forming cell inhibitory concentrations in the adhesive tumor-cell culture system: an *in vitro* method for screening new drugs. Submitted for publication, 1987.

22. VonHoff, D. D., Casper, J., Bradley, E., Sandbach, J., Jones, D. and Makuch, R., Association between human tumor colony-forming results and response of an individual patient's tumor to chemotherapy. *Am. J. Med.* **70**: 1027–1032, 1981.

23. Salmon, S. E., Alberts, D. S., Durie, B. G. M., Meyskens, F. L., Jones, S. F., Soehnien, B., Chen, H. S. G. and Moon, T. E., Clinical correlations of drug

sensitivity in the human tumor stem cell assay. *Recent Results Cancer Res.* **74:** 300–305, 1980.

24. VonHoff, D. D., Clark, G. M., Stogdill, B. J., Sorosdy, M. F., O'Brien, M. T., Casper, J. T., Mattox, D. E., Page, C. P., Cruz, A. B. and Sandbach, J. F., Prospective clinical trial of a human tumor cloning system. *Cancer Res.* **43:** 1926–1931, 1983.

25. Alberts, D. S., Chen, H. S. G and Salmon, S. E., Chemotherapy of ovarian cancer directed by the human tumor stem cell assay. *Cancer Chemother. Pharmacol.* **6:** 279–285, 1981.

26. Fertil, B., Dertinger, H., Courdi, A. and Malaise, E. P., Mean inactivation dose: a useful concept for intercomparison of human cell survival curves. *Radiation Research* **99:** 73–84, 1984.

27. Weichselbaum, R. R., Beckett, M. and Dahlberg, W., Radiobiological parameters of a human tumor parent line and four tumor clones of a human epidermoid carcinoma. 35th Annual Meeting of the Radiation Research Society, Atlanta, Georgia, Feb. 21–26, 1987 Abstract.

28. Tofilon, P. J., Vines, C. M., Baker, F. L., Deen, D. F. and Brock, W. A., Cis-platinum-induced sister chromatid exchanges: an indicator of sensitivity and heterogeneity in primary human tumor cell cultures. *Cancer Res.* **46:** 6156–6159, 1986.

29. Tofilon, P. J., Vines, C. M., Meyn, R. E. and Brock, W. A., Identification of heterogeneity in radiation sensitivity within human primary tumor cell cultures using the SCE assay. Submitted for publication, 1987.

30. Deen, D. F., Kendall, L. E., Marton, L. J. and Tofilon, P. J., Prediction of human tumor cell chemosensitivity using the sister chromatid exhange assay. *Cancer Res.* **46:** 1599–1602, 1986.

11

Glutathione as a Predictor of Tumor Response

James B. Mitchell, Angelo Russo, James Carmichael,
and Eli Glatstein

INTRODUCTION

In conjunction with diagnostic tests and clinical judgment, predictive assays may aid oncologists in choosing the most beneficial course for individual patient treatment. Ideally these assays should identify feature(s) of the patient's tumor that could be easily and accurately determined prior to therapy. The reliability of the assay will depend upon a number of factors; the most important is whether the particular parameter being measured can be exploited such that treatment strategies would prove efficacious to the individual patient. It would also be desirable, particularly for therapies involving systemic treatment, for there to be a differential between normal and tumor tissues in the particular parameter being assayed. Such a differential might allow design of treatment protocols that would result in a greater therapeutic gain.

Biochemical and molecular biology studies performed over the past few years have sought to identify specific genes or molecules present in cells that may modify the cellular response to cytotoxic therapies. A considerable list of biochemical systems has been studied that may have impact on modulating cytotoxicity to drugs and radiation-drug combinations. These include: amplification of specific genes leading to an overproduction of enzymes involved in the metabolism of certain chemotherapy agents,[1] the presence of specific membrane glyco-proteins in drug-resistant cells,[2] and various cellular detoxification systems.[3,4] Among cellular detoxification systems, intracellular glutathione (GSH) and related enzymes have been extensively studied for both drug and radiation related responses.[5,6] This review focuses on GSH

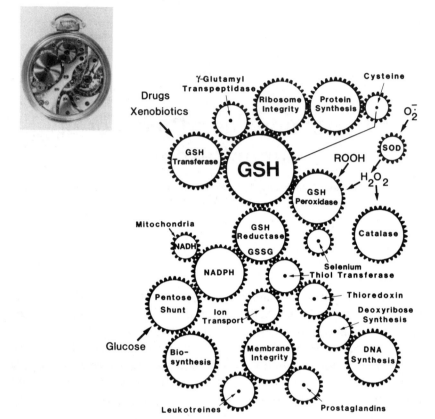

FIG. 11.1. Interrelationship of GSH with other cellular systems. The insert of the clock serves to draw the analogy of the dependency of one system to another as depicted by meshing gears or cogs. GSH is either directly or indirectly involved with many important biochemical systems.

and GSH-related enzymes and how they influence drug and radiation effects. Approaches as to how they may be evaluated in clinical samples for predictive purposes will be emphasized.

THE IMPORTANCE OF CELLULAR GSH

GSH serves many cellular functions. In addition to providing reducing equivalents for biochemical reductive processes, GSH detoxifies oxygen-induced free radicals in conjunction with glutathione peroxidase[3] and electrophilic xenobiotics through glutathione-S-transferases.[7] GSH is intimately involved in a number of biochemical systems, as shown in Figure 11.1. This figure demonstrates the complexity of the interdependency of GSH with other biochemical systems by using the analogy of meshing gears or cogs in a clock. This analogy emphasizes that single entities such as GSH do not stand alone but are related to, and in fact may depend on, other complex biochemical systems in the cell. It is for this reason that care should be taken when attributing a cellular phenomenon to a single molecule or system.

The eludication of the importance of GSH in radiation and drug-induced cytotoxicity has been facilitated by the introduction of agents that "selectively" modulate GSH levels in the cell. Two agents widely used for these studies are buthionine sulfoximine (BSO), which inhibits GSH synthesis[8] and oxothiazolidine-4-carboxylate (OTZ), which stimulates GSH synthesis.[9] These agents are relatively non-toxic and exert their effects on cellular GSH over relatively short time periods.

RADIATION AND DRUG-INDUCED CYTOTOXICITY: EFFECTS OF GSH MODULATION

Radiation

Depletion of cellular GSH levels to low levels (<5%) by BSO pre-treatment results in radiosensitization of both aerobic and hypoxic cells.[10,11] The extent of sensitization has been relatively small (10–20%). In fact, the oxygen enhancement ratio was shown to be unchanged for cells depleted of GSH by BSO pretreatment (compared to control cells), where sensitization of both aerobic and hypoxic cells were approximately the same.[10] When GSH levels are elevated by OTZ pretreatment, some radioprotection has been reported for lymphoid cells.[12] However, for Chinese hamster cells, doubling the normal GSH level provides no aerobic protection and minimal hypoxic protection (30%).[13,14] When GSH levels are increased to even higher levels (200–300% of control) by GSH esters,[15] only modest aerobic protection is observed (10–20%).[16]

Radiation resistance in human ovarian cells made resistant to certain chemotherapeutic drugs has recently been attributed to high intracellular GSH levels.[17] These drug resistant cells are two to three fold higher in GSH than in parental cell lines. However, Mitchell et al. recently demonstrated that there is no difference between the radiosensitivity of Chinese hamster pleiotropic drug-resistant cells and that of the parental cell line—despite a two fold higher level of GSH in the drug resistant line.[18] The discrepancy may be attributed to the mode of drug resistance. The ovarian cell line is resistant to alkylating agents; whereas, the pleotropic drug resistant cell line has a broader but different resistance profile. More work is necessary to either confirm or refute radiation resistance associated with alkylator resistance. While there may continue to be discrepancies in the literature over the extent and mode of involvement of GSH in the radiation response, one thing is clear: GSH is not the *only* intracelluar determinant of radiation sensitivity. In fact, there is increasing evidence that other thiols, particularly protein thiols, may be important.[11] Protein thiol equivalents, which are present in cellular concentrations much higher than that of GSH, warrant further study. Whether the protein-bound thiols are directly involved in radical scavenging or indirectly involved through disturbances of complex biochemical controls such that the normal cellular functions of metabolism, repair, and cell structure are disturbed, remains to be seen. It is possible that no specific biochemical disturbance will prove ultimately responsible for the inability of a cell to divide. Figure 11.1 aptly demonstrates interdependencies of a simple system. The figure could be made much more complicated if multiple sulfhydryl-containing proteins were responsible for various control points in the system. What is certain is that there is a need to learn about these systems and to learn ways to apply this information to the clinical setting.

Radiation and Nitroimidazoles

Various nitroimidazoles sensitize hypoxic cells to ionizing radiation.[19] These sensitizers have been extensively studied in the laboratory and evaluated in world-wide clinical trials. The clinical experience with misonidazole has been somewhat discouraging,[20] with perhaps many factors contributing to the disappointing results.[21] Recently, Phillips and co-workers identified yet another potential problem relating to the ineffectiveness of nitroimidazoles.[22,23] Human tumor cell lines were found to have high intracellular levels of GSH, and an inverse correlation was observed between the GSH level and the extent of hypoxic radiosensitization by SR-2508 (See Fig. 11.2).[22,23] These data may have important clinical implications. If human tumors *in vivo* have high GSH levels, currently achievable plasma levels of SR-2508 (~1mM) would inevitably result in little sensitization. Whether the poor clinical results with misonidazole relate to elevated GSH levels remains to be determined. But in order to preempt poor results and also learn more about the parameters of successful treatment, it would seem reasonable to measure GSH levels in human tumor specimens to determine if there were high levels and perhaps identify those tumors best suited for nitroimidazole therapy. A reciprocal set of experiments have been performed that reinforce the importance of the nitroimidazole/GSH interaction. GSH depletion of human tumor cell lines having high GSH levels potentiates nitroimidazole hypoxic radiosensi-

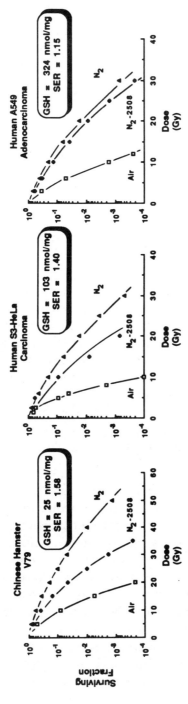

FIG. 11.2. Radiosensitization of hypoxic cells by SR-2508. The three cell lines shown, Chinese hamster V79, human S3-HeLa, and human A549 have different levels of cellular GSH and exhibit different SER's at 1% survival for 1mM SR-2508 treatments (see inserts). Higher intracellular GSH levels resulted in lower SER values. Adapted from 22, 23.

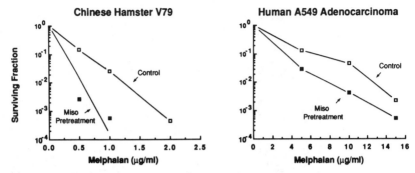

FIG. 11.3. Survival curves of Chinese hamster V79 and human A549 adenocarcinoma cells to melphalan. Cells were pre-incubated for two hours with two mM misonidazole (Miso) under hypoxic conditions, reaerated, rinsed free of Miso, exposed to varying concentrations of melphalan for one hour, and assayed for colony-forming ability. The enhancement in melphalan cytotoxicity by Miso pre-incubation at 1% survival was 2.4 and 1.6 for V79 and A549 cells, respectively. (Data adapted from Mitchell *et al.*, unpublished observations.)

tization.[23] BSO treatment has also been shown to potentiate radiosensitization in rodent tumor models,[24] and is currently being considered for clinical trials not only for use as a means to gain further hypoxic radiosensitization with nitroimidazoles, but also as a chemotherapeutic drug sensitizer.[25–28] Here, too, it would be most useful to have a predictive assay to identify those tumors that would be best suited for BSO modulation. The biochemistry of tumors more than likely differs; some tumors with high GSH levels may also have high turnover rates and thus be best suited to BSO treatment, while others may have slow turnover rates and present difficult pharmacologic problems.

NITROIMIDAZOLES AS CHEMOSENSITIZERS

Hypoxic preincubation with nitroimidazoles has been shown to potentiate the cytotoxicity of some chemotherapeutic drugs.[29] Clinical trials have been initiated to evaluate this means of chemosensitization.[30] In part, the mechanism for nitroimidazole chemotherapy potentiation results from the depletion of GSH by reduced nitroimidazole metabolites.[31,32] An experiment that lends support to this arguement is illustrated in Figure 11.3. Hypoxic preincubation with misonidazole was shown to exhibit less sensitization to melphalan in cell lines high in GSH. These data also emphasize the possible importance of determining GSH levels in human tumors which may be high in GSH prior to clinical protocols that have been designed based on murine models that may not relate to human tumors.

GSH AND CHEMOSENSITIVITY

GSH, by virtue of the possible different chemical reactions it can undergo as well as GSH dependent detoxifying enzymes, affords several different defensive modes for interaction with different types of chemotherapeutic agents.[5,33] Redox active drugs, such as bleomycin and adriamycin are capable of producing hydroxyl radicals, superoxide, and hydrogen peroxide.[34,35] These toxic species may be detoxified by GSH peroxidase and transferase, superoxide dismutase, or catalase. Potentiation of the cytotoxic effects of both adriamycin and bleomycin as GSH levels are depleted (GSH < 5%) by BSO pretreatment have been reported.[36,37] Conversely, when GSH levels are elevated by OTZ pretreatment (GSH = 200%) protection was observed.[36,37]. Such studies serve to demonstrate that GSH may be important in the response of tumors to these redox active agents. Not only are GSH levels important, but the activities of GSH peroxidase and GSH reductase are also important, since GSH must be continually cycled from the oxidized form to the reduced form as H_2O_2 is detoxified (see Fig. 11.1).

The cytotoxicity of certain alkylating agents, such as melphalan and cyclophosphamide has been shown to depend, in part, on intracellular GSH levels.[38–40]. Melphalan cytotoxicity has been lessened by GSH elevation following pretreatment with OTZ.[41] Human ovarian cells made resistant to melphalan have higher GSH levels than parental lines, and GSH depletion by BSO markedly sensitizes these cells.[27]. An example of similar melphalan resistance in multidrug resistant Chinese hamster cells[42] and sensitization of these cells by GSH depletion is shown in Figure 11.4. The GSH levels in the C5 cells was approximately two-fold higher than the parental line. However, complete sensitization back to the parental melphalan response was not achievable, even though most of the GSH (<5%) was removed prior to drug exposure. These studies nonetheless demonstrate that GSH is a major contributor to melphalan resistance in these cells. A likely explanation for the protective role of GSH in melphalan cytotoxicity would be the non-catalyzed nucleophilic reaction of GSH and melphalan to form GSH-melphalan adducts.[43] Such detoxifying reactions would serve to lower the level of melphalan available for cytotoxic interactions. It may be possible to measure the capacity of tumor tissue (perhaps in single cells) to form GSH-melphalan adducts and thus provide a predictive assay that would aid the clinician in his choice of alkylating agent therapy.

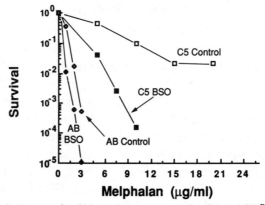

Melphalan (μg/ml)

FIG. 11.4. Survival curves for Chinese hamster ovary AuxB1 and CH^RC5 cells exposed to melphalan for one hour. The CH^RC5 cell line is a multi-drug resistant cell line derived from the parental line AuxB1.[42] Open symbols represent control survival curves and closed symbols represent cells pretreated with BSO such that GSH levels were <5% of control values at the time of melphalan exposure. The CH^RC5 cell line was two-fold higher in inherent GSH levels than the parental line.

TABLE 11.1 *IC$_{50}$ values for Human Lung Cancer Cell Lines Exposed to Adriamycin*

Cell Line	Type	Treatment Status	GSH (nmol/mg protein)	IC$_{50}$ Adriamycin (nM)
Small Cell				
NCI-H187	C-SCLC	UT	41	26
NCI-H209	C-SCLC	UT	56	25
NCI-H678	C-SCLC	UT	32	61
NCI-H719	C-SCLC	UT	54	10
NCI-H526	V-SCLC	UT	54	37
NCI-H 60	C-SCLC	T(CT)	43	171
NCI-H 69	C-SCLC	T(CT)	48	127
NCI-H524	V-SCLC	T(CT)	25	16
NCI-H128	C-SCLC	T(CT)	26	110
Non Small Cell				
NCI-H 23	Adenocarcinoma	UT	103	39
NCI-H125	Adenocarcinoma	UT	100	216
NCI-H522	Adenocarcinoma	UT	80	197
NCI-H520	Squamous	UT	160	411
NCI-H226	Squamous	UT	210	221
NCI-H596	Adenosquamous	T(XRT)	140	813
NCI-H322	Adenosquamous	T(CT)	150	173
NCI-H157	LCC	UT	65	238
NCI-H460	LCC	UT	220	17

Data adapted from Carmichael *et al.*[46]

GSH levels were determined in a panel of human lung cancer cell lines and related to their sensitivity to a number of chemotherapy drugs recently by Carmichael and co-workers.[44–46] Drug sensitivity was assessed by a non-clonogenic colorimetric assay.[47] A portion of these data is shown in Table 11.1. While the correlation is not absolute, there is a tendency for cell lines which are high in GSH to be less responsive to adriamycin cytotoxicity as reeflected by higher IC_{50} values. Interestingly, the sensitivity of this panel of human tumor cell lines to adriamycin (and other cytotoxic drugs not shownn) generally parallels the response of these particular tumors in the clinic; non-small cell carcinomas are more resistant to cytotoxic drugs than small cell lung cancer.[48] Along with the possibility of assessing drug sensitivity of tumor specimens taken directly from the patient using non-clonogenic assays, it will be interesting also to assay GSH levels to ascertain if the correlation between GSH levels and cytotoxicity holds for fresh biopsied tumor samples.

Most of the examples cited in this chapter demonstrate the role of GSH in drug-induced cytotoxicity; however, as seen in Figure 11.1, other enzyme systems may also be significant. GSH transferase and GSH peroxidase levels have been studied in a human breast cancer cell line that had been selected for cross resistance to a wide range of anticancer drugs.[49,50] GSH transferase was found to be 45-fold higher, and GSH peroxidase was 13-fold higher than the parental line.[49,50] While it is not clear at present that the increases seen in these two enzymes are responsible for the drug resistance in these cells, they are certainly likely candidates, since in conjunction with GSH they afford the cell considerable detoxification capacity for organoperoxides and xenobiotics. Further studies are needed to determine if increased levels and activities of these enzymes are associated with drug resistance. Should such correlations exist, assessment by activity, quantity, or molecular probes of these enzymes from biopsied tumors would also be useful in predictive assays.

GSH AS A PREDICTOR OF TUMOR RESPONSE?

The examples discussed in this chapter lend support to the involvement of GSH and perhaps GSH related-detoxification enzymes in drug-induced and radiation/drug cytotoxicity. High levels of GSH or related enzymes observed in many human tumor cell lines may also apply to human tumors *in vivo* and thus be responsible, in part, for resistance encountered in clinical studies. Tumors high in GSH might be sensitized to chemotherapy by drugs that deplete GSH such as BSO. Most of the studies discussed above involved *in vitro* cell systems. A major question is whether or not *in vitro* data apply to *in vivo* human tumors. Considering the complexity of human tumors, the answer to this question will probably be complicated. However, based on supportive evidence, a systematic evaluation of GSH and related enzymes from human tumors seems justified.

A note of caution is in order regarding various factors that might influence the interpretation of the data. It should be appreciated that cells from a tumor biopsy will not represent a homogeneous population. Most assuredly there will be a distribution of cells including cells in exponential growth, plateau phase-like cells, cells out of the growth cycle (G_o), cells that have experienced either acute or chronic hypoxia, and dead cells that are in the process of being removed from the tumor through necrotic or apototic processess. Undoubtly there will be variation in GSH levels from cells experiencing different environmental conditions and growth states within a tumor. In animal models there are large diurnal variations in normal tissues. Whether this occurs in tumors is not known. Further, it is probable that various nutritional states influence GSH levels. Cellular GSH in homogeneous cell lines can vary by an order of magnitude for log versus plateau phase cells, the latter having the lower values (personal observation). A tumor biopsy will probably contain cells from normal tissue, connective tissue, blood vessels, and blood. To illustrate this point, Figure 11.5 shows GSH levels from human tumor xenografts, wherein multiple samples from the same tumor were taken and analyzed.[51] In these studies, no attempt was made to separate the sample into various subpopulations or to eliminate normal cells from the determination. Note that from the same tumor, GSH values vary by two to three-fold. The reasons for this variation may reside in one or more of the considerations discussed above. Yet data such as these, despite the heterogeneity of GSH values in the tumor, may prove useful, if tumor GSH levels are higher than those of normal tissue or if GSH levels can be differentially modulated in tumor as opposed to normal tissues.[41,52]

What may be more important in relating to predictive responses is not the average GSH value for the tumor but rather the cellular distribution of GSH levels in a tumor biopsy. While the average value may be low compared to normal tissues, there may be subpopulations in the sample that are very high in GSH. If these cells with high GSH levels ultimately determine the tumor cure after treatment with certain cytotoxic therapies, assessment of these cells and their relative proportions may not only be instructive but may actually be of determinis-

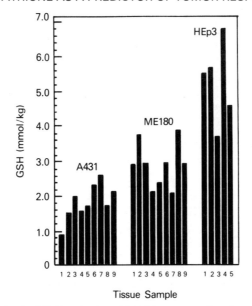

FIG. 11.5. Variation in GSH levels of multiple biopsy samples taken from three different human tumors grown as subcutaneous tumors in nude mice. Each tumor sample was taken from the same tumor. Differences in GSH levels in the same tumor were found to vary up to two- to three-fold. Data from Allalunis-Turner, *et al.*,[51] with permission.

tic importance. An example of this is shown in Figure 11.6.[53] Human ovarian cells (MLS) were sorted on the basis of their GSH content by flow cytometry using a fluorescent compound (monobromobimane).[54] Note that there is a distribution of GSH levels (panel a). The lower and upper 1% of this distribution were further sorted (panels b and c) and exposed to adriamycin. The cell survival curves shown in Figure 11.6 illustrate that the cells with the highest GSH levels were the most resistant to adriamycin. It is not known if comparable situations exist in human tumors, but most certainly study of distributions of cellular GSH before treatment and possibly during and after treatment may prove useful.

Whether or not GSH or GSH-related enzymes will serve as predictors of tumor response will require further careful experimentation and evaluation. Ultimately, the predictive utility of such assays will depend upon how accurately they can be quantitated in *clonogenic* or *potentially* clonogenic tumor cells from biopsy material. There are many difficulties associated with the actual measurement of thiols from biological materials,[55] since thiol groups are extremely reactive and subject to oxidation during sampling procedures. The specificity of agents used

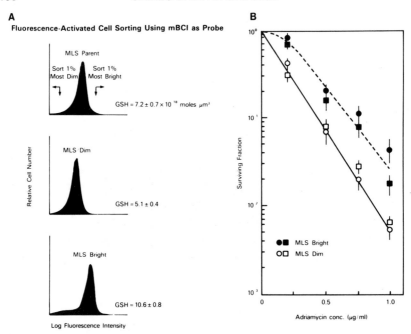

FIG. 11.6. **A.** Fluorescence-activated cell sorting of human ovarian cells (MLS) using monobromobimane as a probe for GSH. The top panel shows the distribution of the GSH levels within the cell population (GSH levels as determined by HPLC analysis is on each panel). From populations of cells with the brightest and most dim fluorescence corresponding to the highest and lowest GSH levels were sorted. The distribution of these populations along with their determined GSH levels are shown in the middle and lower panel. **B.** The latter two populations shown in part A were exposed to Adriamycin for three hours and assessed for colony-forming ability. Those cells with the greater GSH levels were the most resistant to the cytotoxic effects of Adriamycin. Data from Lee *et. al.*,[53] with permission.

to bind thiols and the stability of such conjugates during processing is also of concern.[55] Durand used a number of thiol binding agents that fluoresce at certain wavelengths in conjunction with flow cytometry to rapidly assess thiol levels in cells.[56] Of particular interest were the bimanes introduced by Kosower[54] which covalently bind GSH and other thiol-containing compounds. The alkyl-bimane thioether is highly fluorescent. Yet, monobromobiamane also reacts rapidly with other compounds and also shows significant hydrolysis. Kosower, Pazhenschvsky, and Hershkowitz showed the halogen homolog monochlorobimane to be less reactive by a factor of 43.[54] Rice *et al.* used monochlorobimane to bind specifically GSH and quantitate GSH in cells by flow cytometry.[57] This technique as demonstrated above is

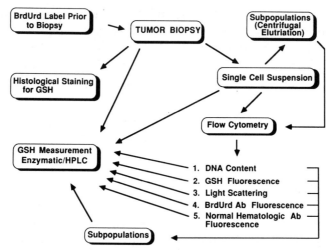

FIG. 11.7. Suggested approach toward the determination of GSH levels in human tumors. The various techniques shown should allow for determination of GSH in various subpopulations of cells taken from a tumor biopsy and thus obtain a more accurate assessment of GSH distribution.

useful in determining GSH levels in various subpopulations that can be discriminated by flow cytometry.

Figure 11.7 illustrates a suggested approach for the measurement of GSH from subpopulations of cells taken from a tumor biopsy. Single cell suspensions are made from tumor biopsies by enzymatic treatment of the tissue. Studies will have to be done to determine the effect the isolation step has on ultimate GSH determinations. It has recently been shown that various combinations of enzymatic cocktails effect the yield of single cells, and GSH levels have been shown to vary with the isolation technique used.[58] Once single cells have been obtained, they can be directly analyzed by flow cytometry by a variety of methods, all of which can provide information about subpopulations. Normal cells can be excluded by differences in their DNA profiles compared to frequently aneuploid tumor cells. Normal hematological cells can be discriminated by use of specific fluourescent monoclonal antibodies. Cells in S phase can be evaluated using a monoclonal antibody that recognizes DNA-containing bromodeoxyuridine (BrdUrd),[59] assuming patients are given a pulse of BrdUrd prior to the biopsy.[60,61] Finally, GSH fluorescense can be assessed directly using the bimane derivatives mentioned above. All of these subpopulations can be sorted and GSH determined using conventional assays.[62,63] Subpopulations can also be obtained from single cell suspensions using centrifugal elutriation.[64] These subpopulations can be assayed directly or further evaluated by flow cytometry. It should be noted that these subpopulations can be assayed for GSH-related enzymes and other redox enzymes. The general approach which may require slight to major alteration, depending on assays performed, will provide an idea about distributions of GSH (and other enzymes) in various subpopulations. However, this information will not reveal the location of GSH in the tumor. A number of available histochemical assays stain tissue sections for GSH.[65–70] Sections of the tumor stained for GSH may yield important information about the distribution of GSH within the tumor.

The assays outlined above are indeed complex and necessitate careful experimentation. These studies will hopefully expand our knowledge of *in vivo* tumor biology to include biochemical parameters relating to cellular/tumor redox states. *In vitro* investigations and limited *in vivo* studies all underscore the importance of GSH in drug and radiation/drug cytotoxicity. Now what is needed is detailed work that will ensure accurate and reproducible measurement of GSH (and related enzymes) in tumor tissues. Once these assays become standardized and are available, there will be a need to initiate prospective clinical trials to determine tumor GSH and related enzyme levels prior to therapy. Ultimately, there will be a need to relate these measurements to the eventual outcome of the therapy. Additionally, should tumors recur, assessment of GSH in these tumors would potentially yield important information regarding biochemical changes in GSH and tumor drug resistance. The planning and accomplishing of a multi-tiered study between the laboratory and the patient will require significant effort and cooperation on the part of clinicians and biologists to determine if GSH will be useful as a predictor of tumor response. If the outcome of these efforts were to demonstrate that GSH measurements are indeed predictive of tumor response, the oncologist will have additional information that will allow better treatment strategies and ultimately a longer and better life for the patient.

REFERENCES

1. Alt, F. W., Kellems, R. E., Bertino, J. R. and Schimke, R. T., Selective multiplication of dihydrofolate reductase genes in methotrexate resistant variants of cultured murine cells. *J. Biol. Chem.* **253**: 1357–1370 1978.
2. Riordan, J. R., Deuchars, K., Kartner, N., Alon, N., Trent, J. and Ling, V., Amplification of P-glycoprotein genes in multidrug-resistant mammalian cell lines. *Nature* **316**: 817–819 1985.
3. Meister, A. and Anderson, M. E., Glutathione. *Annu. Rev. Biochem.* **52**: 711–760 1983.
4. Fridovich, I., The biology of oxygen radicals. *Science* **201**: 875–880 1978.

5. Russo, A., Carmichael, J., Friedman, N., DeGraff, W., Tochner, Z., Glatstein, E. and Mitchell, J. B., The roles of intracellular glutathione in antineoplastic chemotherapy. *Int. J. Radiat. Oncol. Biol. Phys.* **12:** 1347–1354, 1986.

6. Mitchell, J. B. and Russo, A., The role of glutathione in radiation and drug induced cytotoxicity. *Br. J. Cancer.* **55:** 96–104, 1987.

7. Jakoby, W. B and Habig, W. H., Glutathione transferases. In: *Enzymatic Basis of Detoxification* (W. B. Jakoby Ed.), Vol. 2, Academic Press, New York, pp. 63–94, 1980.

8. Dethmers, J. K. and Meister, A., Glutathione export by human lymphoid cells: Depletion of glutathione by inhibition of its synthesis decreases export and increases sensitivity to irradiation. *Proc. Natl. Acad. Sci. USA* **78:** 7492, 1981.

9. Williamson, J. M., Bottcher, B. and Meister, A., Intracellular delivery system that protects against toxicity by promoting glutathione synthesis. *Proc. Natl. Acad. Sci. USA,* **79:** 6246, 1982.

10. Mitchell, J. B., Russo, A., Biaglow, J. E. and McPherson, S., Cellular glutathione depletion by diethylmaleate or buthionine sulfoximine: No effect of glutathione depletion on the oxygen enhancement ratio. *Radiat. Res.* **96:** 422–428, 1983.

11. Biaglow, J. E., Morse-Guadio, M., Varnes, M. E., Clark, E. P., Epp, E. R. and Mitchell, J. B., Non-protein thiols and the radiation response of A549 human lung carcinoma cells. *Int. J. Radiat. Biol.* **44:** 489–495, 1983.

12. Jensen, G. L. and Meister, A., Radioprotection of human lymphoid cells by exogenously supplied glutathione is mediated by γ-glytamyl transpeptidase. *Proc. Natl. Acad. Sci. USA,* **80:** 4714–4717, 1983.

13. Russo, A. and Mitchell, J. B., Radiation response of Chinese hamster cells after elevation of intracellular glutathione levels. *Int. J. Radiat. Oncol. Biol. Phys.* **10:** 1243–1247, 1984.

14. Russo, A., Mitchell, J. B., DeGraff, W., Spiro, I. and Gamson, J., The effects of cellular glutathione elevation on the oxygen enhancement ratio. *Radiat. Res.* **103:** 232–239, 1985.

15. Anderson, M. E., Powrie, F., Puri, R. N. and Meister, A., Glutathione monoethyl ester: Preparation, uptake by tissues, and conversion to glutathione. *Arch. Biochem. Biophys.* **239:** 538, 1985.

16. Astor, M. B., Meister, A. and Anderson, M. E., Intracellular thiol levels and radioresistance: Studies with glutathione and glutathione mono ethyl ester. 35th Annual Meeting Radiation Research Society, Atlanta GA 1987.

17. Louie, K. G., Behrens, B. C., Kinsella, T. J., *et. al.*, Radiation survival parameters of antineoplastic drug-sensitive and -resistant human ovarian cancer cell lines and their modification by buthionine sulfoximine. *Cancer Res.* **45:** 2110–2115, 1985.

18. Mitchell, J. B., Gamson, J., Russo, A., Friedman, N., DeGraff, W., Carmichael, J. and Glatstein, E., Chinese hamster pleiotropic multidrug resistant cells are not radioresistant. *NCI Monogr.* **6:** 187–197, 1988.

19. Breccia, A., Rimondi, C. and Adams, G. E., *Radiosensitizers of Hypoxic Cells.* Elsevier, 1979.

20. Phillips, T. L. and Wasserman, T., Promise of radiosensitizers and radioprotectors in the treatment of human cancer. *Canc. Treat. Rep.* **68:** 291, 1984.

21. Brown, J. M., Clinical trials of radiosensitizers: What should we expect? *Int. J. Radiat. Oncol. Biol. Phys.* **10:** 425–429, 1984.

22. Phillips, T. L., Mitchell, J. B., DeGraff, W., Russo, A. and Glatstein, E., Variation in sensitizing efficiency for SR-2508 in human cells dependent on glutathione content. *Int. J. Radiat. Oncol. Biol. Phys.* **12:** 1627–1635, 1986.

23. Mitchell, J. B., Phillips, T. L., DeGraff, W., Carmichael, J., Rajpal, R. K. and Russo, A., The relationship of SR-2508 sensitizer enhancement ratio to cellular

glutathione levels in human tumor cell lines. *Int. J. Radiat. Oncol. Biol. Phys.* **12**: 1143–1146, 1986.

24. Yu, N. Y. and Brown, J. M., Depletion of glutathione *in vivo* as a method of improving the therapeutic ratio of misonidazole and SR 2508. *Int. J. Radiat. Oncol. Biol. Phys.* **10**: 1265–1269, 1984.

25. Somfai-Relle, S., Suzukake, K., Vistica, B. P. and Vistica, D. T., Reduction in cellular glutathione by buthionine sulfoximine and sensitization of murine tumor cells resistant to L-phenylalanine mustard. *Biochem. Pharmacol.* **1**: 485–490, 1984.

26. Green, J. A., Vistica, D. T., Young, R. C., Hamilton, T. C., Rogan, A. M. and Ozols, R. F., Potentiation of melphalan cytotoxicity in human ovarian cancer cell lines by glutathione delpetion. *Cancer Res.* **44**: 5427–5431, 1984

27. Hamilton, T. C., Winker, M. A., Louie, K. G., Batist, G., Behrens, B. C., Tsuruo, T., Grotzinger, K. R., McKoy, W. M., Young, R. C. and Ozols, R. F., Augmentation of adriamycin, melphalan, and cisplatin cytotoxicity in drug-resistant and -sensitive human ovarian carcinoma cell lines by buthionine sulfoximine mediated glutathione depletion. *Biochem. Pharmacol.* **34**: 2583–2586, 1985.

28. Ozols, R. F., Louie, K. G., Plowman, J., Behrens, B. C., Fine, R. L., Dykes, D. and Hamilton, T. C., Enhanced melphalan cytotoxicity in human ovarian cancer *in vitro* and in tumor-bearing nude mice by buthionine sulfoximine depletion of glutathione. *Biochem. Pharmacol.* **1**: 147–153, 1987.

29. Siemann, D. W. and Mulcahy, R. T., Sensitization of cancer chemotherapeutic agents by nitroheterocyclics. *Biochem. Pharmacol.* **35**: 111–115, 1986.

30. Bleehen, N. M., Roberts, J. T. and Newman, H. F. V., A phase II study of CCNU with benznidazole for metastatic malignant melanoma. *Int. J. Radiat. Oncol. Biol. Phys.* **12**: 1401–1403, 1986.

31. Varnes, M. E., Bigalow, J. E. Koch, C. J. and Hall, E. J., Depletion of nonprotein thiols of hypoxic cells by misonidazole and metronidazole: Implications for cytotoxicity. In: *Radiation Sensitizers. Their use in the Clinical Management of Cancer* (L. Brady, Ed.) pp. 121, 1980.

32. Varghese, A. J. and Whitmore, G. F., Misonidazole-glutathione conjugates in CHO cells. *Int. J. Radiat. Oncol. Biol. Phys.* **10**: 1341–1345, 1984.

33. Reed, D. J., Defense mechanisms of normal and tumor cells. *Int. J. Radiat. Oncol. Biol. Phys.* **12**: 1457–1461, 1986.

34. Goodman, J. and Hochstain, P., Generation of free radicals and lipid peroxidation by redox cycling of adriamycin and daunomycin. *Biochem. Biophys. Res. Comm.* **77**: 797–803, 1977.

35. Suzuki, H., Nagia, K., Yamaki, H., Tanaka, N. and Umezana, H., On the mechanism of action of bleomycin: Scission of DNA strands *in vitro* and *in vivo*. *J. Antibiot.* (Tokyo) **22**: 446–448, 1969.

36. Russo, A. and Mitchell, J. B., Potentiation and protection of adriamycin cytotoxicity by cellular glutathione modulation. *Canc. Treat. Rep.* **69**: 1293–1296, 1985.

37. Russo, A., Mitchell, J. B., McPherson, S. and Friedman, N., Alteration of bleomycin cytotoxicity by glutathione depletion or elevation. *Int. J. Radiat. Oncol. Biol. Phys.* **10**: 1675–1678, 1984.

38. Roizin-Towle, L., Selective enhancement of hypoxic cell killing by melphalan via thiol depletion: *In vitro* studies with hypoxic cell sensitizers and buthionine sulfoximine. *JNCI* **74**: 151–157, 1985.

39. Taylor, C. U., Evans, J. W. and Brown, J. M., Mechanism of sensitization of Chinese hamster ovary cells to melphalan by hypoxic treatment with misonidazole. *Cancer Res.* **43**: 3175–3181, 1983.

40. Carmichael, J., Friedman, N., Tochner, Z., Adams, O. J., Wolf, R., Ihde, D. C., Mitchell, J. B. and Russo, A., Inhibition of the protective effect of cyclopho-

sphamide by pre-treatment with buthionine sulfoximine. *Int. J. Radiat. Oncol. Biol. Phys.* **12**: 1191–1193, 1986.

41. Russo, A., DeGraff, W., Friedman, N. and Mitchell, J. B., Selective modulation of glutathione levels in human normal versus tumor cells and subsequent differential response to chemotherapy drugs. *Cancer Res.* **46**: 2845–2848, 1986.

42. Ling, V., Kartner, N., Sudo, T., *et al.*, Multidrug-resistance phenotype in Chinese hamster ovary cells. *Canc. Treat. Rep.* **67**: 869–874, 1983.

43. Joshi, U. M., Dumas, M. and Meheudale, H. M., Characterization of melphalan-glutathione adducts whose formation is catalyzed by glutathione transferase. *Biochem. Phar.* **35**: 3405–3409, 1986.

44. Carmichael, J., DeGraff, W. G., Gazdar, A. F., Minna, J. D. and Mitchell, J. B., Evaluation of a tetrazolium-based semiautomated colorimetric assay: Assessment of chemosensitivity testing. *Cancer Res.* **47**: 936–942, 1987.

45. Carmichael, J., DeGraff, W. G., Gazdar, A. F., Minna, J. D. and Mitchell, J. B., Evaluation of a tetraxolium-based semiautomated colorimetric assay: Assessment of radiosensitivity. *Cancer Res.* **47**: 943–946, 1987.

46. Carmichael, J., Mitchell, J. B., DeGraff, W. G., Gamson, J., Gazdar, A. F., Johnson, B., Glatstein, E. and Minna, J. D., Chemosensitivity testing of human lung cancer cell lines using the MTT assay. *Br. J. Cancer* **57**: 540–547, 1988.

47. Mossman, T., Rapid colorimetric assay for cellular growth and survival: Application to proliferation and cytotoxicity assays. *J. Immunol. Methods* **65**: 55–63, 1983.

48. Minna, J. D., Higgins, G. D. and Glatstein, E., Cancer of the lung. In: *Cancer Principles and Practice of Oncology* (V.T. DeVita, S. Hellman, and S. A. Rosenberg, Eds.) pp. 396–475. J. B. Lippincott Co., Philadelphia, 1982.

49. Batist, G., Tulpule, A., Sinha, B. K., Katki, A. G., Meyers, C. E. and Cowan, K. H. Overexpression of a novel anionic glutathione transferase in multidrug-resistant human breast cancer cells. *J. Biol. Chem.* **261**: 15544–15549, 1986.

50. Cowan, K. H., Batist, G., Tulpule, A., Sinha, A. B. K. and Meyers, C. E., Similar biochemical changes associated with multidrug-resistance in human breast cancer cells and carcinogen-induced resistance to xenobiotics in rats. *Proc. Natl. Acad. Sc.* (USA) **83**: 9328–9332, 1986.

51. Allalunis-Turner, J., Lee, F. and Siemann, D. W., Comparison of glutathione (GSH) content of tumor cells grown *in vivo* and *in vitro*. *Cancer Res.* **48**: 3657–3660, 1988.

52. Lee, F. Y. F., Allalunis-Turner, M. J. and Siemann, D. W., Depletion of tumor vs. normal tissue glutathione by buthionine sulfoximine. *Br. J. Cancer* **56**: 33–38, 1987.

53. Lee, F. Y. F and Siemann, D. W. Isolation by flow cytometry of the human ovarian tumor cell subpopulation exhibiting a high glutathione content phenotype and increased resistance to adriamycin. *Int. J. Radiat. Oncol. Biol. Phys.* (In press.)

54. Kosower, E. M., Pazhenschvsky, B. and Hershkowitz, E., 1,5-Diazabicyclo[3.3.0]octadienediones (9, 10-Dioxabimanes). Strongly fluorescent syn isomers. *J. Amer. Chem. Soc.* **100**: 6516–6518, 1978.

55. Russo, A. and Bump, E. A., Detection and quantitation of biological sulfhydryls. Methods *Biochem. Anal.* **33**: 165–242, 1988.

56. Durand, R. E. and Olive, P. E., Flow cytometry techniques for studying cellular thiols. *Radiat. Res.* **95**: 456–470, 1983.

57. Rice, G. C., Bump, E. A., Shrieve, D. C., Lee, W. and Kovacs, M., Quantitative analysis of cellular glutathione by flow cytometry utilizing monochlorobimane: Some applications to radiation and drug resistance *in vitro* and *in vivo*. *Cancer Res.* **46**: 6105–6110, 1986.

58. Siemann, D. W., Allalunis-Turner, M. J., Keng, P. C., Lee, F. Y. F. and Alliet, K. L., Assessing tumor properties from biopsies: Influence of sample selection and enzyme dissociation technique. Abstract, Conference on Prediction of Tumor Treatment Response, Banff, Canada April, 1987.
59. Gratzner, H. G., Monoclonal antibody to 5-bromo- and 5-iodo deoxyuridine: A new reagent for detection of DNA replication. *Science* (Washington, D.C.) **218**: 474–475, 1982.
60. Morstyn, G., Hsu, S.-M., Kinsella, T. J., Gratzner, H., Russo, A. and Mitchell, J. B., Bromodeoxyuridine in tumors and chromosomes detected with a monoclonal antibody. *J. Clin. Invest.* **72**: 1844–1850, 1983.
61. Wilson, G. D., McNally, Dunphy, E., Karcher, H. and Pfragner, R., The labeling index of human and mouse tumours assessed by bromodeoxyuridine staining *in vitro* and *in vivo* and flow cytometry. *Cytometry* **6**: 641–647, 1985.
62. Tietze, F., Enzymic method for quantitative determination of nanogram amounts of total and oxidized glutathione. Application to mammalian blood and other tissues. *Anal. Biochem.* **27**: 502–522, 1969.
63. Fahey, R. C. and Newton, G. L. Determination of low molecular weight thiols using monobromobimane fluorescent labeling and high-performance liquid chromatography. *Methods Enzymol.* **143**: 85–96, 1987.
64. Siemann, D. W., Lord, E. M., Keng, P. C. and Wheeler, K. T., Cell subpopulations dispersed from solid tumours and separated by centrifugal elutriation. *Br. J. Cancer* **44**: 100–108, 1981.
65. Asghar, K., Reddy, B. G. and Krishna, G., Histochemical localization of glutathione in tissues. *J. Histochem. Cytochem.* **23**: 774–779, 1975.
66. Murray, G. I., Burke, M. D. and Ewen, S. W. B., Glutathione localization by a novel o-phthaldehyde histofluorescence method. *Histochem. J.* **18**: 434–440, 1986.
67. Harisch, G. and Meyer, W., Studies on tissue distribution of glutathione and on activities of gluathione-related enzymes after carbon tetracholride-induced liver injury. *Res. Commun. Chem. Path. Pharmac.* **47**: 399–414, 1985.
68. Sippel, T. O., The histochemistry of thiols and disulphides. I. The use of N-(4-aminophenyl) maleimide for demonstrating thiol groups. *Histochem. J.* **5**: 413–423, 1973.
69. Sippel, T. O., The histochemistry of thiols and disulphides. II. Methodology of differential staining. *Histochem. J.* **10**: 585–595, 1978.
70. Sippel, T. O., The histochemistry of thiols and disulphides. III. Staining patterns in rat tissues. *Histochem. J.* **10**, 597–609, 1978.

12

In Vitro Assays for Predicting Clinical Response in Human Lung Cancer

Adi F. Gazdar, Chun-Ming Tsai, Jae-Gahb Park, Daniel Ihde,
James Mulshine, James Carmichael, James B. Mitchell, and
John D. Minna

INTRODUCTION

Selection of optimal chemotherapy regimens for individual patients has been a goal of investigators for over 30 years. However, the various methodologies present several theoretical and practical problems, and their applications have been limited to a modest number of experimental studies. In this chapter we discuss our experience, both clinically and in the laboratory, to apply drug sensitivity testing (DST) for selection of individualized therapy for lung cancer patients.

For over 10 years, the Navy Medical Oncology Branch of the National Cancer Institute (originally at the VA Medical Center, Washington, D.C.) has intensively studied the biology of lung cancer, in particular small cell lung cancer (SCLC). As a result of these studies, conditions for the growth of some of the major forms of lung cancer have been established using serum-free (SFM) and serum-supplemented (SSM) media. We have applied our knowledge of the growth and biology of these tumors to devise unique strategies for DST.

TYPES OF LUNG CANCER

Lung cancer is the leading cause of deaths in the USA, with an estimated 145,000 cases occurring every year.[1] Unfortunately, nearly 90% of the patients will eventually die from their disease. According to the WHO classification, there are four major types of lung cancer: (1) squamous cell, (2) large cell, (3) adenocarcinoma, and (4) SCLC. For a number of clinical and biological reasons, lung cancers may be divided into two broad categories: SCLC and non-SCLC (all other

types). SCLC is an aggressive form of tumor that frequently metasta-
sizes prior to diagnosis and is seldom cured by surgical resection alone.
However, it is usually initially responsive to chemotherapy. Unfortunately, most tumors recur, at which time they are usually resistant to
further chemotherapy, including agents to which they were not previously exposed. Because few SCLC tumors are electively resected,
most laboratory studies, including DST, have to be performed on
tumor-containing samples obtained during routine staging procedures,
such as marrow aspirates, malignant effusions, lymph nodes, and subcutaneous nodules. Many of these positive specimens contain relatively
few tumor cells and relatively large numbers of stromal or other non-
malignant cells, which further complicates the performance of DST.

Non-SCLC tumors are relatively resistant to chemotherapy, and we
find surgical resection offers the best prospect for long-term survival.
Specimens available for DST include resections of primary tumors as
well as those obtained by diagnostic procedures performed at the time
of relapse or metastatic spread. They frequently (but not always) contain relatively generous numbers of tumor cells admixed with varying
numbers of stromal cells. Although DST may be performed on a primary tumor, the data are usually not applied clinically until the time
of tumor recurrence many months later.

ENDOCRINE ASPECTS OF LUNG CANCER

While SCLC was originally considered to be an undifferentiated
tumor, it is now recognized to be a tumor related to a widely dispersed
network of endocrine cells.[2] Because these cells share many properties
with neurons, they are referred to as neuroendocrine (NE) cells. The
major function of NE cells is the synthesis, packaging, and secretion
of small peptide and amine hormones. These products are stored in
cytoplasmic dense core granules (DCG) prior to secretion. The DCG
contain a matrix protein referred to as chromogranin A. Amine synthesis requires a specific enzyme, DOPA decarboxylase. Neurons and
NE cells also express an acidic form of the glycolytic enzyme—enolase—known as neuron-specific enolase. SCLC cells may elaborate multiple hormones, but the peptide most commonly expressed, and in
the highest concentrations, is related to amphibian bombesin or its
mammalian homologue, gastrin-releasing peptide. SCLC tumors
expressing all of these neuroendocrine properties and typical morphology are referred to as "classic tumors". Occasional tumors have
altered morphology, rapid growth *in vitro*, and selective loss of some
NE properties. These are referred to as "variant tumors".[3,4] Variant

tumors respond poorly to therapy and are associated with a shorter mean survival time. They frequently represent tumor progression events associated with amplification and over expression of the c-*myc* proto-oncogene.[4] Another lung tumor of low grade malignancy, the rare bronchial carcinoid, also expresses the entire range of NE properties.

While non-SCLC tumors are not considered to be endocrine tumors, about 12% express the partial or complete range of NE properties.[5] These tumors are usually adenocarcinomas or large cell carcinomas. About 5–20% of non-SCLC tumors respond to therapy, and we are currently investigating whether expression of the NE phenotype is associated with chemosensitivity.

ASSAYS FOR DST

For many years, clonogenic assays[6] for DST have attracted the most attention. While it is frequently claimed that such assays measure true tumor stem cells, an equally important reason for their popularity has been the inability of stromal cells (other than hematopoietic) to form clones in semi-solid media. Thus clonogenic cells can be presumed to be of tumor origin, and mixtures of tumor and stromal cells (as exist in fresh tumor specimens) can be assayed. Unfortunately, clonogenic assays suffer from major practical problems: including (1) long assay times, (2) need for disaggregation into strict single cell suspensions, and (3) low clonogenic potential of many tumor samples.[7] Theoretical problems exist also with the stem cell concept.[7]

Initially, we evaluated a clonogenic assay as applied to SCLC.[8] Carney et al.[8] reported that while some colonies were observed from 69/80 (80%) of tumor-containing specimens, the number yielding sufficient colonies to test even three drugs at a single concentration was only 18/80 (23%). In a retrospective correlation of DST and patient response, the clonogenic assay accurately predicted sensitivity in 73% and resistance in 100% of the tests, thus confirming its potential clinical relevance. Even SCLC lines clone inefficiently,[4] especially newly-established classic lines from untreated patients. While we have utilized the clonogenic assay for many biologic studies of SCLC, its clinical applications in this disease are limited at the present time.

For these reasons, we explored a dye exclusion assay devised by Weisenthal.[9] Its virtues include speed, relative simplicity, relatively small inoculum number, and ability to cytologically distinguish between tumor and stromal cells. In the assay, tumor cells are disaggregated, incubated with drugs for one hour or continuously, incubated

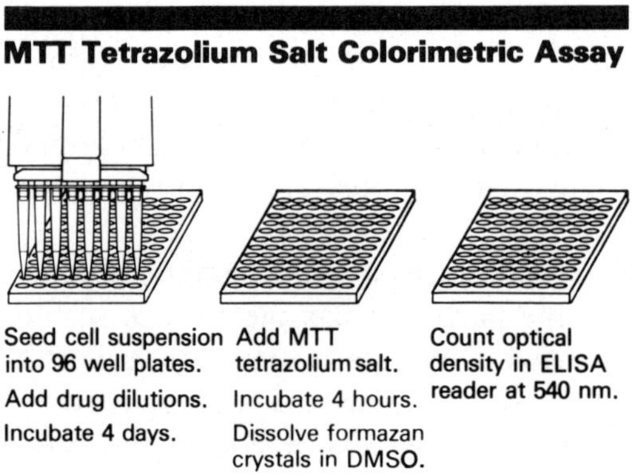

MTT Tetrazolium Salt Colorimetric Assay

Seed cell suspension into 96 well plates. Add drug dilutions. Incubate 4 days.

Add MTT tetrazolium salt. Incubate 4 hours. Dissolve formazan crystals in DMSO.

Count optical density in ELISA reader at 540 nm.

FIG. 12.1. Cartoon depicting the semi-automated MTT tetrazolium salt colorimetric assay.

at 37° in growth medium for four days, nucleated duck, red blood cells and the dyes fast green and/or nigrosin added, and cytospin samples prepared and counterstained with hematoxylin/eosin. Live cells (stained with hematoxylin/eosin) can be distinguished from dead or dying cells (stained green, grey, or black). The ratio of surviving tumor cells to the eliptical nucleated duck cells is determined and compared to the ratio of control tubes. A drug is considered active if there is less than 50% cell survival at a preselected concentration. These concentrations were determined by testing a large number of fresh lung tumor samples and were selected to yield results that correspond to the clinical efficacy of the individual drugs.

While preliminary data suggest that the Weisenthal test yields clinically relevant data (see below), it also presents major problems. It is subjective, highly laborious, requires professional input, and cell clumping occurs with some tumor types, especially SCLC (a modest degree of clumping is acceptable). Despite these problems, we have used this assay for our lung cancer clinical trials, but not for extensive biological studies.

Recently, we have explored a third assay, the MTT tetrazolium dye assay[10] as modified by us.[11,12] It is semi-automated, rapid, objective and highly reproducible (Fig. 12.1). Its major drawback is its inability to distinguish tumor from stromal cells. Thus, it can only be applied to cell lines or other populations of "pure" tumor cells. In the assay, cells are seeded into 96 well plates and incubated with drugs for four days. MTT tetrazolium dye (yellowish color) is added, and converted by a mitochondrial dehydrogenase to purple-violet colored formazan crystals. Some of the media is removed and replaced by DMSO, which dissolves the crystals. The absorbance of each well is measured at 540 nm in an automatic plate reader coupled to a computer, which stores the data and performs calculations. The data are plotted and the concentrations of drug required to reduce absorbance by 50% (IC_{50}) is calculated.

SELECTIVE GROWTH OF LUNG CANCERS IN SERUM FREE MEDIA

As previously mentioned, tumors contain varying numbers of stomal cells, and in routine staging biopsies, the latter may be in great excess. The culture of tumors in routine SSM frequently results in overgrowth or persistence of stromal cells. Some years ago, Sato and co-workers determined that different tumor types had specific growth factor requirements, and that tumors could be cultured selectively in fully-defined medium.

Following this lead, we have developed media for the selective growth of SCLC (HITES medium,[14]) and adenocarcinoma (ACL-4 medium[15,16]). The growth requirements for squamous cell carcinomas have been partially identified.[15] As large cell carcinomas are really undifferentiated forms of the other types of lung cancer, especially adenocarcinomas, and because the incidence of squamous cell carcinomas is declining rapidly, we have media for the selective culture of most lung cancers.

Selective media have two major roles in DST. They permit the rapid selection of pure tumor cell populations. Thus, assays that cannot distinguish tumor from stromal cells can be applied within a relatively short time of obtaining a tumor sample admixed with a large number of stromal cells. In addition, we have pioneered the use of fully defined media (SFM) as applied to DST. As the *in vitro* cytotoxicity of some drugs (MTX, 5-FU) is partially inhibited in SSM, the use of SFM circumvents this problem.

DESIGN OF CLINICAL PROTOCOLS

We currently have active clinical protocols based on individualized chemotherapy for extensive stage SCLC and non-SCLC (all stages). In the former, tumor-containing specimens are obtained during routine staging procedures or by biopsy of easily accessible subcutaneous or node metastases. DST is performed on "cell lines" initiated from these samples. For practical reasons, we define a cell line as selective amplification of tumor cell number sufficient to permit adequate DST. The time required may vary from one day to up to several weeks. In fact, most of these short-term cultures develop into fully-established continuous cell lines. Because the therapy of newly diagnosed SCLC patients cannot be delayed for several weeks, the patients are given front line therapy with VP-16 and cisplatin (PLA) while DST data are being obtained. The patients are restaged at week twelve. Those in complete remission (CR) continue with VP-16/PLA therapy. Those who have progressive disease (PD) or partial response (PR) are switched to the three drug *in vitro* best regimen (IVBR) at week thirteen, if DST data are available. If DST data are not available, a combination of VCR/ADR/CYT is administered.

For non-SCLC, the clinical possibilities are more complex. Patients undergoing potentially curative resections of primary tumors may never require chemotherapy. In case of recurrence, DST data may not be applied until many months after they have been performed. In cases presenting with unresectable or metastatic disease, DST data may be applied as soon as it is available. However, unlike SCLC, a delay of several weeks can frequently be tolerated. Finally, some non-SCLC tumors express NE markers. Our approach to this subgroup is discussed later in this chapter.

THE USE OF CELL LINES FOR DST

There are certain advantages and disadvantages to using cell lines for DST (Table 12.1). Tumor specimens contain relatively few tumor cells admixed with stromal cells, repeat testing is difficult or impossible, and test variability is high. Their major advantage is that DST data are available within a short time. Cell lines offer pure populations of relatively large numbers of tumor cells, repeat testing is feasible, and assay variability is low. Their major disadvantage is that DST is delayed. Of course, the clinical relevance of DST of both tumors and cell lines remains to be determined.

TABLE 12.1. *Relative Advantages and Disadvantages of DST of Tumors and Cell Lines*

	Tumors	Cell Lines
Tumor cells	Few	Many
Stromal cells	Present	Absent
Intra-assay variability	High	Low
Repeat testing	Difficult	Easy
Specimen to assay time	Immediate	Delayed
Clinical relevance	?	??

TABLE 12.2. *Relative Chemosensitivity of Human Tumor Cell Lines Derived from Previously Untreated Human Tumors.*

Tumor Type	VP-16	PLA	ADR	MEL
SCLC	1	1	1	1
Non-SCLC	31	4	8	9
Colon	68	8	30	12

In an effort to determine the potential clinical value of the use of cell lines, we performed DST on a relatively large number of continuous cell lines derived from untreated human tumors (Table 12.2). SCLC lines were more sensitive than non-SCLC lines, and colon carcinomas were the most uniformly resistant.[17,18] These findings, of course, correlate with our clinical experience with these diseases.

FEASIBILITY OF CLINICAL PROTOCOLS BASED ON DST

Our first task was to demonstrate the feasibility of successfully culturing and performing DST on tumor samples from a sufficient percentage of patients entered on protocol. We have entered 63 patients into our extensive stage SCLC protocol, and have obtained at least one specimen from 62 (98%). An average of 2.7 specimens were received per patient, of which 41% contained tumor cells. Twenty-two cell lines were established from 21 patients. This represents 46% of patients from whom a tumor-containing specimen was received and represents 33% of all patients.

Of the first 83 patients entered onto the non-SCLC protocol, DST was performed on 21 (25%) and recently we have improved this rate to about 40%. Thus, for both SCLC and non-SCLC, DST can be obtained for 25-40% of all patients entered on protocol. These figures are close to those projected prior to the start of these studies. However, both protocols are exceedingly labor-intensive, with many negative samples having to be processed and cultured.

DST DATA FROM LUNG CANCER LINES

We tested SCLC lines against seven drugs having known clinical activity. There was considerable heterogeneity, both of individual lines to the drugs as well as among the various drugs. VP-16 was the most effective drug *in vitro,* both as far as being active (i.e., less than 50% survival) as well as being among the top three drugs irrespective of activity. Vincristine and methotrexate were the least active. We tested 21 non-SCLC lines against 13 drugs with known or suspected clinical activity. While we have not fully analyzed our data, 24% of individual drug assays were "active". Certain drugs present specific problems. These problems and their possible solutions are presented in Table 12.3.

TABLE 12.3. *Drug Sensitivity Testing: Problems with Individual Agents*

Drug	Problem	Comment
CYT	Inactive *in vitro*	Substitute active alkylating agent
MTX, 5FU	Reduced activity in serum containing media	Use serum-free media
Nitrosoureas	Reduced solubility	Use organic solvents
VCR, MTX	"Flat" DST curves	Calculate area under the curve

CLINICAL CORRELATIONS

At present, clinical correlations between DST and patient responses are available only for the SCLC protocol. There was an excellent correlation between DST of SCLC lines and the response to front line therapy. In 14/15 (93%) of lines from patients who were in complete or partial response at week 12, two or more drugs were "active", and 45% of all individual assays yielded < 50% survival at the test concentration. In contrast, in none of four lines from patients who failed to respond were two or more active agents identified, and only 1/25 (4%) of the individual assays resulted in < 50% survival. These differences are highly significant.

Thirty patients received second line therapy (VIN/ADR/CYT) after failing to respond or relapsing after front line therapy. Of these patients, there were only two complete responses (7%). Among 12 similar patients whose second line therapy was the IVBR, there were three complete responses (25%), suggesting a modest benefit to individualized drug selection.

ADAPTATION OF THE MTT ASSAY TO CLINICAL PROTOCOLS

As previously mentioned, the highly labor-intensive Weisenthal assay is not suitable for extensive laboratory use, and we have limited its application to protocol studies. We have used the semi-automated MTT assay for other laboratory investigations involving continuous cell lines. Currently, we are attempting to utilize the assay for clinical

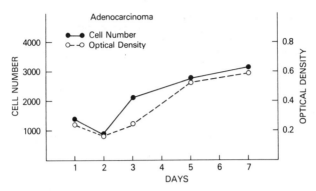

FIG. 12.2. MTT assay: relationship between cell number and absorbance. A lung adenocarcinoma cell line was tested in serum-free ACL-4 medium.

testing, but before this can be done, further modifications of the assay are required.

Initially we determined that DMSO was a more desirable solvent than the one originally utilized.[11] We have also demonstrated that over a wide range, optical density is linear with cell number (Fig. 12.2). We then determined that most lung cancer lines could be tested in SFM (HITES medium for SCLC and ACL-4 medium for non-SCLC) (Table 12.2). However, for optimal growth, we add 0.2% bovine albumin to both defined media. Under these conditions, most lung lines grow in microtiter wells at least as well as in SSM. The activities of MTX and 5FU are enhanced considerably in SFM, while most other drugs yield similar results in SFM and SSM. However, some drugs, such as VCR and MTX, yield "flat" DST curves. Thus a slight deviation on repeat testing may result in a relatively large alteration in the IC_{50} value. Alternative means of comparing sensitivity to these drugs are being explored, such as area under the curve measurements. Finally, the problem of selecting active drugs has not been fully resolved. One method is to test a large panel of lines of one tumor type. The response of a test line to an agent is compared to the reference panel and the relative activity of each of the drugs determined and compared. Alternative methods include *in vitro* area under the curve measurements with correlation with the values clinically achievable. We are also trying to determine an *in vitro* therapeutic index, comparing the relative sensitivities of the patient's tumor, bone marrow, and other normal cells.

RELATIVE CHEMOSENSITIVITY OF NON-SCLC LINES EXPRESSING NE PROPERTIES

As previously mentioned, about 12% of non-SCLC tumors and cell lines express multiple NE markers. We refer to them as NSCLC-NE tumors and lines. Usually, these tumors are large cell or adenocarcinomas, with NE properties rarely being expressed by squamous carcinomas. Of interest is the fact that 5–20% of non-SCLC tumors are responsive to chemotherapy. Thus, we wished to determine whether the responsive subgroup corresponded with those expressing NE markers. In our non-SCLC protocol, tumor samples are tested for four NE markers. Tumors expressing one or more markers are labelled NSCLC-NE tumors and those patients are treated with a six-drug combination of proven effectiveness against SCLC. We have established six cell lines expressing multiple NE markers. The sensitivity patterns of five of these NSCLC-NE were similar to those of untreated SCLC lines and were more sensitive than other untreated NSCLC lines when compared by rank order. These differences were statistically significant. Thus, prediction of chemosensitivity of non-SCLC tumor and lines may be associated with expression of NE markers. However, the results of our clinical trial will be required to confirm these *in vitro* studies.

SUMMARY AND FUTURE APPLICATIONS

From the data presented, it is obvious that current clonogenic assays have little or no application to the clinical DST of lung tumors, and that many samples require selective amplification of tumor cell number prior to testing. The use of cell lines appears to be closely correlated with clinical studies, both retrospectively and prospectively. Thus, SCLC lines are usually more sensitive than non-SCLC lines and colon lines are highly resistant. DST data of SCLC lines are highly correlated with the clinical response to front line therapy. Finally, there may be a modest benefit from using DST to select second line therapy for SCLC patients not completely responding to front line therapy.

These data are encouraging enough to enable us to be more aggressive in obtaining clinical samples (such as by elective mediastinoscopy, open liver biopsy, etc.) and to perform DST as early as possible. With these techniques, we may be able to apply DST data to a larger percentage of patients and, perhaps, use the IVBR as front line instead of second line therapy.

It is obvious that the MTT assay provides us with a powerful tool for biological studies such as testing synergism of drug combinations, preclinical screening of the selective antitumor effects of new agents, individualized selection of the most active phase II agent, etc. Some of these applications are currently in use at our hospital. While certain problems remain in applying this assay to clinical specimens, we hope to resolve these difficulties within a short time. Finally, the relative chemosensitivity of NSCLC-NE lines is an exciting observation, suggesting that biochemical properties can be used to predict response to therapy. We are investigating the use of molecular probes as more accurate and sensitive markers of NE expression.

REFERENCES

1. Minna, J. D., Higgins, G. A. and Glatstein, E. J., Cancer of the Lung. In: *Cancer Principles and Practice of Oncology*, 2nd ed. (V.T. DeVita, S. Hellman, and S. A. Rosenberg, eds.) pp. 507–597. J. B. Lippincott, Philadelphia, PA 1985.
2. Gazdar, A. F., The biology of endocrine tumors of the lung. In: *The Endocrine Lung in Health and Disease* (K. L. Becker and A. F. Gazdar, eds.), pp. 448–459. W. B. Saunders, Philadelphia, PA 1984.
3. Carney, D. N., Gazdar, A. F., Bepler, G., Guccion, J. G., Marangos, P. J., Moody, T. W., Zweig, M. H. and Minna, J. D., Establishment and identification of small cell lung cancer cell lines having classic and variant features. *Cancer Res.* 45: 2913–2923, 1985.
4. Gazdar, A. F., Carney, D. N., Nau, M. M. and Minna, J. D., Characterization of variant subclasses of cell lines derived from small cell lung cancer having distinctive biochemical, morphological and growth properties. *Cancer Res.* 45: 2924–2930, 1985.
5. Gazdar, A. F., Advances in the biology of non-small cell lung cancer. *Chest* 89: 277S–283S, 1986.
6. Hamburger, A. W. and Salmon, S. E., Primary bioassay of human tumor stem cells. *Science* 197: 461–463, 1977.
7. Weisenthal, L. M. and Lippman, M. E., Clonogenic and nonclonogenic *in vitro* chemosensitivity assays. *Cancer Treatment Rep.* 69: 615–632, 1985.
8. Carney, D. N., Gazdar, A. F., Cuttitta, F. and Minna, J. D., *In vitro* studies of the biology of lung cancer. In: *Lung Cancer: Causes and Prevention* (Mizell and Correa, eds.) pp. 247–261. Verlag Chemice International, 1984.
9. Weisenthal, L. M., Morsden, J. A., Dill, P. L. and Macaluso, C. K., A novel dye exclusion method for testing *in vitro* chemosensitivity of human tumors. *Cancer Res.* 43: 749–757, 1983.
10. Mossman, T., Rapid colorimetric assay for cellular growth and survival: Application to proliferation and cytotoxic assays. *J. Immunol. Methods* 65: 55–63, 1983.
11. Carmichael, J., DeGraff, W. G., Gazdar, A. F., Minna, J. D. and Mitchell, J. B., Evaluation of a tetrazolium-based semiautomated colorimetric assay: Assessment of chemosensitivity testing. *Cancer Res.* 47: 936–942, 1987.
12. Carmichael, J., DeGraff, W. G., Gazdar, A. F., Minna, J. D. and Mitchell, J. B., Evaluation of a tetrazolium-based semiautomated colorimetric assay: Assessment of radiosensitivity. *Cancer Res.* 47: 943–946, 1987.
13. Barnes, D. and Sato, G. Serum-free cell culture: A unifying approach. *Cell* zz, 649–655, 1980.
14. Simms, E., Gazdar, A. F., Abrams, P. and Minna, J. D., Growth of human small cell (oat cell) carcinoma of the lung in serum-free growth factor supplemented medium. *Cancer Res.* 40: 4356–4363, 1980.

15. Gazdar, A. F. and Oie, H. K., Cell culture methods for human lung cancer. *Cancer Genet. Cytogenet.* **19**: 5–10, 1986.
16. Gazdar, A. F. and Oie, H. K., Growth of cell lines and clinical specimens of human non-small cell lung cancer in a serum-free defined medium. Letter to the editor, *Cancer Res.* **46**: 6011–6012, 1986.
17. Carmichael, J., Mitchell, J. B., DeGraff, W. G., Gamson, J., Gazdar, A. F., Johnson, B. E., Glatstein, E. and Minna, J. D., Chemosensitivity testing of human lung cancer cell lines using the MTT assay. Submitted for publication, 1987.
18. Park, J. G., Kramer, B. S., Steinberg, S. M., Carmichael, J., Collins, J. M., Minna, J. D. and Gazdar, A. F., Chemosensitivity testing of human colorectal carcinoma cell lines using a tetrazolium-based colorimetric (MTT) assay. Submitted for publication, 1987.

13

Commentary on Part III: Tumor Cell Response *in vitro*

Ronald N. Buick, Ralph Weichselbaum and Edmond Malaise

Exposure of human cells to X-rays or chemical agents may lead to DNA damage resulting in mutations, malignant transformation, or cell death. In the treatment of malignant disease, mechanisms that result in tumor cell mortality are of greatest interest. Variability in treatment outcome relating to tumor physiology and microenvironment (such as tumor cell hypoxia and reoxygenation following radiotherapy) has been widely studied in animal tumor systems. In Part III emphasis has been placed upon the predictive information to be gained from study of cell viability after exposure to drugs or radiation *in vitro*, i.e., measurement of the intrinsic sensitivity of tumor cells.

The notion of correlating *in vivo* clinical response with indices of *in vitro* cell survival is not a new one; attempts have been made over a number of decades, initially involving endpoints of "well-being" in tissue culture and, subsequent to the development of radioactive precursors for DNA synthesis, more direct proliferation measurements. In the late 1970s, in part stimulated by the notion of a stem cell compartment within tumors, clonogenic assays were applied vigorously to this task. More recently, however, in light of the extreme technical demands and limitations of this procedure, emphasis has been placed on the practicality of measurement, and simple assessments of total tumor cell viability (eg., dye exclusion, MTT reduction) have been reinvestigated and improved upon by a number of investigators. Thus, over the last two decades, a number of independent approaches have been taken to predict response using assays of *in vitro* viability. The most extensively tested of these for utility in clinical settings are clonogenic growth potential in semi-solid medium, the ATCCS, ^{3}H-TdR uptake, MTT reduction, and dye-exclusion. The major question of course remains; can we identify chemo/radio-resistant cells in a timely and reliable fashion, and will this information allow for advances in treatment efficacy?

Two chapters emerging from this conference, one by Brock *et al.*, and one by Gazdar, *et al.*, highlight a number of important points about the current status of this field of research. Firstly, Brock *et al.* provide data on the characteristics of a relatively new procedure for the assessment of tumor cell viability based on an adhesive tumor cell culture system (ATCCS). In this procedure, small numbers of tumor cells, disaggregated from solid tumors, can be selectively grown attached to tissue culture plates pre-coated with a matrix material. Evidence was presented in poster C-7 that indicate the procedure allows the growth of a high proportion of tumors of a variety of histological types and does select for the growth of tumor cells in the mixed populations obtained from solid tumor biopsies. Both clonal counts and bulk indices of cell number could be used as endpoints of cell growth. Brock *et al.* demonstrate the usefulness of this tissue culture procedure in assessing cell mortality associated with both drug and radiation treatment *in vitro*. Ajani *et al.* (C-6) describe the use of this procedure to predict chemotherapy response. As has been the finding with all such methods relying on assays of *in vitro* cell survival, the procedure can apparently predict sensitivity with—60% accuracy and resistance with > 90% accuracy. Interesting results are presented by Tofilon *et al.* (C-8) who employed the ATCCS assay in combination with the sister chromatid exchange assay to detect platinum resistant (and apparently radioresistant) cell populations.

The high quality of the dose response curves to ionizing radiation has allowed Brock and his colleagues to classify individual tumor types as to radio-sensitivity by measuring survival at 2 Gy. This classification of primary tumor biopsies leads to similar conclusions about histopathology-related radiosensitivity which has been previously shown for cell lines. In addition, the range in sensitivities seen in the individual tumors of each histological type has encouraged these investigators to initiate a trial of the predictive value of this important information in squamous carcinomas of the head and neck. Preliminary results of this correlative test have now been published.[1]

The quality of the does-response data presented by Brock *et al.* in Chapter 10 of this volume, is of particular importance because of the fact that clonogenic assays relying on growth of cells in semi-solid medium have been found, in general, to be incapable of measuring, with any reasonable precision or high reproducibility, the radiosensitivity of tumor cells derived directly from large series of human tumor biopsies.

Malaise (C-11) compared the results obtained by the ATCCS method to those obtained by traditional clonogenic methods. The survival levels at 1.5 to 2 Gy were compared for 77 established tumor cell lines (clonogenic assay) with those from 30 primary mass cultures. In general, mass cultures elicited higher survival levels than clonogenic methods for a given radiation dose. However, in both systems melanomas were the least radiosensitive, and myelomas and lymphomas were the most sensitive to radiation.

Steel and Horwich (C-13) presented data which showed that low dose-rate radiation discriminates better than high dose-rate radiation between radio-sensitive and radioresistant tumor cells, although the extent of repair of low dose rates varies widely among human tumor cell lines. These authors suggest that the use of low dose-rate radiation may be an accurate method to discriminate between radioresistance and radiosensitive human tumor cells. The authors state that low dose-rate treatment is radiobiologically advantageous with some tumors and not with others.

The data presented by Brock and colleagues has been the result of the application of a new technology to a variety of histological subtypes of tumors. The work of Gazdar *et al.*, however, exemplifies a different approach. Over the last number of years this group has taken a multi-disciplinary approach to the biology of human lung cancer, which has led to a sophisticated view of classification, growth requirements, and molecular abnormalities related to carcinogenesis in this tissue. These insights allow existing procedures for treatment to be tailored to the biology of a particular tumor. Gazdar and colleagues have in the past demonstrated the lack of utility of clonogenic assay procedures and dye-exclusion studies for lung cancer biopsies, and in his Chapter describes the use of an MTT-reduction assay, coupled with the use of specialized media, for the selective growth of SCLC cells. This approach to testing the properties of individual tumor cell types has also been applied to myeloid leukemias over the last few years (because of the advances in knowledge of specific growth regulatory molecules for myeloid cells) and will undoubtedly be applied to other tumor types as knowledge of tissue-specific cellular growth control increases.

Other presentations dealt with several other issues relating to the use of these assays of cell viability. For instance, the important notion of therapeutic index has been approached in work described by Valeriote and Corbett (C-1), Kimler *et al.* (C-21) and Spitzer *et al.* (C-5) which used either clonogenic or ATCCS procedures to compare or normalize the tumor cell sensitivity to the sensitivity of hemopoietic progenitor cells. It is hoped that such knowledge will allow more successful drug screening and realistic prediction of therapeutic effect in the face of dose-limiting toxicity to normal tissue.

The criteria for use of an MTT assay for prediction of clinical response was approached by Wasserman and Twentyman (C-17) using the well-established transplantable animal tumor models RIF-1 and EMT6. This careful study of validation of procedures in animal tumors prior to clinical implementation was noteworthy and the concept was endorsed by other researchers. It was felt by many that more reliance on traditional strategies for assay development was required in this area of research.

The relative merits of the various cell viability assays which have been used for prediction of human tumor response was raised as a discussion point. Although it can be argued that those assays depending on multiple cell division (clonogenic, ATCCS) might be biologically more relevant with respect to stem cell concepts, it must be conceded that the speed and the improving specificity for tumor cells shown by the current MTT and dye-exclusion assays might, in selected situations, be equally efficient at predicting response. Indeed, the predictive powers of the multiple assays in various clinical trials of chemotherapy response have been remarkably similar in publications stretching back over the last two decades. Significantly, however, although retrospective and prospective studies have demonstrated a predictive power of *in vitro* essays, no study to date has demonstrated benefit to a patient population in a randomized prospective trial.

Another major question which was raised during conference was the issue of the parameters used to express drug and radiation sensitivity/ resistance. Clearly, since dose-response curves to radiation can be produced for cells from large numbers of primary tumors (see Brock, *et al.*, Chapter 10), it is appropriate that some discussion be made of methods of data presentation and comparability between laboratories. The issue of parameters of the radiation survival curve was particularly significant. Malaise proposed that mean inactivation dose, $\bar{D}$, is an accurate parameter to characterize tumor cell radiosensitivity. The $\bar{D}$ has been calculated by Malaise *et al.* (C-11) from published *in vitro* survival curves obtained from human tumor tissue. In general, tumors classified within histological categories which are difficult to cure with radiotherapy (melanoma, glioblastoma) have a higher $\bar{D}$ than do tumor cells derived from tumors less difficult to cure by radiotherapy (breast carcinoma, medulloblastoma). Weichselbaum et al.[2] studied inherent cellular radioresistance (D_O) and repair of X-ray damage (n, SLDR, and PLDR) in 19 early passage squamous cell carcinoma lines derived from head and neck cancer patients with known clinical results following radiotherapy. Human tumor cells that were radioresistant $D_O >$ 180, and/or proficient in the accumulation/repair of X-ray damage were cultured from patients unsuccessfully treated with radiotherapy. This is the first demonstration of the presence of radiation-resistant and repair-proficient cells in human tumors with known clinical follow-up, and suggests the possibility of predictive assays based on *in vitro* radiobiological parameters. Weichselbaum proposed the 24 hour PLDR surviving fraction, designated as the maximum recovery potential or MRP, which is a function of initial damage (D_O, n) as well as recovery over time (PLDR) as the best predictor of radiotherapy failure. This led to further discussion as to whether $\bar{D}$ (mean lethal dose) the surviving fraction of 2 Gy or calculation of D_O and n are the best ways to present radiobiological data. Vijayyakumar et al. (C-3) suggested that the $\bar{D}$ reflects the true characteristics of the survival curve. However, this generated much discussion, since Weichselbaum et al.[2] found all radiobiological parameters to be important in clinical outcome.

The discussion also focused on what endpoints should be used to compare chemotherapy and radiotherapy assays. For example, cellular response to chemotherapeutic agents is generally characterized by the ICD-50 and/or ICD-90 survival; i.e., the inhibitory or lethal doses to generate 50 or 90% survival. On the other hand, radiobiologists generally present full survival curves with shoulder (N or α) and slope (D_O or β) parameters. There is also a tendency in the literature for chemotherapeutic response to be calculated without the benefit of full dose response curves, e.g., based on single point survival after *in vitro* exposure. This stems from the large cell number requirements of several predictive assays (e.g., clonogenicity measurement typically require of the order of 10^5 cells per individual measurement). One major advantage demonstrated by the ATCCS assays is the apparent requirement for fewer cells, allowing much more sophistication to be applied to dose-response relationships.

The conference clearly produced some heated discussion, which was indicative of the importance of this field of research. Based on the points-of-view of those attending, there seems now to be a healthy awareness of the issues of quantitation and data quality control. The introduction of measurements of intrinsic radio-sensitivity and the optimization of procedures to take advantage of individual tumor-type biology are both viewed as important steps in the development of *in vitro* predictive assays.

REFERENCES

1. Peters, L. J., Baker, F. L., Goepfer, H., Campbell, B. H., Rich, T. A. and Brock, W. A., Prediction of tumor radiation response from radiosensitivity of cultured biopsy specimens. In: *Radiation Research* Vol. 2, 1987 (eds.), E. M. Fielden, J. F. Fowler, J. H. Hendry, and D. Scott, pp. 831–836 (Taylor & Francis— London).
2. Weichselbaum, R. R., Pahlberg, W., Beckett, M., Karrison, T., Miller, D., Clark, J. and Ervin, T., Radioresistant and repair proficient human tumor cells maybe associated with radiotherapy failures in head and neck cancer patients. *Proc. Natl. Oncol. Sci.* (USA) **83**: 2684–2688, 1986.

POSTERS

(C-1) A New Assay for Leukemia-Selective Anticancer Agents, F. Valeriote and T. Corbett. Division of Hematology-Oncology, Wayne State University, Detroit, Michigan 48201.

(C-2) Comparison of Cisplatin and its Analogs at Equivalent *In Vitro* Myelotoxic Doses in a Primary Adhesive Human Tumor Cell Culture Assay (ATCCS). D. Fan, F. Baker, A. R. Khokhar, R. A. Newman, G. Spitzer, B. Tomasovic, J. A. Ajani, W. A. Brock, M. Finders, A. Kelly, and T. Joe. The University of Texas System Cancer Center, M.D. Anderson Hospital and Tumor Institute, Houston, Texas 77030.

(C-3) Mean Inactivation Dose (D): A Neglected Parameter—A Critical Analysis. S. Vijayakumar, T. C. Ng, A. W. Majors, N. J. Baldwin, I. Koumoundouros, F. J. Thomas, and T. F. Meaney. Department of Radiation Therapy, Division of Radiology, Cleveland Clinic, 9500 Euclid Avenue, Cleveland, Ohio 44106.

(C-4) Measurements of the Initial Slope of Cell Survival Curves, B. Palcic. B.C. Cancer Research Centre and Pathology, University of British Columbia, Vancouver, British Columbia, Canada V5Z 1L3.

(C-5) *In Vitro* Comparison of Antitumor Efficacy of Investigational and Standard Drugs at the Equitoxic concentrations in the Adhesive Tumor Cell culture system (ATCCS), An *In Vitro* Method of Drug Screening, G. Spitzer, J. Ajani, F. Baker, W. Brock, D. Fan, and B. Tomasovic. The University of Texas M.D. Anderson Hospital and Tumor Institute, Houston, Texas 77030 and LifeTrac, Irvine, California 92715.

(C-6) *In Vitro* Drug Response of Primary Human Tumor Cells in the Adhesive Tumor Cell Culture System (ATCCS) Predicts for Clinical Response, J. Ajani, F. Baker, A. Kelly, G. Spitzer, W. Brock, B. Tomasovic, T. Joe, and D. Fan. The University of Texas M.D. Anderson Hospital and Tumor Institute, Houston, Texas 77030 and LifeTrac, Irvine, California 92715.

(C-7) Assay of Primary Human Tumor Cells for Drug Sensitivity Using the Adhesive-Tumor-Cell Culture System (ATCCS), F. L. Baker, G. Spitzer, J. A. Ajani and W. A. Brock. The University of Texas M.D. Anderson Hospital and Tumor Institute, Houston, Texas 77030 and LifeTrac, Irvine, California 92715.

(C-8) Detection of Heterogeneity in Drug and Radiation Sensitivity Within Primary Human Tumor Cell Cultures Using the SCE Assay, P. J. Tofilon, R. E. Meyn, and W. A. Brock. M.D. Anderson Hospital and Tumor Institute, Department of Experimental Radiotherapy, Houston, Texas 77030.

(C-9) Neuroblastoma Microspheroids: An *In Vitro* Model of *In Vivo* Tumors, M. D. Aja, Indiana University School of Medicine, Indianapolis, Indiana 46223.

(C-10) Intrinsic Resistance of Multicell Spheroids to Mitoxantrone Is Not Solely Due to Restricted Drug Penetration, T. J. Bichay and W. R. Inch. Department of Biophysics, University of Western Ontario and the London Regional Cancer Center, London, Ontario, Canada N6A 4G5.

(C-11) Comparison of Two Tissue Culture Methods (Clonogenic Assay and Mass Culture For Assessing the Intrinsic Radiosensitivity of Human Tumor Cells, E. P. Malaise, B. Fertil, N. Chavaudra, and W. A. Brock. U. Inserm 247, Villejuif, France and U. Inserm 194, Paris, France and M.D. Anderson Hospital and Tumor Institute, Houston, Texas 77030.

(c-12) Variation in Measurement of Drug Response by Human Glioblastoma Cells Using Three Tumor Clonogenic Assays, M. E. Berens, J. R. Giblin, D. V. Dougherty, H. Kleppe Hoifodt, and M. L. Rosenblum. Brain Tumor Research Center, University of California at San Francisco, San Francisco, California 94143.

(C-13) The Dose-Rate Effect in Human Tumor Cells, G. G. Steel and A. Horwich. The Institute of Cancer Research, Sutton, Surrey SM2 5PX England.

(c-14) Influence of Oxygen on the *In Vitro* Chemosensitivity of Cancer Cells in the Soft-Agar Clonogenic Assays, S. Fan, P. Staton, L. R. Morgan, and D. Fan. Baylor College of Medicine, Houston, Texas 77030 and Florida International University, Miami, Florida 33199 and Louisiana State University Medical Center, New Orleans, Louisiana 70119 and The University of Texas System Cancer Center, M.D. Anderson Hospital and Tumor Institute, Houston, Texas 77030.

(C-15) Synergism Between Prednimustine and Tamoxifen in the Human Breast Cancer Line MCF-7, B. Hartley-Asp, and A. B. Leo, Research Laboratories, Box 941, S-251 09 Helsingborg, Sweden.

(C-16) Use of a Rapid Colorimetric Assay for *In Vitro* Chemosensitivity Testing, M. F. Sarosdy. Division of Urology, UTHSC, San Antonio, Texas 78284–7845.

(C-17) Use of a Colorimetric Microtiter (MTT) Assay with *In Vivo* Tumors, T. H. Wasserman and P. Twentyman. MRC Unit and University Department of Clinical Oncology and Radiotherapeutics, Hills Road, Cambridge CB2 2QH, England and the Mallinckrodt Institute of Radiology, Washington University, St. Louis, Missouri.

(C-18) Ability of Dye-Exclusion Assay to Identify Cells Exposed to Agents Under Different Levels of Oxygenation, D. L. Kirkpatrick, M. Duke, and T. S. Goh. University of Regina and Allan Blair Memorial Clinic, Regina, Saskatchewan, Canada S4S 0A2.

(C-19) Heat Enhancement of CIS-DDP Cell Killing in RIF-1 Cells Grown *In Vivo* and *In Vitro*, A. A. Jacoby, R. Rowley, and J. R. Stewart. University of Utah Health Sciences Center, Salt Lake City, Utah 84132.

(C-20) Thermal Enhancement of Response to Radiation and Chemotherapeutic Agents in Human Maligant Glioma Cell Lines, G. P. Raaphorst, V. F. Da Silva, and M. M. Feeley. Ontario Cancer Foundation, Ottawa Civic Clinic, Department of Neurosurgery, Ottawa, Ontario, Canada K1Y 4K7.

(C-21) The Human Bone Marrow Colony Assay as a Predictor of Response, B. F. Kimler, C. H. Park, and R. G. Evans. Departments of Radiation, Oncology and Medicine, University of Kansas Medical Center, Kansas City, Kansas 66103.

(C-22) Growth Chamber Assay for Measuring Sensitivity of Tumor Cells to Drugs *In Vitro*, M. E. Key, J. Gut, and O. D. Holton. Earl-Clay Laboratories, Novato, California 94947.

(C-23) Radioresistant Leukemic Lymphocytes, Intractable Chronic Lymphocytic Leukemia, R. Schrek. Research Service, VA Hospital, Hines, Illinois 60141.

PART IV

TUMOR CELL
RESPONSE
IN VIVO

14

Human Tumor Xenografts in Development of Predictive Assays of Tumor Treatment Response

Einar K. Rofstad

INTRODUCTION

Clinical investigations have shown the response to radio- and chemotherapy of human tumors to differ significantly among individual patients. Treatment response can depend upon histological type and differentiation status, but histology is probably not a major determinant of responsiveness. In fact, different tumors of the same origin and with similar histological appearance may require totally different radiation doses to be locally controlled. Moreover, histologically similar tumors may respond differently to the same chemotherapy regimen; one treatment protocol that gives beneficial results for one patient may be ineffective on another, and vice versa for another treatment protocol. Thus, optimum radio- and chemotherapy of malignant disease will probably require an individualized treatment strategy. Consequently, there is a need for predictive assays to assess the clinical responsiveness of individual tumors to different treatment regimens.

Murine and rat tumors have been used by many investigators in studies aimed at improving the radio- and chemotherapy of human cancer. Valuable information on the biology of solid tumors has been obtained. However, it has not been possible to explain the underlying mechanisms for inter-tumor differences in response to radio- and chemotherapy, and to develop predictive assays of treatment response for different types of human tumors from such studies.

A simple experimental model for *in vivo* studies of human tumors may in some ways be preferable to rodent tumor systems. Recently, new and improved procedures for immune-suppression of conventional mice and subsequent heterotransplantation of human tumors have been developed.[1] In addition, congenitally athymic nude mice have been shown to be useful as hosts for human tumor xenografts.[2] No pretreatment of these mice is necessary, although the "take" rate of some tumors may be improved after whole-body irradiation or treatment with immune-suppressive chemical agents.

The main purpose of this chapter is to discuss the potential usefulness of human tumor xenografts in the development of laboratory assays for prediction of clinical tumor treatment response. The first part will deal with the clinical relevance of treatment response data obtained from human tumor xenografts. This discussion is based partly on studies of biological characteristics of xenografts and partly on studies of therapeutic response of xenografts as measured *in vitro* and *in vivo*. Then the usefulness of the human tumor xenograft model in prediction of treatment response of individual patients is discussed, both used directly and in development and calibration of different short term *in vitro* assays of present interest.

TREATMENT RESPONSE

Relevant questions in an evaluation of the usefulness of human tumor xenografts in development of predictive assays are: (a) whether the growth and treatment response of xenografts are seriously influenced by host-tumor immunological interactions, (b) whether the treatment response of xenografts can be measured with sufficient accuracy, and (c) whether the treatment response of xenografts reflects the clinical responsiveness of the parent tumors in the donor patients. In this section of the chapter, I will discuss some immunological reactions against heterotransplanted tissue and possible consequences for the treatment response of xenografts. Furthermore, I will evaluate the endpoints most commonly used in studies of murine tumors and their applicability for assessment of the treatment response of xenografts. Then, I will briefly review the most relevant studies comparing the treatment response of xenografts and tumors in man.

Host-Tumor Immunological Interactions

The acceptance of human tumor xenografts in congenitally athymic mice has been attributed to the lack of development of T lymphocytes in the absence of thymic influence. However, some human tumors fail to grow in adult athymic mice. The "take" rate of others is enhanced in newborn mice and in adult mice given sublethal whole-body irradiation or treatment with anti-lymphocyte serum, suggesting that some host defense mechanisms are active against heterotransplanted tumor tissue. Thus, it has been shown that athymic mice exhibit an unusually high level of natural killer cells[3] and elevated macrophage activity,[4] compared with conventional mice. Recent studies have also shown that certain lymphoid cells in athymic mice express surface antigens characteristic of mature T lymphocytes.[5] The role played by each of these cell types in the rejection of non-accepted heterotransplanted tumor tissue is not well understood.

Natural killer cells, macrophages as well as "T-like" cells may interact with human tumor cells and hence artificially enhance the response to therapy of xenografts. There is some evidence that this indeed is the case in both congenitally athymic mice and immune-suppressed mice. Steel and Peckham[6] have reviewed reports where local control of xenografts by chemotherapy has been described. They concluded that local control was sometimes observed at surprisingly low dose levels (i.e., dose levels which often caused only minor growth delays in non-cured mice), and suggested that this might be due to participation of host defense mechanisms. In our laboratory, local control following single dose irradiation of a melanoma xenograft was found to occur at considerably lower doses than predicted from the *in vitro* survival curve of cells from the same melanoma irradiated *in vivo*,[7] as described in detail below. Since the "take" rate of small implants of this melanoma was enhanced in whole-body irradiated athymic mice, we suggested that an immune response by the host was involved when the radiation response was measured as local control. Immune responses by the host may therefore be a potential source of artefacts in therapeutic studies of xenografts, especially when local tumor control is used as the endpoint.

Endpoints for Treatment Response

Single cell survival assayed *in vitro* using conventional cell culture techniques is a useful endpoint for many rodent tumors treated *in vivo* with radiation or with chemotherapeutic agents. Much effort has been expended on the development of similar colony assays applicable to human tumors. Recently, Courtenay *et al.*[8] published a new soft agar colony assay based on observations of the growth requirements of cells isolated directly from tumors. The most important feature of this assay is the use of tissue-mimicking oxygen concentrations in the gas phase, together with the admixture of rat erythrocytes and the replenishment of the nutrients in the agar by

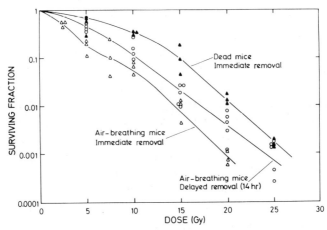

FIG. 14.1. Survival curves for cells from a human melanoma xenograft (E.E.) irradiated as solid tumors *in vivo* and assayed *in vitro*.[10] The tumors were irradiated in air-breathing mice ($\triangle$, $\bigcirc$) or in asphyxiated mice ($\blacktriangle$), and were removed from the mice either immediately ($\triangle$, $\blacktriangle$) or 14 hours ($\bigcirc$) after irradiation. Each point is based on one tumor. Air-breathing mice, immediate removal: $D_0 = 2.27\pm0.19$ Gy. Air-breathing mice, delayed removal: $D_0 = 2.90\pm0.25$ Gy. Asphyxiated mice: $D_0 = 2.47\pm0.23$ Gy. PLD-repair factor is about 1.3. Hypoxic fraction is 5–10%.

added liquid medium. Comparative studies have indicated that the Courtenay assay is superior to other colony assays commonly used in studies of human tumors. Radiobiological studies of cells from human tumor xenografts have provided survival curves of similar shape to those obtained with established cell lines. Following treatment *in vivo*, this assay has been used to determine the chemo- and radiosensitivity, the fraction of hypoxic cells, and the capacity for PLD-repair of human tumor xenografts of many histological categories (Fig. 14.1).[9,10] However, although the Courtenay assay is useful for many xenograft lines, it cannot be used for all types of xenografts, either because the plating efficiency is too low or because of difficulties in obtaining a single cell suspension of sufficient quality (i.e., with a high yield of viable cells and without clumps and aggregates).

Tumor growth delay is the only available conventional endpoint for some human tumor xenografts. This endpoint is easy to use in practice, and discriminates adequately between the effect of different treatment doses for a given xenograft line (Fig. 14.2). However, there is no generally accepted way of analyzing growth delay data in order to compare the treatment sensitivity of xenograft lines with different volumetric growth rate. Specific growth delay, i.e., actual growth delay divided by the volume-doubling time of untreated controls, has been suggested to be a useful parameter for ranking

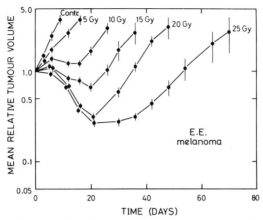

FIG. 14.2. Regrowth curves for a human melanoma xenograft (E.E.) irradiated with single doses of 5–25 Gy.[11] Each curve is based on 15 to 25 tumors. The vertical bars represent standard errors.

tumor lines according to treatment sensitivity. Good correlations have been found between specific growth delay and cell surviving fraction measured *in vitro* for human melanoma xenografts.[11,12] However, in order to base comparisons of treatment sensitivity on differences in specific growth delay, it is a strict prerequisite that the average doubling time of the surviving clonogenic cells equal that of the clonogenic cells in untreated tumors. There is good evidence from studies of melanoma xenografts that the doubling time of the clonogenic cells is shortened during the repopulation period. Some data have suggested that actual growth delay divided by potential doubling time may also be a useful parameter for comparing treatment sensitivity of xenograft lines.[13] Further studies involving many xenograft lines need to be carried out before the most appropriate method of analyzing growth delay data can be assessed.

Local tumor control following treatment has been occasionally observed for many human tumor xenografts, but has not often been used as an endpoint. In our laboratory, tumor control following single dose irradiation has been studied for a melanoma xenograft.[7] The TCD_{50} was found to be 27.4 ± 0.6 Gy (Fig. 14.3). These tumor control data and the single cell survival data in Figure 14.1 were obtained using the same xenograft line and, consequently, the two endpoints can be compared. Assuming that (a) the survival curve measured *in vitro* at high doses has the form $S = n \exp(-D_o/D)$, (b) the tumors can recur from one cell, and (c) N is the number of clonogenic cells in the tumors, the theoretical TCD_{50} is expressed by the equation:

TABLE 14.1. *Potential Predictive Assays of Treatment Response*

a. Measurement of the intrinsic treatment sensitivity of the tumor cells
   Cell survival (e.g., after 2.0 Gy)
   PLD-repair capacity
   Chromosome aberrations
   Micronuclei
   DNA strand breaks and repair
b. Measurement of the proliferative and ploidy state of the tumor cells
   DNA-content (ploidy pattern)
   Labeling index
   Fraction of cells in S (flow cytometry)
   Potential doubling time (BUdR antibody)
c. Measurement of tumor pathophysiological conditions
   PO_2-distribution (microelectrodes)
   Hypoxic fraction (labeled nitroaromatic compounds)
   Lactate and pyruvate levels
   Capillary density
   HbO_2 saturation in capillaries (cryospectrophotometry)
   Tumor metabolism (^{31}P NMR spectroscopy and positron emission tomography
   (PET))

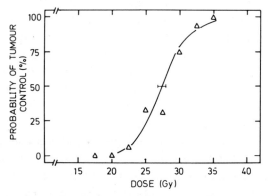

FIG. 14.3. Local control curve for a human melanoma xenograft (E.E.) irradiated with single doses of 17.5–35.0 Gy.[7] Each point is based on 15 to 20 tumors. TCD_{50} = 27.4±0.6 Gy (horizontal bar).

$$TCD_{50} = D_o \left[\ln n - \ln \frac{\ln 2}{N} \right]$$

Since N from the clonogenicity of the cells in soft agar has been estimated to be higher than 1×10^7, the TCD_{50}, based on the survival curve measured *in vitro* when allowing the PLD-repair (D_o = 2.90 Gy; n = 4), can be estimated to be greater than 50 Gy. This calculated TCD_{50} is considerably higher than the measured TCD_{50} of 27.4±0.6 Gy. First, the number of clonogenic cells in the tumors *in vivo* may be lower than that estimated from *in vitro* studies, perhaps as a result of radiation-induced vascular damage. Secondly, an immune response by the host may have contributed to the production of long-term tumor control, even though the fraction of cells inactivated by radiation was relatively low. If the discrepancy between the *in vivo* and the *in vitro* data was due largely to host defence mechanisms, the treatment response of human tumor xenografts, when local control is used as an endpoint, may not necessarily be representative for tumors in humans.

Response to Chemotherapy

The literature dealing with the response to chemotherapy of human tumor xenografts and similarities/dissimilarities to the clinical chemotherapeutic response is expansive, and has recently been reviewed by several authors.[14,15] Most such studies have involved few xenograft lines, and the main purpose has often been to test the efficiency of well-established drugs on different histological types of tumors or to screen potentially new chemotherapeutic agents. Comparative studies of the chemotherapeutic response of xenografts and the source tumors in the donor patients are rare. However, a few comprehensive studies on this subject, performed under carefully-defined conditions, have recently been reported and deserve special mention in this chapter.

Steel and his collaborators, using immuno-suppressed mice, studied the response to chemotherapy of a large number of human tumor xenografts originating from nine different anatomical sites, with the main emphasis on malignant melanomas and colorectal, pancreas, breast, lung, and testicular carcinomas. About 25 single drugs and drug combinations were investigated, and tumor growth delay as well as single cell survival *in vitro* were used as endpoints. Wide differences in chemotherapeutic response were observed among individual xenografts of the same histological type, as well as among the different histological categories. Testicular teratomas and small-cell lung tumors generally responded well, breast tumors showed modest response, whereas melanomas, colorectal tumors, and non-small-cell lung tumors generally responded poorly. Moreover, comparison of the xenograft response with the donor patient response to chemotherapy was possible for a few colorectal carcinomas, bronchial carcinomas (including small-cell, large-cell, squamous and adenocarcinomas), as well as for malignant melanomas. A consistent agreement between xenograft and patient responses was found. Steel *et al*[9] drew the general conclusion that their data supported the hypothesis that human tumor xenografts broadly maintain the level of chemotherapeutic responsiveness of the source tumors in humans.

Giovanella et al.[16] studied the response to chemotherapy of three panels of xenografts consisting of 14 human tumors each: (1) one panel of melanomas, (2) one of colorectal carcinomas, and (3) one of breast carcinomas. The response to nine different single drugs was measured for each of the 42 xenograft lines, using the subrenal capsule assay in congenitally athymic mice. The responsiveness data were compared with published results of various clinical trials with the same histological categories of tumors, and a close correlation was found. This panel study detected nine out of ten effective drugs; six for breast carcinomas, one for colorectal carcinomas, and two for melanomas, giving only two false-positive results. The authors drew the general conclusion that their data strongly support the validity of heterotransplants of human tumors in the athymic mouse as a predictive system for testing new anticancer agents and in determining optimal treatment schedules and combinations of known drugs.

Discrepancies between the response to chemotherapy of human tumor xenografts and tumors in man have also been reported in the literature. However, the results from the majority of the studies are in close agreement with the general conclusions drawn by Steel et al.[9] and Giovanella et al.[16]

Response to Radiotherapy

Well-documented comparative studies of the radiation response of human tumor xenografts and the source tumors in the donor patients have not been reported, to date. However, several studies of the radiation response of cell suspensions prepared directly from xenografts as well as of xenografts irradiated in vivo and assayed in vitro or in vivo have been carried out. Some relevant studies are reviewed later in this chapter and are discussed in relation to experiences from clinical radiotherapy.

Growth delay studies of xenografts following single dose irradiation have been carried out at several institutes and include different histological types of tumors. Steel[17] has summarized the data in a recent review (Fig. 14.4) from which two interesting conclusions can be drawn. First, the radiation response varied considerably among the xenografts. Secondly, there is some evidence that the radiation response correlated with the clinical radioresponsiveness of tumors of corresponding histology. The small-cell bronchial carcinoma and the testicular teratoma xenografts appeared to be relatively radiosensitive,

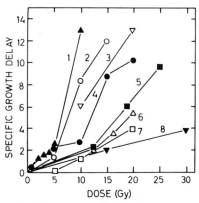

FIG. 14.4. Specific growth delay curves for human tumor xenografts given single radiation doses.[17] Testicular teratoma (1), pancreatic carcinoma (2), small-cell bronchial carcinoma (3), glioma (4), melanoma (5), osteosarcoma (6), bladder carcinoma (7), and bronchial adenocarcinoma (8).

and these tumor types are known to be radiosensitive clinically, whereas the osteosarcoma, the bronchial adenocarcinoma, and the bladder carcinoma xenografts appeared to be radioresistant, as these tumor types often are clinically.

Malignant melanoma is the tumor type that has been subjected to the most extensive radiation studies as xenografts.[10,18-21] Single cell survival measured *in vitro* has been the most commonly used endpoint; also after irradiation *in vivo*. Clinically, melanomas are known to constitute an extremely heterogeneous tumor category with highly variable radioresponsiveness. This heterogeneity is reflected in the radioresponsiveness of the melanoma xenografts. Thus, in a recent study of five melanoma xenograft lines in our laboratory,[11] the specific growth delays for the two most sensitive lines were similar to those for the small-cell bronchial carcinoma in Figure 14.4, whereas the two most resistant lines showed about the same specific growth delays as the bladder carcinoma and the bronchial adenocarcinoma. The D_o for the melanoma xenografts studied so far has been found to range from 2.27 to 5.85 Gy, i.e., they varied within a factor of about 2.6. When cells from the same xenografts were irradiated under aerobic conditions *in vitro*, the D_o varied within a factor of 2.8. Similarly, melanoma xenografts have been found to demonstrate a large variability in hypoxic fraction, reoxygenation pattern, capacity for PLD- and SLD-repair, and intercellular contact effect.[18] Moreover, cell subpopulations isolated from a single tumor of a melanoma xenograft were shown to be heterogeneous in response to radiation and hyperthermia, both *in vitro* and *in vivo*.[22,23]

Selby and Steel[24] have measured the radiosensitivities *in vitro* of a melanoma xenograft and of cryopreserved cells isolated from the parent tumor. They found levels to be quite similar. Although the data for the cryopreserved cells were sparse, both data sets indicated broad-shouldered survival curves. In our laboratory, the radiosensitivity of cell populations isolated directly from 11 melanoma surgical specimens and from seven melanoma xenografts have been studied using exactly the same experimental procedure.[25] The cell survival curves measured for the xenografts and the surgical specimens were similar in shape, covered the same range of survival levels, and gave no indications that xenografted melanomas and melanomas in humans might be different in radioresponsiveness.

Deacon *et al.*[26] have studied the radiobiology of a human neuroblastoma xenograft using cell survival *in vitro* as well as growth delay as endpoints. The xenograft was found to be highly radiosensitive with limited repair capacity, similar to the high clinical radiosensitivity of neuroblastomas.

Lindenberger *et al.*[27] have studied two human squamous cell carcinoma xenografts using single dose as well as fractionated irradiation. They found α/ß ratios in the range 6.4–16.0, depending on the experimental conditions. These values were considered to be in good agreement with clinical α/ß ratios for skin cancer.

PREDICTIVE POTENTIAL

Since there is significant evidence that the radio- and chemotherapeutic response of human tumor xenografts reflects that of the parent tumors in the donor patients, one potential use of heterotransplanted tumors could be the testing of an individual patient's tumor for responsiveness to alternative treatments, e.g., different cytotoxic drugs, as suggested by Povlsen.[28] This possibility has since been studied by several investigators, and severe limitations of the human tumor xenograft system in clinical sensitivity testing have been revealed. First, the time interval between implantation of a surgical specimen and treatment results becoming available is too long for many patient categories. Bailey *et al.*[29] showed that this period was seldom shorter than 30 weeks and usually in excess of 50 weeks. Secondly, the "take" rate of heterotransplanted surgical specimens is low, usually in the 10–30% range, implying that the proportion of patients who might benefit would be low. Thirdly, treatment sensitivity testing using the xenograft model system would involve considerable expense. The costs of a multiple drug sensitivity testing experiment were estimated by Bailey et al.[29] to be in the order of \$3,000 (in 1984).

For these reasons, human tumor xenografts used directly as test systems are unlikely to be of value in individual patient treatment sensitivity testing. However, human tumor xenografts may, on the other hand, be very useful in development and calibration of short-term in vitro predictive assays, as discussed later in this chapter.

DEVELOPMENT OF *IN VITRO* PREDICTIVE ASSAYS

Much effort has recently been concentrated on development of predictive assays of treatment response based primarily on biological properties of tumors. These assays could be roughtly classified in three distinctive groups, i.e.: (1) assessment of the intrinsic treatment sensitivity of the tumor cells, (2) measurement of the proliferative and ploidy state of the tumor cells, and (3) assessment of the tumor pathophysiological conditions. Some of the most promising predictive assays currently under investigation are listed in Table 14.1. The potential usefulness of human tumor xenografts in the evaluation and calibration of these three categories of possible predictive assays is discussed later in this chapter.

Intrinsic Cellular Treatment Sensitivity

During the last decade, several colony assays have been developed for human tumor treatment sensitivity testing. Such assays have to some extent been used in attempts to predict the response of tumors to chemotherapeutic agents and hence to prescribe the optimal treatment. Several authors have claimed that the differences in intrinsic cellular radiosensitivity among human tumors are too small to account for the differences in radioresponsiveness observed among tumors in the clinic. However, the interest in cellular radiosensitivity as an important parameter for clinical radioresponsiveness has increased gradually as more data have become available. Fertil and Malaise[30,31] analyzed published survival curves for human tumor cell lines and found evidence that the cell survival at 2.0 Gy, as well as the mean inactivation dose ($\bar{D}$) for a given cell type, were correlated to the 95% control dose for tumors of corresponding histology. Deacon et al.[32] reanalyzed the same survival curves using an altogether different approach and also found a positive correlation between the initial slope of the cell survival curves and the clinical radioresponsiveness. Similarly, Weichselbaum et al.[33] have suggested that differences in PLD-repair among cell lines in vitro may reflect differences in clinical radiocurability among tumors of corresponding histology.

Human tumor xenografts may be of significant importance in evaluating the usefulness of predictive assays based on the intrinsic treatment sensitivity and the repair capacity of tumor cells for several reasons. As discussed above, there is significant evidence that the intrinsic chemo- and radiosensitivity of tumor cells are maintained during serial heterotransplantation. The chemo- and radioresponsiveness of human tumor xenografts treated *in vivo* can be assessed with considerable accuracy by using growth delay and/or cell survival measured *in vitro* as endpoints. The intrinsic treatment sensitivity and repair capacity of the same cells, obtained by disaggregation of xenografts, can be measured easily *in vitro* by using the Courtenay soft agar colony assay for many tumor types.

Rofstad and Brustad[12] have thus used human melanoma xenografts to investigate whether the radioresponsiveness *in vivo* of tumors given clinically relevant fractionated irradiation might be correlated with the initial slope of the *in vitro* cell survival curves, as suggested by Fertil and Malaise[30,31] and by Deacon *et al.*[32] Five different melanomas were studied, and specific growth delay as well as cell survival *in vitro* were used as endpoints after treatment *in vivo*. Superfractionation (three fractions of 2.0 Gy with four hour intervals each day) as well as conventional fractionation (one fraction of 2.0 Gy each day) were used. The total dose was varied within the range of 12–30 Gy and 10–30 Gy, respectively. The rankings of the melanomas in radioresponsiveness were found to be almost identical, irrespective of the endpoint and the fractionation regimen applied. The cellular radiosensitivity was studied under aerobic conditions *in vitro* at conventional and at low dose rate. The radioresponsiveness *in vivo* was found to be positively correlated to the initial slope of the *in vitro* cell survival curves, i.e., the α and the surviving fraction at 2.0 Gy (conventional dose rate; 3.0 Gy/min) and the D_0 (low dose rate; 1.25 cGy/min) (Fig. 14.5). It was concluded that the differences in radioresponsiveness among the melanomas were governed mainly by the intrinsic repair capacity of the tumor cells. This work, thus strongly supported the suggestion of Fertil and Malaise[30,31] and Deacon *et al.*[32] that the initial slope of the *in vitro* cell survival curve may be a useful parameter for predicting the clinical radioresponsiveness of a tumor. Moreover, Rofstad *et al.*[25,34] have demonstrated that survival curves for tumor cells isolated directly from patients may

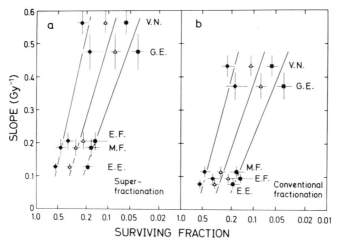

FIG. 14.5. Radioresponsiveness of human melanoma xenografts *in vivo*, measured as the slope of specific growth delay curves, as a function of cell surviving fraction at 2.0 Gy (single dose irradiation) (●), 2 × 2.0 Gy (split dose irradiation) (■), and 4.0 Gy (low dose rate irradiation) (△). All three parameters were measured after irradiation of single cells *in vitro*.[12] The dose per fraction *in vivo* was 2.0 Gy: (a) superfractionation and (b) conventional fractionation (see text). The bars represent standard errors.

be determined by using the Courtenay assay for some tumors, and thus suggested that similar clinical studies like their xenograft study should be undertaken using malignant melanomas.

Tumor Cell Proliferation and Ploidy

Tumors characterized by high DNA indices and high proliferative activity are often biologically more aggressive and may show an altogether different treatment response than diploid tumors. Rapidly regenerating tumors, e.g., tumors with potential doubling times of less than about five days, are likely to be controlled better by accelerated than by conventionally fractionated irradiation. It has therefore been suggested that flow cytometric parameters such as DNA-content, fraction of cells in S-phase, and potential doubling time, measured by using the BUdR antibody, may be used to predict response to therapy and therefore to better individualize treatment regimens. The question then arises: Would it be profitable to use human tumor xenografts to evaluate the potential predictive value of such flow cytometric parameters?

TABLE 14.2. *Volume-Doubling Times* (T_d) *for Human Melanoma*
Xenografts

Melanoma	T_d (days)	
	(V = 50 mm^3)	(V = 200 mm^3)
B.E.	12.7	22.5
E.E.	3.0	4.4
E.F.	8.6	21.6
E.K.	15.3	64.6
G.E.1	10.0	36.5
G.E.2	3.1	4.2
G.R.E.	6.1	12.7
K.A.	4.4	6.0
K.F.	3.4	7.7
K.J.A.	6.8	10.1
M.F.	7.6	20.0
R.A.	16.5	25.3
T.H.	2.8	3.8
V.N.	3.7	6.2

Human tumor xenografts frequently increase their rate of volume growth during the first three to five passages in mice, possibly as an adaptation to the new environment. Changes in DNA index have also been observed during the first few adaptation passages. On subsequent transplantations, many xenograft lines have been found to retain relatively constant growth rates, even for several years. The growth characteristics of 14 human melanoma xenografts have been studied in our laboratory.[35,36] After the growth rate had stabilized, the xenografts showed individual and characteristic volume-doubling times, ranging from 2.8 to 16.5 days at a volume of 50mm^3 and from 3.8 to 64.6 days at a volume of 200mm^3 (Table 14.2). Similar volume-doubling times have also been reported for other histological types of xenografts,[37,38] indicating that inherent properties of tumors are significant to their growth rate as xenografts. However, the volume-doubling times of the majority of the xenografts were less than 20 days and thus considerably shorter than those reported for most tumors in humans. Detailed studies of the cell proliferation kinetics have shown that the discrepancy between the volume-doubling times is mainly a consequence of a reduced cell loss factor in the xenografts. The distribution of cells in the cell cycle, the growth fraction, and the duration of the cell cycle phases all seem to be similar in xenografts and in tumors in humans.[35,39]

The relatively short volume-doubling time of many xenograft lines may limit their usefulness as models in studies aimed at evaluating the predictive value of proliferative and ploidy parameters. However, a panel of xenografts of a given histological category would generally cover a wide range of growth rates, compared to a panel of murine tumors, and hence might give some valuable information not obtainable from conventional experimental tumor systems.

Tumor Pathophysiological Conditions

Some malignant tumors are reported to be inadequately vascularized, resulting in abnormal physiological conditions and local areas with hypoxic and necrotic tissues. The vascular architecture of tumors may be of significance to their response to therapy. Chemotherapeutic agents are partly distributed by the vascular system, and the inactivation of tumor cells following exposure to some agents may depend on the oxygen concentration. Moreover, it is often assumed that the response of tumors to radiotherapy depends on the fraction of hypoxic cells and the rate of reoxygenation. Clinical observations that reduction in hemoglobin level is associated with higher rates of local tumor control failures and that local control can be improved in some tumors by treatment in hyperbaric oxygen or with the hypoxic cell radiosensitizer misonidazole, support this assumption. Much effort has therefore been concentrated on the development of methods for assessing the pathophysiological conditions in tumors, especially the oxygenation status. The most promising assays include direct measurement of pO_2 with microelectrodes, assessment of the morphology and functionality of the vasculature (e.g., measurement of HbO_2 saturation in capillaries by cryospectrophotometry), identification of hypoxic cells by use of isotope or fluorescence-labeled nitroaromatic compounds, and detection of anaerobic metabolism (e.g., measurements of lactate and pyruvate levels). Non-invasive methods for characterization of tumor metabolism, such as high resolution ^{31}P nuclear magnetic resonance (NMR) spectroscopy, and positron emission tomography (PET) techniques are particularly interesting. The important question in the present discussion is to what extent human tumor xenografts may be useful in assessing the potential of such physiological assays in predicting clinical tumor treatment response.

Tumor cells implanted in mice have the ability to promote neovascularization, probably via endogeneous tumor angiogenesis factors. The vascular system and the supporting stromal elements of human tumor xenografts thus originate from the host, whereas only the tumor parenchyma is of human origin. Immune-fluorescence studies have shown that for some xenografts in immune-suppressed mice, murine cells can constitute up to 35% of the volume of the tumors.[40] Moreover, microvascular changes may occur in tumors during treatment and hence change the pathophysiological conditions. The vascular density in a human melanoma xenograft following single dose irradiation has been studied in our laboratory, and the length of vessels with diameters 5-15 μm was found to decrease significantly during the first week after exposure to 15 Gy and then to increase. Beyond two weeks after irradiation, the length of these vessels was greater than in untreated tumors. These changes were due to several factors, including (1) vessel occlusion, (2) thrombosis, (3) stasis, (4) changes in tumor volume and, (5) neovascularization.[41] The vulnerability of murine endothelial cells and vascular structures to treatment may be different from that of vascular structures of human origin. Consequently, since the vascular network in human tumor xenografts is of murine origin, and since the capillary density may change with time after irradiation, the pathophysiological conditions in human tumor xenografts before and during treatment may possibly not reflect that of tumors in man.

On the other hand, the vascular architecture of human tumor xenografts is not determined by the murine host only, but is also—at least in part—determined by the human parenchymal tumor cells. This is evident from a study of the microvasculature in five melanoma xenografts by Solesvik et al.[42] Total vessel length, surface, and volume per unit histologically intact tumor volume for the melanomas are presented in Table 14.3. These data demonstrate that the five xenograft lines, implanted exactly at the same site in the hosts, exhibited individual characteristic microvascular structures.

TABLE 14.3. *Total Vessel Length (L), Surface (S), and Volume (V) per Unit Histologically Intact Tumor Volume for Human Melanoma Xenografts*

Melanoma[a]	L (mm/mm^3)	S (mm^2/mm^3)	V (mm^3/mm^3)
E.E.	46±2	2.5±0.2	0.015±0.002
E.F.	32±2	1.6±0.1	0.009±0.001
G.E.	55±1	3.1±0.1	0.021±0.001
M.F.	36±2	2.2±0.1	0.015±0.001
V.N.	80±4	3.8±0.2	0.022±0.002

[a] Mean ± standard errors.

Tumor pathophysiological conditions are not only a result of the efficiency of the vascular supply. Genetic and biochemical properties of the tumor cells are also of extreme importance. Studies of monolayer cell cultures and multicellular spheroids under well-defined growth conditions have demonstrated significant differences among cell lines in response to and ability to survive under hypoxic stress and/or deprivation of glucose and other nutrients. Human tumor cells may be different from rodent tumor cells in that respect, implying that pathophysiological studies of human tumor xenografts may give tumor-specific, clinically relevant information not obtainable from murine tumors.

Few studies of human tumor xenografts have dealt with the potential value of tumor pathophysiological parameters in predicting treatment response. Rofstad and Brustad[11] found that the radiation response of human melanoma xenografts given single dose irradiation was correlated to the pretreatment vascular density, i.e., the most sensitive lines were best vascularized. However, when the same melanoma lines were given fractionated irradiation (2.0 Gy per fraction), no correlations were found between the radiation response and the vascular density.[12] The radiation response did not correlate with the fraction of radiobiologically hypoxic cells, nor with the volume fraction of necrosis.

In conclusion, although the pathophysiological conditions in human tumor xenografts may be different from those of tumors in man due to the murine origin of the vascular bed and the supporting stroma, pathophysiological studies using xenografts may give clinically relevant information not achievable from rodent tumor systems. More studies are needed to evaluate in which way and to what extent the pathophysiological conditions in xenografts may deviate from those of tumors in man. A conclusive standpoint to the potential usefulness of human tumor xenografts in development of predictive assays of treatment response based on tumor pathophysiological conditions should therefore also deserve further experimentation.

CONCLUSIONS

The use of human tumor xenografts as an *in vivo* method for clinical treatment sensitivity testing of tumors of individual patients will be limited by the speed of the assay and the rate of success, and is therefore not a realistic prospect. However, xenografts may be very useful in the development and calibration of short-term *in vitro* assays. The treatment response of xenografts can often be measured with a high degree of accuracy. Moreover, there is significant evidence that the response to radio- and chemotherapy of xenografts generally correlates well with clinical responsiveness. At least three main disadvantages may limit the usefulness of xenografts in attempts to develop *in vitro* predictive assays of treatment response. First, the volume doubling time is usually shorter for xenografts than for tumors in humans. Secondly, the vascular system and the supporting stromal elements of xenografts originate from the host. Thirdly, host defense mechanisms may be active against xenografts. These disadvantages may represent a serious problem for assays based on tumor growth and pathophysiological parameters, but are probably less important for assays based on the intrinsic treatment sensitivity of the tumor cells.

ACKNOWLEDGMENTS

Financial support was from The Norwegian Cancer Society, The Norwegian Research Council for Science and the Humanities and The Nansen Scientific Fund.

REFERENCES

1. Steel, G. G., Courtenay, V. D., and Rostom, A. Y., Improved immunesuppression techniques for the xenografting of human tumours. *Br. J. Cancer* 37: 224–230, 1978.
2. Rygaard, J., *Thymus and Self. Immunobiology of the Mouse Mutant Nude*, F.A.D.L., Copenhagen, 1973.
3. Herberman, R. B., Natural cell-mediated cytotoxicity in nude mice. In: *The Nude Mouse in Experimental and Clinical Research* (J. Fogh and B. C. Giovanella, eds.), Vol. 1, pp. 135–166. Academic Press, New York, 1978.
4. Sharp, A. K. and Colston, M. J., Elevated macrophage activity in nude mice. In: *Immune-Deficient Animals* (B. Sordat, ed.), pp. 44–47. Karger, Basel, 1984.
5. MacDonald, H. R., Phenotypic and functional characteristics of "T-like" cells in nude mice. In: *Immune Deficient Animals* (B. Sordat, ed.), pp. 2–6. Karger, Basel, 1984.
6. Steel, G. G. and Peckham, M. J., Human tumor xenografts: A critical appraisal. *Br. J. Cancer* 41: Suppl. IV, 133–141, 1980.
7. Rofstad, E. K. and Brustad, T., Tumour control following single-dose irradiation of a human melanoma xenograft. *Eur. J. Cancer Clin. Oncol.* 19: 1127–1131, 1983.
8. Courtenay, V. D. and Mills, J., An *in vitro* colony assay for human tumours grown in immune-suppressed mice and treated *in vivo* with cytotoxic agents. *Br. J. Cancer* 37: 261–268, 1978.
9. Steel, G. G., Courtenay, V. D., and Peckham, M. J., The response to chemotherapy of a variety of human tumour xenografts. *Br. J. Cancer* 47: 1–13, 1983.
10. Rofstad, E. K., Human tumour xenografts in radiotherapeutic research. *Radiother. Oncol.* 3: 35–46, 1985.
11. Rofstad, E. K. and Brustad, T., Tumour growth delay following single dose irradiation of human melanoma xenografts. Correlations with tumour growth parameters, vascular structure and cellular radiosensitivity. *Br. J. Cancer* 51: 201–210, 1985.
12. Rofstad, E. K. and Brustad, T., Radioresponsiveness of human melanoma xenografts given fractionated irradiation *in vivo*—Relationship to the initial slope of the cell survival curves *in vitro*. *Radiother. Oncol.*, 9: 45–56, 1987.
13. Rofstad, E. K., Radioresponsiveness of human tumor xenografts: Growth delay and vascular damage. In: *Rodent Tumor Models in Experimental Cancer Therapy* (R. F. Kallman, ed.), pp. 209–213. Pergamon Press, Oxford, 1987.
14. Sharkey, F. E. and Fogh, J., Considerations in the use of nude mice for cancer research. *Cancer Metastasis Rev.* 3: 341–360, 1984.

15. Giovanella, B. C. and Fogh, J., The nude mouse in cancer research. *Advances Cancer Res.* **44**: 69–120, 1985.

16. Giovanella, B. C., Stehlin, J. S., Shepard, R. C., and Williams, L. J., Correlation between response to chemotherapy of human tumors in patients and in nude mice. *Cancer* **52**: 1146–1152, 1983.

17. Steel, G. G., Therapeutic response of human tumour xenografts in immune-suppressed mice. In: *Immune-Deficient Animals* (B. Sordat, ed.), pp. 395–404. Karger, Basel, 1984.

18. Rofstad, E. K., Radiation biology of malignant melanoma. *Acta. Radiol. Oncol.* **25**: 1–10, 1986.

19. Chavaudra, N., Guichard, M., and Malaise, E. P., Hypoxic fraction and repair of potentially lethal radiation damage in two human melanomas transplanted into nude mice. *Radiat. Res.* **88**: 56–68, 1981.

20. Guichard, M., Dertinger, H., and Malaise, E. P., Radiosensitivity of four human tumor xenografts. Influence of hypoxia and cell-cell contact. *Radiat. Res.* **95**: 602–609, 1983.

21. Spang-Thomsen, M., Visfeldt, J., and Nielsen, A., Effect of single-dose X irradiation on the growth curves of a human malignant melanoma transplanted into nude mice. *Radiat. Res.* **85**: 184–195, 1981.

22. Rofstad, E. K. and Brustad, T., Differential responses to radiation and hyperthermia of cloned cell lines derived from a single human melanoma xenograft. *Int. J. Radiat. Oncol. Biol. Phys.* **10**: 857–864, 1984.

23. Rofstad, E. K., Heterogeneous responses to radiation and hyperthermia of cell subpopulations of a human melanoma xenograft. In: *Immune-Deficient Animals in Biomedical Research* (J. Rygaard, N. Brünner, N. Graem, and M. Spang-Thomsen, eds.), pp. 329–334. Karger, Basel, 1987.

24. Selby, P. J. and Steel, G. G., Clonogenic cell survival in cryopreserved human tumour cells. *Br. J. Cancer* **43**: 143–148, 1981.

25. Rofstad, E. K., Wahl, A., Tveit, K. M., Monge, O. R., and Brustad, T., Survival curves after X-ray and heat treatments for melanoma cells derived directly from surgical specimens of tumours in man. *Radiother. Oncol.* **4**: 33–44, 1985.

26. Deacon, J. M., Wilson, P. A., and Peckham, M. J., The radiobiology of human neuroblastoma. *Radiother. Oncol.* **3**: 201–209, 1985.

27. Lindenberger, J., Hermeking, H., Kummermehr, J., and Denekamp, J., Response of human tumour xenografts to fractionated X-irradiation. *Radiother. Oncol.* **6**: 15–27, 1986.

28. Povlsen, C. O., Status of chemotherapy, radiotherapy, endocrine therapy, and immunotherapy studies of human cancer in the nude mouse. In: *The Nude Mouse in Experimental and Clinical Research* (J. Fogh and B. C. Giovanella, eds.), Vol. 1, pp. 437–456. Academic Press, New York, 1978.

29. Bailey, M. J., Jones, A. J., Shorthouse, A. J., Raghaven, D., Selby, P., Gibbs, J., and Peckham, M. J., Limitations of the human tumour xenograft system in individual patient drug sensitivity testing. *Br. J. Cancer* **50**: 721–724, 1984.

30. Fertil, B. and Malaise, E. P., Inherent cellular radiosensitivity as a basic concept for human tumor radiotherapy. *Int. J. Radiat. Oncol. Biol. Phys.* **7**: 621–629, 1981.

31. Fertil, B. and Malaise, E. P., Intrinsic radiosensitivity of human cell lines is correlated with radioresponsiveness of human tumors: Analysis of 101 published survival curves. *Int. J. Radiat. Oncol. Biol. Phys.* **11**: 1699–1707, 1985.

32. Deacon, J., Peckham, M. J., and Steel, G. G., The radioresponsiveness of human tumours and the initial slope of the cell survival curve. *Radiother. Oncol.* **2**: 317–323, 1984.

33. Weichselbaum, R. R., Schmit, A., and Little, J. B., Cellular repair factors influencing radiocurability of human malignant tumours. *Br. J. Cancer* **45**: 10–16, 1982.
34. Rofstad, E. K., Wahl, A., and Brustad, T., Radiation sensitivity *in vitro* of cells isolated from human tumor surgical specimens. *Cancer Res.* **47**: 106–110, 1987.
35. Rofstad, E. K., Fodstad, Ø., and Lindmo, T., Growth characteristics of human melanoma xenografts. *Cell Tissue Kinet.* **15**: 545–554, 1982.
36. Rofstad, E. K., Wahl, A., and Brustad, T., Radiation and heat sensitivity of cells from two slowly growing human melanoma xenografts. *Br. J. Cancer* **49**: 745–752, 1984.
37. Houghton, J. A. and Taylor, D. M., Growth characteristics of human colorectal tumours during serial passage in immune-deprived mice. *Br. J. Cancer* **37**: 213–223, 1978.
38. Mattern, J., Wayss, K., Haag, D., Toomes, H., and Volm, M., Different growth rates of lung tumours in man and their xenografts in nude mice. *Eur. J. Cancer* **16**: 289–291, 1980.
39. Kopper, L. and Steel, G. G., The therapeutic response of three human tumor lines maintained in immune-suppressed mice. *Cancer Res.* **35**: 2704–2713, 1975.
40. Warenius, H. M., Identification and separation of mouse and human components of heterotransplanted human tumours. In: *Immuno-Deficient Animals for Cancer Research* (S. Sparrow, ed.), pp. 207–220. MacMillan Press, London, 1980.
41. Solesvik, O. V., Rofstad, E. K., and Brustad, T., Vascular changes in a human malignant melanoma xenograft following single-dose irradiation. *Radiat. Res.* **98**: 115–128, 1984.
42. Solesvik, O. V., Rofstad, E. K., and Brustad, T., Vascular structure of five human malignant melanomas grown in athymic nude mice. *Br. J. Cancer* **46**: 557–567, 1982.

15

Determination of DNA, Micronuclei and Vascular Density in Human Rectum Carcinomas

Christian Streffer, Dirk van Beuningen, Eberhard Gross, Friedrich-Wilhelm Eigler, and Tamara Pelzer

INTRODUCTION

The last few decades of radiobiology research have led to a better understanding of the action of ionizing radiation on cells *in vitro* and on tumors in situ. From these data, models and treatment schedules have been developed which have influenced clinical tumor therapy. The studies have been performed with comparatively few transplantable animal tumors. On the other hand, it is well known that human tumors show a high inter-individual heterogeneity with respect to many biological parameters. It is therefore important to study parameters in human tumors which have been found relevant by radiobiological investigation and to compare these results with clinical data for survival time, tumor regression, recurrence, etc. in the same patient. One aim of each study is to develop assays for specific biological factors from which a prognosis for the patient is possible or from which a selection of the therapy modality can be made for the individual tumor.[1]

It has been well-established that the radiosensitivity of cells and tissues strongly depends on cell proliferation.[2,3] Radiation damage is expressed faster in rapidly proliferating cell populations and, in this connection, the distribution of cells in the cell generation cycle is significant. Such information can be obtained from flow cytometric determinations of the DNA content.[4] Tumor growth can be estimated from measurements of cell proliferation and cell loss.[5] Cells with a micronucleus are known as dying cells and their determination can yield a rough estimate for all cell loss.[6,7] After irradiation, the number of cells with micronuclei increases in a cell population,[8] and this effect correlates with cell death.[9,10] Therefore, such measurements might be useful as a measure of tumor cell loss.

Radiobiological investigations with experimental tumors have demonstrated that hypoxia in a tumor decreases the radiation response and can cause a serious problem for tumor control through radiation.[11] In this connection, the density of small blood vessels, from which oxygen diffuses into the tissues, is of great importance. It has been demonstrated in cervix carcinomas that the vascular density correlates with the therapeutic success.[12] Using these three parameters, cytofluorimetric DNA determinations, measurements of micronuclei, and the density of arterial capillaries, correlations with treatment outcome were performed in human rectal carcinomas.

METHODS AND MATERIALS

Biopsies from human rectal carcinomas were obtained before the start of therapy. In some cases, biopsies were performed before and after preoperative radiotherapy. Single cell suspensions were prepared and cytofluorometric DNA determinations were made after staining with ethidium bromide. DNA histograms and the frequencies of micronuclei were also measured.[6,7] The vascular density was determined after staining the arterial sides of capillaries by the histochemical reaction of alkaline phosphatase. Details of this method have been published earlier by Mlynek *et al.*[13]

RESULTS AND DISCUSSION

DNA Measurements

DNA histograms were obtained from tumor cell suspensions of rectal carcinoma from more than 150 patients. About 40% of these tumors contained cells with diploid DNA content (n = 1.0). The other tumors (more than 50%) contained cells with a hyperploid DNA content (n>1.0) with a maximal frequency of n equal to 1.6–1.8. Most of the tumors were in the stage pT_3. However, the distribution of diploid and hyperploid tumors was not different in the other stages (pT_2 or pT_4). Patients with a hyperploid tumor had a worse prognosis with respect to survival than did patients with diploid tumors.[7] This difference was statistically significant when calculated according to the method of Kaplan and Meier.[14] A similar result was also obtained with colon carcinomas[15] and bladder cancers.[16] On the other hand, it was found with cervix carcinomas that the prognosis of patients with hyperploid tumors was better than for patients with diploid tumors.[17] With astorcytoma, patients with tetraploid tumors survived longer than did those patients with diploid tumor cells (unpublished results). From these data, it can be concluded that the DNA content of the tumor cells is a prognostic factor. However, no one rule can be applied to all tumor types.

TABLE 15.1. *DNA content (diploid = 1.0) and number of S-phase cells (percent) in primary rectum carcinomas (DNA$_p$: S$_p$)*

Patient	DNA$_p$	S$_p$	DNA$_M$	S$_M$	Localization of the Metastases
Di	1.7	36	1.7	24	Liver
Ho	1.5	23	1.5	20	Liver
Ga	1.0	19	1.0	16	Liver
Ba	1.9	52	1.9	37	Liver
Is	2.0	29	2.0	23	Liver
Br	2.5	39	2.8	21	Liver
We	1.0	22	1.0	23	Retrop.
Sch	1.7	28	1.5	—	Liver

With the rectal carcinomas, generally only one tumor cell line was found. This observation was different for colon carcinomas and for bronchial carcinomas where several hyperploid tumor cell lines were frequently observed (unpublished data). With several patients, it was possible to measure the DNA content in the primary rectal carcinoma and in one or even several of the metastases. In the overwhelming number of cases, the same DNA content found in cells from the primary tumor were found in cells from metastases at different locations within the same patient (Table 15.1). In this study, metastases were mainly found in the liver. These data show that rectal carcinomas are apparently less heterogenous with respect to DNA content than are other tumors. This finding agrees very well with the concept of monoclonal tumor growth.[18]

Determination of S-Phase Cells

In most cases, the percentage of S-phase cells could be calculated from the DNA histograms, and this parameter demonstrated a wide variability between individual tumors. Generally, the percentage of S-phase cells was higher in hyperploid tumors than in diploid tumors.[6,19] However, certain problems exist in this connection: (1) in tumors with a diploid tumor cell line, it is not possible to distinguish between the tumor cells and normal stromal cells by cytometric DNA determination alone. In these cases, the percentage of S-phase tumor cells cannot be corrected for the stromal cells. (2) By the technique of cytofluorometric DNA determination, a distinction between DNA synthesizing cells and resting S-phase cells is not possible. This can complicate the interpretation of data, especially for measurements made after tumor treatment. (3) Measurements from one small tumor biopsy might be representative of only a small region of the tumor. On the other hand, in several rectal carcinomas, it was possible to measure the percentage of S-phase cells in several regions of the tumor after tumor resection. In these cases, it was demonstrated that the percentage of S-phase cells varied in the range of ±20% or less.[19] Taking all these complications into account, an estimation of the range for the percentage of S-phase cells appears reasonable.

TABLE 15.2 *DNA content (diploid = 1.0) (D.I. and number of S-phase-cells (S) (%) in rectal carcinomas and in rectal mucosa of the same patients. Biopsies were taken directly from the tumor and from the marginal rectal mucosa about 1 and 5cm from the tumor border (Marg.).*

	Tumor		Marg. (1cm)		Marg. (5cm)	
	D.I.	S	D.I.	S	D.I.	S
Pat. 1	1.5	21	1.0	25	1.0	12
Pat. 2	2.6	33	2.6	41	1.0	11
Pat. 3	1.6	20	1.0	26	1.0	10
Pat. 4	1.9	32	1.0	18	1.0	13
Pat. 5	1.5	32	1.0	18	1.0	17
Pat. 6	1.3	28	1.0	11	1.0	15
Pat. 7	1.2	27	1.0	13	1.0	11
Pat. 8	1.7	14	1.0	9	1.0	7
Pat. 9	1.0	20	1.0	23	1.0	11
Pat. 10	1.0	26	1.0	34	1.0	10
Pat. 11	1.0	19	1.0	7	1.0	8
Pat. 12	1.0	16	1.0	9	1.0	9
Pat. 13	1.0	25	1.0	23	1.0	17
Pat. 14	1.0	15	1.0	12	1.0	11
Pat. 15	1.0	12	1.0	7	1.0	8

In 15 patients, DNA histograms were determined from biopsies of tumor and from biopsies of adjacent rectal mucosa. The biopsies of the rectal mucosa were obtained from about 1cm and 5cm from the tumor border (where the tumor was resected). As can be seen from Table 15.2, in several patients the percentage of S-phase cells increased in the rectal mucosa from the normal value of 6–12%. This effect was observed especially at a distance of 1cm from the tumor border, but in some patients, it also occurred at larger distances. Apparently, the

Number of S-Phase Cells
before and after Radiotherapy (18.9 Gy)

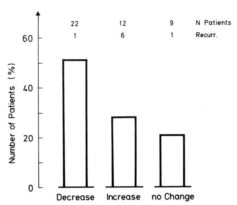

FIG. 15.1.   Comparison of the number of S-phase cells before and after preoperative radiotherapy in rectum carcinomas. In 22 patients S-phase cells were lower, in 12 patients higher after irradiation than before.

tumor can cause some irritation in the normal tissue, which leads to a stimulated cell proliferation. It will be interesting to determine whether local recurrences occur in those patients which showed the largest increases of S-phase cells in the rectal mucosa. Time of follow-up has been too short for answers resulting from these studies. In one of the patients, tumor cells were even observed in a region which appeared tumor free during the resection (Pat. 2, Table 15.2).

In some patients, it was possible to measure the number of S-phase cells before and after preoperative radiotherapy. Preliminary results have been reported earlier and demonstrated that in some patients, the percentage of S-phase cells increased rapidly after radiotherapy and that the frequency of local recurrences was high in that group of patients.[7] The patients had received hyperfractionated radiotherapy of three times 2.1 Gy per day on three consecutive days (total dose 18.9 Gy). Surgical resection of the tumor took place one to three days after the last radiation dose. Figure 15.1 illustrates data from 43 patients in this study. The percentage of S-phase cells decreased in 22 patients with one local recurrence; it increased after radiotherapy in 12 patients with 6 local recurrences; and it did not change in 9 patients with one local recurrence. Apparently, rapid cell repopulation occurred in those tumors which also showed an increase in micronuclei (see Fig. 15.2). Micronuclei measurements were performed with a fluorescence micro-

Rectum Carcinomas p T$_3$; N = 49

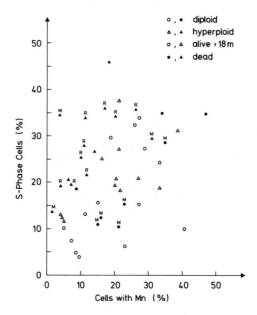

FIG. 15.2. Number of S-phase cells and cells with micronuclei (Mn) in 49 individual rectum carcinomas; (O, ●) diploid, (△, ▲) hyperploid tumor cell lines; (O, △) patients who are alive for more than 18 months after therapy: (●, ▲) patients who have died. Cause of death: (M) metastasis, (R) local recurrence.

scope after staining with ethidiumbromide, since determination by flow cytometry was not feasible. After preoperative radiotherapy, an increase of micronuclei was observed in most tumors.[7] This was especially the case in those tumors which showed significant regression. In this connection, it is important to have some information about the cell kinetics of the same cell population, as radiation-induced micronuclei are only expressed by those mitotic cell divisions which occur after the radiation exposure.[20]

VASCULARIZATION OF RECTUM CARCINOMAS

In 32 rectal carcinomas, the density of blood capillaries was determined after histochemically staining the endothelial cells by the enzymatic reaction of alkaline phosphatase.[13] Vascular density was determined in the rectal carcinomas as well as in the normal mucosa of the same patient, and the ratio of these two measurements was defined as the vasculariziation index. This index was determined in 15 patients without radiotherapy and in 17 patients with radiotherapy (one to three days p.r.). A wide range of the vascularization index (0.12–1.1) was

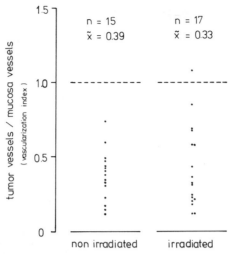

FIG. 15.3 Vascularization index (ratio tumor vessels/vessels in rectal mucosa) in rectum carcinomas. Some patients received radiotherapy[15] others did not.[17]

observed between individual patients (Fig. 15.3). Five histological sections from different regions of the tumor and mucosa of each patient were analyzed so these data should be representative. No differences were observed between irradiated and nonirradiated patients (see Fig. 15.3).

In the same rectal carcinomas, the percentage of S-phase cells and cells with micronuclei were determined. No correlation was found between the percentage of S-phase cells and the vascularization index. In this connection, it is important that the cytometric determinations of S-phase cells were obtained from large samples of tumors, after destruction of the morphological structure, and probably represent an average of cell proliferation in that tumor region. Also, no direct correlation was observed between the number of cells with micronuclei and the vascularization index, but it was interesting to note that tumors with a high vascularization index (0.6) had comparatively low numbers of micronuclei (Fig. 15.4). Further, the disseminated tumors generally had a lower vascularization index with a lower number of micronuclei than did the tumors with only local disease.

In 14 patients, micronuclei were determined both before and after preoperative radiotherapy. Generally, the radiation response increased with the vascularization index (Fig. 15.5). An arbitrary regression line is drawn in Figure 15.5 which represents the data from 9 of the 14 patients in the study. In four patients, the radiation response was higher than expected, and in one patient, it was lower than would be expected

Micronuclei and Vascularization in Rectum Carcinomas

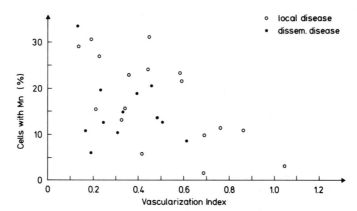

FIG. 15.4. Cells with micronuclei (Mn) and vascularization index in individual rectum carcinomas; (O) local disease; (●) disseminated disease (lymph nodes or distant metastases.

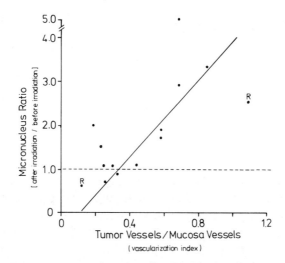

FIG. 15.5. Ratio of cells with micronuclei (Mn) before and after preoperative radiotherapy plotted against the vascularization index in individual rectum carcinomas; (R) patients with local recurrences.

from this regression line. The latter patient had a local recurrence. A further local recurrence occurred in the patient with the lowest vascularization index (Fig. 15.5). These data show that in most patients the extent of radiation response follows the general rule that well-oxygenated tumors respond better to radiation than do hypoxic tumors.[11] The tumors which do not follow this rule might be interesting from the clinical viewpoint. In this respect, the vascularization index might be a useful indicator for prediction of tumor response.

The data are not conclusive up to now, as the number of patients in the study is too small and the time of follow-up should be longer. The data, however, are promising. They give some indication that it might be possible by such comparatively simple and rapid assays to improve the prediction of the prognosis for individual patients before or during the therapeutic treatment.

SUMMARY

Cytometric DNA measurements were performed on more than 150 colorectal carcinomas. Only one tumor cell line apparently appeared in these tumors. About 40% of the tumors had a diploid DNA content. The prognosis for these patients was better than for patients with hyperploid tumors. Metastases usually showed the same tumor cell line as the primary tumors. S-phase cells were determined from the DNA histograms. The percentage of S-phase cells was frequently increased in the rectal mucosa around the tumor, and in some patients, the percentage of S-phase tumor cells increased rapidly after preoperative radiotherapy. Local recurrences were found with high probability in this group of patients.

Cells with micronuclei indicate the degree of cell loss in the carcinomas. A wide inter-individual variability was found for S-phase cells and micronuclei as well as for the density of small blood vessels. After radiotherapy, the number of micronuclei frequently increased. This increase correlated, in most cases with the vascularization index. Radiation response could be generally predicted from the vascularization index and from the radiation-induced increase of micronuclei.

ACKNOWLEDGMENT

The investigations were supported by the Deutsche Forschungsgemeinschaft, SFB 102. We thank Mrs. Jutta Müller for her help preparing the manuscript.

REFERENCES

1. Peters, L. J., Brock, W. and Johnson, T., Predicting radiocurability. *Cancer (Suppl.)* 55: 2118–2122, 1985.
2. Alper, T., *Cellular Radiobiology.* Cambridge University Press, Cambridge—London—New York—Melbourne, 1979.
3. Hall, E. J., *Radiobiology for Radiologist,* 2nd edn. Harper and Row Publishers, Hagertown—New York—Evanston—San Francisco—London, 1978.

4. Barlogie, B., Drewinko, B., Schumann, J., Göhde, W., Dosik, G., Latreille, J., Johnston, D. A., and Freieich, E. J., Cellular DNA content as a marker of neoplasia in man. *Am. J. Med.* **69**: 195–203, 1980.

5. Steel, G. G., Cell loss from experimental tumours. *Cell Tissue Kinet.* **1**: 193–207, 1968.

6. Streffer, C., van Beuningen, D., Bamberg, M., Eigler, F.-W., Gross, E. and Schabronath, J., An approach to the individualization of cancer therapy. Determination of DNA, SH-groups and micronuclei. *Strahlentherapie* **160**: 661–666, 1984.

7. Streffer, C., van Beunigen, D., Gross, E., Schabronath, J., Eigler, F. W. and Rebmann, A., Predictive assays for the therapy of rectum carcinoma. *Radiother. Oncol.* **5**: 303–310, 1986.

8. Heddle, J. A., A rapid *in vivo* test for chromosomal damage. *Mutat. Res.* **18**: 187–198, 1973.

9. Midander, J. S. and Revesz, L., The micronucleus (MN) in irradiated cells as a measure of survival. *Br. J. Cancer* **41**: 204, 1980.

10. van Beuningen, D., Streffer, C., and Bertholdt, G., Mikronukleusbildung im Vergleich zur Überlebenstrate von menschlichen Melanomzellen nach Röntgen-, Neutronenbestrahlung und Hyperthermie. *Strahlentherapie* **157**: 600–606, 1981.

11. Suit, H. D., Radiation biology: A basis for radiotherapy. In: *Textbook of Radiotherapy* (G. H. Fletcher ed.) 2nd edition, Philadelphia: Lea Febiger, pp 75–121, 1973.

12. Revesz, L., Siracka, E. and Balmukhanov, S., Gefäßdichte in Tumoren: Ihr möglicher prognostischer und therapeutischer Wert. *Strahlentherapie und Onkol.* **162**: 639–641, 1986.

13. Mlynek, M. L., van Beuningen, D., Leder, L. D. and Streffer, C., Measurement of the grade of vascularisation in histological tumor sections. *Brit. J. Cancer* **52**: 945–948, 1985.

14. Kaplan, E. S. and Meier, P., Nonparametric estimation from incomplete observation. *Am. Stat. Assoc. J.* **53**: 457–480, 1958.

15. Wolley, R. C., Schreiber, K., Koss, L. G., Karas, M. and Sherman, A., DNA distribution in human colon carcinomas and its relationship to clinical behaviour. *J. Natl. Cancer Inst.* **69**: 15–22, 1982.

16. Tribukait, B. and Gustafson, H., Impulscytophotometrische DNS-Untersuchungen bei Blasenkarzinomen. *Onkologie* **6**: 278–288, 1980.

17. Dyson, J. E. D., Joslin, C. A. F., Rothwell, R. J., Quirke, P., Khoury, G. G. and Bird, C. C., Flow cytofluorometric evidence for the differential radioresponsiveness of aneuploid and diploid cervix tumours. *Radiother. Oncol.* **8**: 263–272, 1987.

18. Fialkow, P. J., Clonal origin of human tumours. *Cancer Reviews* **458**: 283–321, 1976.

19. Streffer, C., van Beuningen, D., Gross, E. and Eigler, F. W., DNA-Messungen und Prognose von Rektum-karzinomen. *Strahlentherapie und Onkol.* **162**: 629–632, 1986.

20. Molls, M., Streffer, C. and Zamboglou, N., Micronucleus formation in preimplanted mouse embryos culture *in vitro* after irradiation with X-rays and neutrons. *Int. J. Radiat. Biol.* **39**: 307–314, 1981.

16

Heterogeneity of Tumor Cell Sensitivities: Implications for Tumor Response

Bonnie E. Miller, Fred R. Miller, and Gloria H. Heppner

INTRODUCTION

Heterogeneity of solid tumors in regard to sensitivity to chemotherapeutic drugs has become a well-accepted concept.[1] A logical extension is the idea that the assessment of the drug sensitivity profiles of individual tumor cell subpopulations would allow for prediction of the therapeutic response of the original, mixed tumor of which the subpopulations were a part. We have tested this hypothesis in a mouse mammary tumor model system that consisted of a series of subpopulation lines originally derived from a single tumor.[2–4] The tumor subpopulations were separated by various techniques, including differential trypsinization, and were not selected for any kind of drug resistance. From the parental lines of the series, we developed a set of companion lines that contained selectable markers and allowed us to accurately quantitate the proportion of individual subpopulations growing within mixed tumors before and after treatment.[5,6]

Our model system exhibited the characteristics necessary for an investigation of the implications of tumor heterogeneity on the prediction of therapeutic response: (1) the individual subpopulations are differentially sensitive to chemotherapeutic drugs *in vitro*, (2) the individual subpopulations are differentially sensitive to chemotherapeutic treatment *in vivo*, and (3) the *in vitro* assays can predict *in vivo* response of the individual subpopulations. We have used this model system to assess the influence of heterogeneity on the response of tumors to chemotherapy *in vivo*.

IN VITRO SENSITIVITY OF INDIVIDUAL SUBPOPULATIONS TO CHEMOTHERAPEUTIC DRUGS

We have tested the sensitivity of our mammary tumor lines by several *in vitro* methods, including colony forming assays on collagen and on plastic[7,8], inhibition of growth in monolayer[7,9], and inhibition of growth of collagen gel cultures.[7,8] We have tested several drugs, including doxorubicin, melphalan, methotrexate, and 5-fluorouracil. In general, similar results were obtained with all four assays. Pooled data from several experiments which tested the ability of several of the tumor subpopulation lines to form colonies on plastic in the presence of these drugs are summarized in Table 16.1. There were reproducible, small (up to seven-fold) differences in the intrinisic sensitivities to the first three drugs among some of the cell lines. All four lines were similarly sensitive to 5-fluorouracil.

TABLE 16.1 *Response of Subpopulations to Cytotoxic Drugs* In Vitro

Cells from culture were plated at 150 to 2,000 cells per 60mm tissue culture dishes, and cytotoxic drugs in a range of concentrations yielding 0 to 99% inhibition were added immediately. Medium was not changed, so drug exposure was continuous, for seven to nine days of culture, until plates were fixed and stained, and colonies counted. Throughout the range tested, the inhibition of colony formation by increasing concentrations of drugs followed an exponential curve for all drugs. Data from three to six experiments were pooled for each value given.

Cell subpopulation line	I.C.$_{90}$ for Colony Formation (uM)[a]			
	Doxorubicin	Melphalan	Methotrexate	5-Fluorouracil
168	0.074 ± 0.003[b]	3.2 ± 0.5	0.023 ± 0.001	0.51 ± 0.04
66	0.027 ± 0.003	11 ± 2	0.09 ± 0.02	0.49 ± 0.01
410	0.010 ± 0.001	3.1 ± 0.8	0.021 ± 0.003	0.68 ± 0.04
410.4	0.026 ± 0.002	6 ± 2	0.014 ± 0.001	0.64 ± 0.08

[a] Drug concentration at which colony formation was 10% of controls,
[b] Mean ± S.E.

IN VIVO SENSITIVITY OF INDIVIDUAL SUBPOPULATIONS TO CHEMOTHERAPEUTIC DRUGS

Syngeneic mice were injected subcutaneously with 10^5 to 3×10^5 cells of one or another of our mammary tumor lines. Treatment was begun soon after injection, according to protocols previously established as being optimal for each drug. The results of these experiments are shown in Table 16.2. These *in vivo* assays also detected differences among the subpopulations in intrinsic sensitivity to these drugs.

TABLE 16.2. *Response of Subpopulations to Cytotoxic Drugs* in vivo

10^5 or 3×10^5 cells of each cell line were injected s.c. into syngeneic mice. Drug treatment was given as noted. Tumors were measured twice a week with calipers, and the time for tumors to reach a mean diameter of 10 mm was determined. Growth delay was determined as the difference in the median values of the parameter for treated and control groups. Each value represents one experiment.

Cell subpopulation line	Growth Delay after Drug Treatment (days)			
	Doxorubicin[a]	Melphalan[b]	Methotrexate[c]	5-Fluorouracil[d]
168	2	5[e],10[f],18[g]	4,1,3	8[f],4[f],3
66	2	3,4[e]	3,0	4[f],1
410	10[f]	NT[h]	NT	NT
410.4	0	2	8[f],10[f],15[f], 10[f],12[f]	1,14[f],3,–3

[a] 3 i.p. injections of 2.5 mg/kg, on days one, five, and nine after cell injection.
[b] 3 i.p. injections of 12 mg/kg, on days two, nine, and 16 after cell injection.
[c] 3 i.p. injections of 38 mg/kg, 3.5 hour apart on day one after cell injection.
[d] 1 i.p. injection of 90 mg/kg, on day one after cell injection.
[e] Significant growth delay by Wilcoxon two-sample test; $p < 0.05$.
[f] Significant growth delay by Wilcoxon two-sample test: $p < 0.01$.
[g] Significant growth delay by Wilcoxon two-sample test; $p < 0.001$.
[h] Not tested.

PREDICTION OF *IN VIVO* RESPONSE FROM *IN VITRO* ASSAYS

Comparison of the data of Tables 16.1 and 16.2 indicates reasonable correlation between the two types of assays. Line 410, most sensitive to doxorubicin *in vitro*, was the only line to be significantly sensitive *in vivo*. Line 168, most sensitive to melphalan *in vitro*, was most sensitive to melphalan *in vivo*. Line 410.4, most sensitive to methotrexate *in vitro*, was the *only* line sensitive to methotrexate *in vivo*. There was little 5-fluorouracil sensitivity *in vivo*, and the occasional response seen was scattered among all cell lines tested.

RESPONSE OF HETEROGENEOUS TUMORS TO CHEMOTHERAPY

We have previously shown that when tumor subpopulations are mixed and grown together, the characteristics of an individual subpopulation, such as growth rate *in vitro*,[10] growth rate *in vivo*,[11] and metastatic capability[12] can be altered by the presence of another subpopulation. The drug sensitivity of one subpopulation can be altered by the presence of another subpopulation as well. By using 6-thioguanine-resistant lines selected from our parental subpopulation lines, we have shown that in mixtures with sensitive cells, 6-thioguanine-resistant cells become sensitive to that drug through the process of metabolic cooperation.[5,6] We have also shown that *in vitro*, line 410.4 interacts with certain of the other less sensitive subpopulations in the presence of methotrexate, so that the methotrexate sensitivity of the less sensitive line is increased.[9] This interaction is not through a process of metabolic cooperation, since it does not require cell contact. However, this interaction cannot be reproduced by conditioned medium and the mechanism still remains unknown to us. We have also shown that the cyclophosphamide sensitivity of line 410 (relatively insensitive) tumors growing subcutaneously in mice is greater when the mice also bear line 168 (relatively sensitive) tumors on the opposite flank. This increase in cyclophosphamide sensitivity may have resulted from greater activation of cyclophosphamide in mice bearing line 168 tumors, since the toxic dose (LD50) of cyclophosphamide is less in these mice than in normal mice or in mice bearing 410 tumors.[9]

Thus, it is clear that interactions among mixed cell populations can influence individual drug sensitivity by a number of different mechanisms. These interactions may be of importance in the development of techniques to predict therapeutic response. We have now tested a series of paired mixtures of our cell subpopulation lines for methotrexate sensitivity *in vivo*, to assess whether the therapeutic response of the mixture is predictable based upon a knowledge of the sensitivity of the individual populations making up the mixture. We used mixtures in which at least one line contained an independent, selectable marker, so that after noncurative therapy, we could determine the proportions of cells in the tumor.

Figures 16.1–16.5 present a series of experiments in which mixtures of cells were injected subcutaneously into mice which were then treated with methotrexate. In Experiment 1 (Fig. 16.1), we injected a mixture of line 66 (methotrexate-insensitive) and line 44FTO—a line derived from line 410.4 which retains methotrexate sensitivity and which is hypoxanthine-guanine phosphoribosyltransferase (HGPRT) deficient and, therefore, resistant to thioguanine.[6] The tumors arising from mixtures were just as sensitive to methotrexate as were the tumors arising from the sensitive line alone, as determined by growth delay. However, when the growth of the untreated tumors arising from the mixtures was compared to the growth of untreated line 66 and line 44FTO tumors, it appeared that the mixture grew faster than either line when not mixed, suggesting that one effect of methotrexate may have been to abrogate the growth stimulatory effect seen in the mixture.

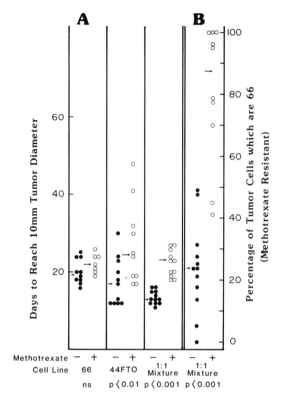

FIG. 16.1.   Effect of methotrexate on 66 and 44FTO cells and on 1:1 mixtures *in vivo*. Each cell line and the mixture were injected s.c. at 10^5 total cells per mouse. Methotrexate treatment was 3 injections of 40 mg/kg given i.p., 3.5 hour apart, on day one after cell injection. Panel A: Tumor growth of each group with and without methotrexate. Panel B: Percentage of line 66 tumor cells in each tumor arising from the mixture, determined by removing tumors, preparing single cell suspensions, and assaying for colony formation in HAT medium and in medium containing 6-thioguanine. In both panels, each point represents a single tumor. Arrows indicate the median in each group. P values indicating the probability that differences between groups were due to chance were determined by the Wilcoxon two-sample test. ns = not significantly different.

All tumors were removed at a size of 10×10 to 15×15mm, enzymatically digested to a single cell suspension, and assayed for colony-formation in medium containing thioguanine and in medium containing hypoxanthine, aminopterin, and thymidine (HAT). Line 66 and other HGPRT-positive cell lines will grow in HAT, whereas line 44FTO and other HGPRT-negative cell lines will not. We calculated the proportions of the two cell lines in the tumor cell suspensions from colony-forming data in these two media as previously described.[13] In

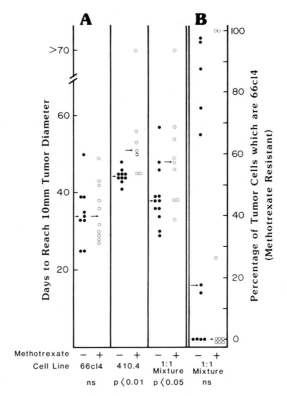

FIG. 16.2.   Effect of methotrexate on 66cl4 and 410.4 cells and on 1:1 mixtures *in vivo*. Injections of cells and methotrexate treatment as in Figure 16.1.

this experiment (Fig. 16.1), the proportion of methotrexate-insensitive cells (line 66) was increased after methotrexate therapy.

In Experiment 2, we injected a mixture of cells from line 66cl4 (methotrexate-insensitive, HGPRT-negative) and line 410.4. As shown in Figure 16.2, again the mixture was as sensitive to methotrexate as was line 410.4 alone. In this case, the growth of mixtures did not exceed the growth of either cell line alone. Analysis of the proportion of each tumor cell line in the mixed tumors demonstrated that line 66cl4 comprised from 0 to 100% of the cells in both treated and untreated tumors, and seemed to cluster at both these extremes. Methotrexate treatment did not significantly affect the proportion of line 66cl4 vs 410.4 cells in this experiment.

In Experiment 3, we injected a mixture of cells from lines 168FAR (methotrexate resistant, 2,6-diaminopurine resistant, grows in HAT) and 44FTO. In this experiment, we used a lower dose of methotrexate, to which line 44FTO did not significantly respond. However, the mix-

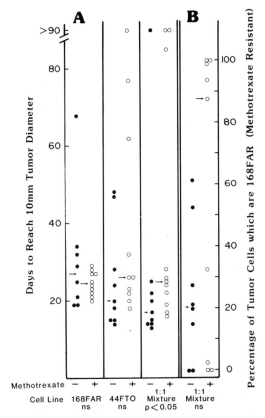

FIG. 16.3.   Effect of methotrexate on 168FAR and 44FTO cells and on 1:1 mixtures *in vivo*. 168FAR and 44FTO were each injected s.c. at 10^5 cells per mouse. The mixture was injected at 2×10^5 cells per mouse. Methotrexate treatment was three injections of 30 mg/kg given i.p., 3.5 hour apart, on day one after cell injection.

ture did respond significantly to this dose of methotrexate (Fig. 16.3). In this case, although the median proportion of line 168FAR was increased, the shift towards more methotrexate resistant cells after treatment was not significant.

In Experiments 4 and 5, we injected mixtures of line 168 and line 4TO7 (a HGPRT-negative line selected from line 44FTO). Line 4TO7 strongly suppresses the growth of line 168 in untreated controls (Fig. 16.4). We have confirmed this in other experiments, and have shown that line 4TO7 can strongly suppress the growth of line 168, even when line 168 is injected in 100-fold excess (Miller, Miller, and Heppner, manuscript in preparation). Figure 16.4 shows that line 168 tumors respond slightly—yet significantly—with a four-day growth delay to the more vigorous methotrexate treatment given. Line 4TO7 tumors

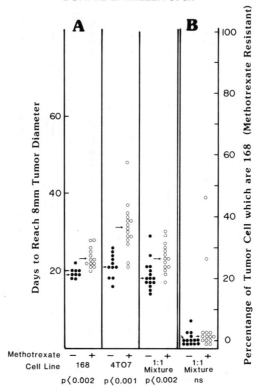

FIG. 16.4.   Effect of methotrexate on 168 and 4TO7 cells and on 1:1 mixtures *in vivo*. Each cell line was injected s.c. at 3×10^5 cells per mouse; the mixture was injected at 6×10^5 total cells per mouse. Methotrexate treatment was three injections of 37.5 mg/kg given i.p., 3.5 hours apart, on day one after cell injection, and again on day 15.

respond with a 10-day growth delay. In this experiment, in contrast to the three previous experiments, the mixture, responding with a 4.5 day growth delay, was not as sensitive as was the more sensitive cell line making up the mixture. In two of the 14 treated tumors arising from mixtures, more than 10% of the tumor cells were line 168, as compared to none of 14 untreated tumors (Fig. 16.4).

In order to compensate for the suppressive effect of 4TO7 tumors on 168 tumors, in Experiment 5 (Fig. 16.5) we injected mixtures of 168 and 4TO7 in which 168 was in excess. Again, line 168 responded significantly to methotrexate (five day delay) as did 4TO7 (nine-day delay). Both groups of tumors arising from mixtures also responded significantly to methotrexate with eight-day growth delays. In this experiment, there was a shift towards having a higher proportion of the less sensitive cells in the methotrexate-treated tumors, but this

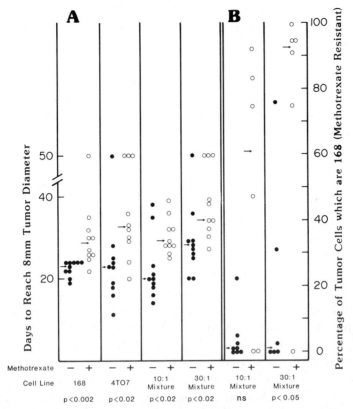

FIG. 16.5.   Effect of methotrexate on 168 and 4TO7 cells and on 10:1 mixtures and 30:1 mixtures *in vivo*. Each cell line and mixture was injected s.c. at 3×10^5 cells per mouse; methotrexate treatment was three injections of 35 mg/kg given i.p., 3.5 hours apart, on day one after cell injection, repeated on day eight and day 15.

shift was significant only in the group injected with 30:1 168:4TO7 mixtures.

For all experiments, we examined the degree of correlation between delayed tumor growth and the proportion of each cell line in tumors within each treatment group by regression analysis. There was never a strong association between time to reach a given size and cell proportion; i.e., the slowest-growing tumors after treatment were not necessarily those which contained the highest proportion of less sensitive cells.

SUMMARY

In summary, it is apparent that tumor subpopulation interactions can affect response to chemotherapy *in vivo*. In four out of five experiments, tumors formed from mixtures of methotrexate-resistant and sensitive cells were at least as responsive as were tumors formed from cells of the more sensitive line alone. Interactions affecting tumor growth and interactions affecting sensitivity to drug per se may both be involved in these results. In some cases, therapy enriches for the resistant subpopulation, but in other cases, it does not. The shift to a higher proportion of resistant cells may be most pronounced when the difference in methotrexate sensitivity is greatest (as in 66/44FTO combinations).

In one experiment, mixed tumors responded like the less sensitive line. In this paired combination, the more sensitive line (4TO7) overgrew the less sensitive (168) in untreated controls, so that line 4TO7 predominated at the time of tumor harvest. Although methotrexate treatment shifted the proportion of cells toward line 168 in two of 14 tumors, treatment did not overcome the strong inhibitory effect of line 4TO7 on line 168 in the remaining 12 tumors. When this same cell combination was injected with a higher proportion of line 168 (10:1 and 30:1, Experiment 5) the inhibitory effect of 4TO7 was somewhat weakened, so that median tumors of both controls and treated groups contained a higher proportion of line 168 cells. In the 30:1 group, the shift towards line 168 caused by methotrexate was large enough to be statistically significant.

We have seen that a consequence of the interactions between subpopulations in heterogeneous tumors is that assessment of the drug sensitivity profiles of individual subpopulations may not be predictive of the therapeutic response of the tumors from which they arise. If these interactions also take place in human tumors, the usefulness of *in vitro* testing is clearly limited. Unfortunately, one cannot conclude from our studies that these interactions might lead to therapy being more efficacious than would be predicted. In intact tumors, a number of different interactions occur simultaneously among many subpopulations. Interactions that affect growth and metastatic potential can impact on interactions that affect drug sensitivity per se.

We have also seen that, at least when intrinsic differences between subpopulations in sensitivity to chemotherapeutic drugs are small, noncurative therapy may or may not result in a higher proportion of resistant cells. In our experiments, in five out of six treated groups the median proportion of tumor cells was shifted towards the more resistant subpopulation, but the shift was statistically significant in only two of the five groups. The magnitude of therapeutic response *in vivo* gave no indication of whether or not such a shift was occurring. There has been a general acceptance of tumor heterogeneity as an explanation for the failure of chemotherapy, based on the assumption that the emergence and overgrowth of drug-resistant subpopulations is responsible for the ultimate lack of therapeutic control. This assumption has seldom been tested directly. Our data suggest that the cellular composition of treated tumors may not be directly reflective of response to therapy and that other explanations may be of greater relevance to treatment failure.

ACKNOWLEDGMENT

This work was supported by USPHS grant CA27419 from the National Cancer Institute.

REFERENCES

1. Heppner, G. H. and Miller, B. E., Tumor heterogeneity: biological implications and therapeutic consequences. *Cancer Metastasis Rev.* 2: 5–23, 1983.
2. Dexter, D. L., Kowalski, H. M., Blazar, B. A., Fligiel, Z., Vogel, R. and Heppner, G. H., Heterogeneity of tumor cells from a single mouse mammary tumor. *Cancer Res.* 38: 3174–3181, 1978.
3. Heppner, G. H., Dexter, D. L., DeNucci, T., Miller, F. R. and Calabresi, P., Heterogeneity in drug sensitivity among tumor cell subpopulations of a single mouse mammary tumor. *Cancer Res.* 38: 3758–3763, 1978.
4. Blazar, B. A., Laing, C. A., Miller, F. R. and Heppner, G. H., Activity of lymphoid cells separated from mammary tumors in blastogenesis and Winn assays. *J. Natl. Cancer Inst.* 65: 405–410, 1980.
5. Miller, B. E., Roi, L. D., Howard, L. M. and Miller, F. R., Quantitative selectivity of contact-mediated intercellular communication in a metastatic mouse mammary tumor line. *Cancer Res.* 43: 4102–4107, 1983.
6. Miller, B. E., McInerney, D., Jackson, D. and Miller, F. R., Metabolic cooperation between mouse mammary tumor subpopulations in three-dimensional collagen gel cultures. *Cancer Res.* 46: 89–93, 1986.
7. Miller, B. E., Miller, F. R. and Heppner, G. H., Assessing tumor drug sensitivity by a new *in vitro* assay which preserves tumor heterogeneity and subpopulation interactions. *J. Cell. Physiol. Suppl* 3: 105–116, 1984.
8. Miller, B. E., Miller, F. R. and Heppner, G. H., Factors affecting growth and drug sensitivity of mouse mammary tumor lines in collagen gel culture. *Cancer Res.* 45: 4200–4205, 1985.
9. Miller, B. E., Miller, F. R. and Heppner, G. H., Interactions between tumor subpopulations affecting their sensitivity to the antineoplastic agents cyclophosphamide and methotrexate. *Cancer Res.* 41: 4378–4381, 1981.
10. Heppner, G. H., Miller, B., Cooper, D. N. and Miller, F. R., Growth interactions between mammary tumor cells. In: *Cell Biology of Breast Cancer* (C. McGrath, M. Brennan and M. Rich, eds.), pp. 166–172, Academic Press, New York, 1980.
11. Miller, B. E., Miller F. R., Leith, J. and Heppner, G. H., Growth interaction *in vivo* between tumor subpopulations derived from a single mouse mammary tumor. *Cancer Res.* 40: 3977–3981, 1980.

12. Miller, F. R., Tumor subpopulation interactions in metastasis. *Invasion Metastasis* **3**: 234–242, 1983.
13. Miller, B. E., Miller, F. R. and Heppner, G. H., Drug sensitivities of subpopulations are not independent: interactions in tumors formed from mixtures of methotrexate-sensitive and resistant cells. In: *Neo-Adjuvant Chemotherapy* (C. Jacquillat, M. Weil, D. Khayat, eds.), pp. 75–81, John Libbey Eurotext Ltd., London, 1986.

17

Immunotherapy of Metastatic Disease

James E. Talmadge

INTRODUCTION

Biological response modifiers (BRMs) are those agents that influence the relationship between the tumor and host by modifying the hosts response to tumor cells with resultant therapeutic activity.[1] In this chapter, we discuss a series of studies with recombinant cytokines designed to better understand their immunomodulatory and therapeutic properties, including studies with recombinant murine interferon-gamma (rM IFN-g), recombinant human tumor necrosis factor (rH TNF), recombinant human interleukin-2 (rH IL-2), and recombinant murine colony-stimulating factor-gm (rM CSF-gm). These cytokines have disparate mechanisms of therapeutic activity as well as different optimal therapeutic protocols. Our approach has been to determine and optimize the immunomodulatory and therapeutic properties of BRMs and to utilize this information to form testable clinical and preclinical hypotheses.

Despite the appeal of immunotherapy, clinical trials have generally been disappointing with inferior results compared to those obtained in a variety of animal models.[2] Positive results in experimental systems often result from the initiation of therapy in normal animals with minimal tumor burden.[2] Clinically, metastasis has often occurred at the time of diagnosis; therefore, the major problem in cancer treatment, as well as in the development of therapeutic protocols with BRMs, is not the elimination of the primary tumor mass, but rather the control of metastasis.

One approach involves determining the optimal immunomodulatory dose (OID) and protocol (OIP), both in clinical trials[3,4] and in preclinical studies.[5,6] The OID has been found, at least preclinically, to correlate directly with the optimal therapeutic dose (OTD), both of which differ from the maximum tolerated dose (MTD).[5,6,7] Similarly, clinical studies with rH IFN-g have revealed that the OID is disparate from the clinical MTD.[3,4,8,9] In addition to the dose administered, the route and nature of administration can have an important role in defining the OIP. For example, preclinically, the continuous infusion of low levels of IL-2 has been found to have significant immunomodulatory and therapeutic activity with minimal toxicity.[10] Recent clinical trials have confirmed this observation, including studies of continuous infusion in the presence[11,12] or absence of lymphokine-activated killer (LAK) cells[13-15] The development of an optimal therapeutic protocol (OTP) appears to depend upon a complex combination of parameters, including dose, frequency of administration, duration of administration, route of administration and, in the case of combination chemoimmunotherapy, the sequence and timing of administration.

THERAPEUTIC ACTIVITY OF rH IL-2

The treatment of experimental or spontaneous metastases with rH IL-2 (generously provided by Biogen, Boston, MA) has a biphasic therapeutic response curve.[13] The OTP depends upon the dose and schedule of administration (Table 17.1). The greatest therapeutic activity in mice bearing spontaneous B16 metastases occurs with daily i.p. administration of 50 or 100,000 units of rH IL-2 per animal, as compared with the saline control. In contrast, intermediate doses or less frequent administration of rH IL-2 has less or no therapeutic activity. The MTD of rH IL-2 is >300,000 units/animal. Thus, less toxic, lower levels of rH IL-2, when given with an OTP, can have significant therapeutic activity. The low dose therapeutic optimum varies from approximately 50 units/animal to 1,000 units/animal, depending on the length of the hosts exposure to the tumor (i.e., immunologic priming). The successful treatment of experimental metastases (brief tumor exposure) requires higher doses of rH IL-2 (100 to 1,000 units/animal) than the therapeutic optimum dose of 25 to 100 units/animal for the spontaneous metastasis model, in which animals have borne tumors for approximately a month prior to the initiation of therapy.

Because of the differing pharmacokinetics of IL-2 following i.p. versus i.v. injection[10,16] and the observation that i.v. administration has significantly less therapeutic activity, the activity of rH IL-2 was investigated following continuous infusion. Alzert osmotic pumps (14 day) were placed in the peritoneal cavities of syngeneic tumor-bearing mice.

TABLE 17.1. *Treatment of Spontaneous Metastases by i.p. Injection of rH IL-2*[a]

Agent	Dose[b] (units/animal)	Median number of metastases (range)	Significance[c]
Saline	—	150 (19– > 300)	—
rH IL-2	100,000	4 (0–73)	<0.001
rH IL-2	10,000	>300 (8– > 300)	0.43
rH IL-2	1,000	161 (23– > 300)	0.72
rH IL-2	100	61.5 (0– > 300)	0.007
rH IL-2	50	27 (0–200)	<0.001

[a] Syngeneic C57BL6 mice were injected in a posterior footpad with 5×10^4 B16–BL6 cells. Twenty-nine days later, when the tumors were 1 cm in diameter, the tumor-bearing leg was resected and therapy was initiated twenty-four hours later. The mice were necropsied 35 days postresection (N = 10).
[b] Mice received saline or rH IL-2 by i.p. injection five times per week for four weeks.
[c] Difference in the median number of spontaneous metastases (Mann-Whitney U-test).

Significant therapeutic activity was observed with the infusion of approximately 14,000 units of rH IL-2 per 24 hour period (approximately 600 units/animal/hour). This level of activity was significantly greater than that observed at either a log higher or lower dose of rH IL-2. Thus, the chronic infusion of rH IL-2 has therapeutic activity at doses lower than the MTD, as determined by histopathology and clinical toxicology. Furthermore, when given either i.p. or by continuous infusion, rH IL-2 must be chronically administered. Regardless of dose, no therapeutic activity is observed following one or two weeks of daily administration, whereas four weeks of administration results in significant therapeutic activity.

One of the most intriguing aspects of the therapeutic activity of rH IL-2 is its biphasic dose response. The low dose therapeutic activity is associated with T cells with the dosage optimum paralleling the adjuvant activity of rH IL-2 for effector T cell activity.[10] Further, the association of a low rH IL-2 dose therapeutic activity and T cell augmentation is supported by the absence of low dose therapeutic activities in nude mice.[10] In contrast, high dose therapeutic activity is present in nude mice at the same doses required to activate natural killer (NK) cells or LAK cells in normal mice.[10] The observation that intermediate doses suppress the development of cytotoxic T effector cells suggest that helper T cells respond to a rH IL-2 dose (low) that differs from the effective dose for augmentation of suppressor T cells (high). Although clinical therapeutic activity and toxicity have been noted when rH IL-2 was administered with an aggressive dosage and schedule, most notably in combination with LAK cells,[17,18] the preclinical observation of therapeutic activity at low doses suggests that rH IL-2 might be therapeutically effective using a less toxic protocol.[10] The hypothesis that moderate, nontoxic doses of rH IL-2 have therapeutic activity when administered by continuous infusion[10] has been studied by West et al.[11] Their studies have shown therapeutic activity when rH IL-2 was administered by continuous infusion in combination with LAK cells. Indeed, in this preliminary report,[11] responses were observed in 9 of 16 evaluable melanoma patients. Sandel et al. have shown that continuous infusion of rH IL-2 initially produces leukopenia and later results in lymphoid hyperplasia in the peripheral blood and increased LAK cell activity ex vivo.[13] This observation has been confirmed by Creekmore and colleagues.[14,15,19] The Biological Response Modifiers Program, NCI-USA (BRMP) has also developed such a protocol and has noted biologic activity following continuous infusions of 100,000 units/M²/hr of IL-2 (Ron Steis and Jeffrey Clark, personal communication). In the Loyola study, weekly and twice weekly infusion of rH IL-2 resulted in clinical activity and tolerable toxicity.[14] In addition, dramatic increases in circulating LAK cells[15] and Leu 19+ cells[19] were observed. To date, rH IL-2 has been administered clinically using a wide variety of doses and routes. However, most of these studies have involved a short duration of drug administration via an i.v. push. Both of these factors may affect therapeutic or immunomodulatory activity, since immunotherapy, at least in rodents, requires chronic administration for significant responses. Thus, the observation of immune modulation and responses following the continuous infusion of 3×10^6 units of rH IL-2/day/M² qd or 3×10^7 units of rH IL-2/day/M² once a week,[14,15,19] is very encouraging. These are better-tolerated protocols that use lower cumulative doses than those used to date in the aggressive therapeutic protocols where approximately 100,000 units/kg is administered intravenously, tid for four days ($\sim$20 million units/day/patient)[17,18] The pharmacokinetics of rH IL-2 administered by continuous infusion results in increased toxicity, as compared on a equadose basis with i.v. bolus. The clinical impression, however, has been that significantly less toxicity and greater immunomodulation is observed in patients receiving continuous infusions of rH IL-2 at approximately 3×10^6 units/day qd or a weekly twenty-four hour infusion of 30×10^7 units/day, as compared with high dose i.v. administration tid. Nonetheless, it remains to be determined in the laboratory whether or not LAK cells are required in combination with rH IL-2,

TABLE 17.2. *Treatment of Experimental Melanoma Metastases with rM IFN-g*[a]

Agent	Dose/Animal (U)	Schedule	Route	Median number of metastases (range)	p[b]
Saline	—	tiw	i.v.	>300 (57– > 300)	—
rM IFN-g	10,000	tiw	i.v.	262 (29– > 300)	N.S.
rM IFN-g	50,000	biw	i.v.	292 (6– > 300)	N.S.
rM IFN-g	50,000	tiw	i.v.	46 (8– > 300)	0.008
rM IFN-g	50,000	qd[c]	i.v.	78 (3- > 300)	0.008
rM IFN-g	100,000	tiw	i.v.	>300 (8- > 300)	N.S.

[a] Syngeneic mice (C57BL6) received 50,000 B16-BL6 tumor cells by i.v. injection, and immunotherapy was initiated 48 hours later. The treatment consisted of i.v. injections using various routes and schedules (tiw = three times per week) of rM IFN-g for four consecutive weeks. Necropsies were performed on day 35, and the extent of experimental metastasis determined (N = 10).
[b] Probability of no difference in the number of lung nodules compared to mice that received saline control, as determined using the Mann-Whitney U-test. N.S. is not significant.
[c] qd was daily administration five days per week.

whether i.v., i.p., or continuous infusion will have the greatest therapeutic activity with the least toxicity, and what dose will result in the greatest therapeutic efficacy.

THERAPEUTIC ACTIVITY OF rM IFN-g

One study to determine the OTP for rM IFN-g (generously provided by Genentech, S. San Francisco, CA) against experimental B16 metastases is shown in Table 17.2. The greatest therapeutic activity is observed when 50,000 units/animal of rM IFN-g is administered i.v. three times per week or daily. In contrast, the i.v. administration of 100,000 units of rM IFN-g per animal produced no therapeutic activity in this experiment, and has consistently shown significantly less therapeutic activity than the injection of 50,000 units/animal. Moreover, therapeutic activity is absent when rM IFN-g is injected at 50,000 units/animal twice a week or 10,000 units/animal three times a week. This bell-shaped dose-response curve has been a consistent observation, with the therapeutic optimum observed when rM IFN-g is administered i.v. at 30,000 or 50,000 units/animal tiw.[7] Thus, it appears that rM IFN-g has a very narrow window of therapeutic activity that is dose, route, and schedule-dependent.

Studies have also examined which effector cells are responsible for the therapeutic activity of rM IFN-g.[6] In these studies, cohorts of animals were examined at various times, and effector cell activities in the blood, tumor-bearing organ, and spleen were determined. These effector cell activities include cytotoxic T lymphocyte (CTL) activity, NK cell activity, LAK cell activity, and macrophage tumoricidal activity. These studies by Black et al.[6] have revealed that the pulmonary macrophage tumoricidal activity and pulmonary CTL activity correlates significantly with a reduction in the median number of metastases and the median survival time. In contrast, alveolar macrophage activity, splenic and peripheral blood CTL activity, splenic, pulmonary, and peripheral blood NK cell activity, as well as pulmonary and splenic LAK cell activity did not correlate with either of the above parameters. This has allowed us to conclude that the effector cells responsible for the therapeutic activity of rM IFN-g are macrophages and cytotoxic T lymphocytes, at least for the treatment of experimental B16 metastases. It is unfortunate that the peripheral blood activities monitored in these studies did not correlate with therapeutic activity, which suggests that new methods of immune analysis may need to be developed in order to monitor clinical trials with rH IFN-g. Regardless, clinical trials to date have determined an optimal immunomodulatory dose for rH IFN-g for monocyte activation as monitored by monocyte hydrogen peroxide[3] or tumoricidal activity.[4] Unfortunately, there has been no reasonable analysis for clinical CTL activity, so the study of this effector cell activity has not been undertaken.

Clinical trials examining immunomodulation with rH IFN-g have revealed a bell-shaped dose-response curve for the activation of macrophages or NK cells following administration, via various routes.[3,8,9] The immune monitoring in these clinical trials was based on the bell-shaped dose-response curve to rM IFN-g discussed earlier in this chapter.[7] The bell-shaped immunomodulation response curve has been observed clinically with rH IFN-g or -a in studies by Ernstoff et al.,[9] Edwards et al.[8] and Kleinerman et al.[3] as well as in studies undertaken by the BRMP.[4] These studies have stressed a variety of monocyte function assays, including hydrogen peroxide production, FC receptors, HLA-DR expression, and macrophage tumoricidal activity. The absence of clinical therapeutic activity with rH IFN-g may be associated with the administration of doses near the MTD as opposed to the OID. The results of these clinical trials have suggested that rH IFN-g OID is approximately 0.1 mg/M^2 administered either tiw or daily. Therefore, the BRMP, in conjunction with the Cancer Therapy Evaluation Program, is now undertaking a phase III clinical trial to test the therapeutic properties of rH IFN-g at the OID.

TABLE 17.3. *Treatment of Spontaneous Melanoma Metastases with rH TNF*[a]

Agent	Dose/animal	MST[b]	Median number of metastases (range)	p[c]
Saline	—	>29	11 (16–27)	—
poly(I,C)-LC	10 ug	>29	1 (0–4)	0.000
rH TNF	1,000,000 U	3	0 (0–1)	0.000
rH TNF	500,000 U	17	0 (0–65)	0.027
rH TNF	50,000 U	>29	0 (0–36)	0.034
rH TNF	5,000 U	>29	1 (0–36)	0.020
rH TNF	500 U	>29	25 (0–65)	0.496

[a] B16–BL6 tumor cells were injected into the posterior footpad of each mouse. When the tumors reached a 0.9 cm diameter, the tumor-bearing limb was resected at midfemur to include the popliteal lymph node. Therapy was initiated one day later with tiw i.v. injections for four weeks. Necropsies were performed on day 29, one day after the last injection (N = 10 mice).

[b] MST is median survival time.

[c] Probability of no difference in the number of pulmonary tumor nodules compared to mice that received saline control, as determined using the Mann-Whitney U-test.

THERAPEUTIC ACTIVITY OF rH TNF

The results of a study which examined the treatment of spontaneous metases with tiw i.v. injections of various doses of rH TNF (generously provided by Genentech, S. San Francisco, CA) are shown in Table 17.3. When rH TNF was administered to tumor-bearing mice by i.v. injection, 1,000,000 units/animal was toxic and 500,000 units/animal was slightly above the MTD. However, significant therapeutic activity was observed when 50,000 or 5,000 units/animal was administered by i.v. injection (Table 17.3). In contrast, none of the doses produced significant therapeutic activity when administered i.p. (Table 17.4). The low level of serum activity observed following i.p. administration[7] may explain the decrease in therapeutic activity when rH TNF is administered via this route. It has been observed that rH TNF's therapeutic activity is greater against spontaneous metastases than against experimental metastases. Thus, the observation of increased therapeutic activity following immunological priming related to primary tumor growth in the spontaneous metastasis model and the T cell adjuvant activity of rH TNF suggests that this may be an important mechanism for therapeutic activity.

When rH TNF is admixed with suboptimal doses of rM IFN-g, a significant increase in therapeutic activity is observed. The additive therapeutic activity is shown in Table 17.4 in an experiment in which rM IFN-g was administered i.p. This is a suboptimal route of adminis-

TABLE 17.4. *Combination Immunotherapy of Experimental Metastases with rM IFN-g and rH TNF*[a]

rH TNF U/A	rM IFN-g U/A	Schedule	Route	Metastasis Median	Metastasis Range	P vs Saline[b]	P vs rM IFN- g[c]
HBSS	—	qd	i.p.	55	(0– > 300)	—	0.003
—	50,000	qd	i.p.	7	(0–54)	0.003	—
500,000	—	qd	i.p.	26	(0–81)	0.09	0.043
50,000	—	qd	i.p.	29	(5–141)	0.35	0.047
5,000	—	qd	i.p.	29	(0–257)	0.16	0.05
50,000	50,000	qd	i.p.	1	(0–5)	0.0009	0.01

[a] C57/BL6 mice were injected i.v. with 5×10^4 B16–BL6 tumor cells, and immunotherapy was initiated two days later. Therapy consisted of the injection of each cytokine for four consecutive weeks. Necropsies were performed 35 days following tumor challenge, and the extent of experimental metastasis was determined with the aid of a dissecting microscope. (N = 10/mice).
[b] Probability of no difference in the number of nodules compared to mice that received the HBSS control, as determined using the Mann-Whitney U-test.
[c] Probability of no difference in the number of nodules compared to mice that received rM IFN-g alone ($P > 0.01$), as determined using the Mann-Whitney U-test.

tration for rM IFN-g, but when administered in combination with rH TNF it produces a significant increase in therapeutic activity. Unfortunately, when rH TNF and rM IFN-g are injected at doses which are individually nontoxic, an increased level of toxicity is also observed.[20] Histopathological studies of the toxicity from the combination of rM IFN-g and rH TNF demonstrated systemic multifocal thrombi with secondary ischemic necrosis. This suggested that one mechanism of rH TNF and rM IFN-g toxicity might involve the coagulation system. Further studies revealed that the toxicity of rH TNF and rM IFN-g, as measured by lethality, could be decreased with the injection of aspirin (thirty minutes before and four hours after BRM administration). Similar results are obtained with corticosteroids and other cyclo-oxygenase inhibitors.[20] In addition, studies examining the therapeutic properties of rH TNF and rM IFN-g in the presence or absence of aspirin to treat subcutaneous or intradermal B16-BL6 or Meth A tumors have revealed that therapeutic activity is maintained regardless of the administration of aspirin. Indeed, there has been a nonsignificant trend for increased therapeutic activity in animals receiving rH TNF, rM IFN-g and aspirin (Fig. 17.1). This has considerable potential for clinical utilization, since rH TNF has shown mild-to-moderate hepatic toxicity and hypotension—which may be at least partially decreased by the administration of cyclo-oxygenase inhibitors.

TREATMENT OF ID BL-6

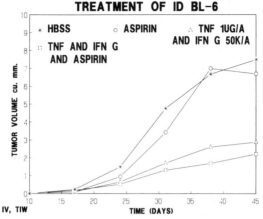

FIG. 17.1. Mice received an intradermal injection of 100,000 B16–BL6 tumor cells in a volume of 0.05 ml. Once the tumors became palpable (approximately one to two mm in diameter) on day 10, treatment was initiated which consisted of the three times per week i.v. administration of TNF at one μg/animal and rM IFN-gamma at 50,000 units/animal. Additional groups received aspirin alone or aspirin, rH TNF and rM IFN-g. The aspirin was injected at 50 mg/kg 30 minutes before and four hours following the administration of rH TNF and rM IFN-g. Tumor diameters were measured weekly using electronic calipers at the widest dimensions and at right angles to the widest dimension. Tumor volume was determined based on the formula for a prolated sphere. The mean volumes from ten animals are shown in Figure 17.1. By 45 days, 50% of the saline-treated animals had died, although none of the rH TNF and rM IFN-g-treated animals had. Therefore, further tumor volumes are not shown, since insufficient saline control animals were available for an accurate comparison.

THERAPEUTIC POTENTIAL OF rM CSF-gm AS A SINGLE AGENT AND FOR CHEMOIMMUNOTHERAPY

CSFs are glycoproteins that control the production and function of granulocytes, macrophages, and other hematopoietic cells. Not too surprisingly, rM CSF-gm has shown no significant therapeutic activity as a single agent (Table 17.5). As shown in Table 17.5, the i.v. or i.p. administration of rM CSF-gm (generously provided by Immunex, Seattle, WA) at doses ranging from 10 μg/A to 0.1 μg/A administered either three times per week (i.v.) or daily (i.p.) had no significant therapeutic activity, whereas the positive control poly (I, C)-LC did. We conclude therefore, that in agreement with the low immunomodulatory properties of rM CSF-gm *in vivo* and *in vitro* for the augmentation of effector cells, that this cytokine has minimal therapeutic potential as a single agent. However, as shown in Figure 17.2, rM CSF-gm not only has the ability to accelerate recovery from lethal irradiation, but it could also protect against lethal irradiation.

TABLE 17.5. *Immunotherapy of B16 Experimental Metastases with rM CSF-gm*[a]

BRM	Dose μg/A	Schedule	Route	Median range	P values[b]
HBSS	—	tiw	i.p.	81 (10–>300)	—
pICLC	10.0	tiw	i.v.	13 (0–174)	0.041
rM CSF-gm	10.0	qd[c]	i.p.	62 (0–>300)	0.760
rM CSF-gm	1.0	qd	i.p.	113 (0–>300)	0.596
rM CSF-gm	0.1	qd	i.p.	89 (8–>300)	0.940
rM CSF-gm	10.0	tiw	i.v.	39 (0–300)	0.569
rM CSF-gm	5.0	tiw	i.v.	94 (12–>300)	0.762
rM CSF-gm	1.0	tiw	i.v.	82 (0–>300)	0.879
rM CSF-gm	0.1	tiw	i.v.	70 (6–>300)	0.940

[a] Syngeneic mice (C57BL6) received 50,000 B16–BL6 tumor cells by i.v. injection, and immunotherapy was initiated forty-eight hours later. The treatment consisted of i.v. injections of each, using various routes and schedules for four consecutive weeks. Necropsies were performed on day 32, and the extent of experimental metastasis was determined with the aid of a dissecting microscope (N = 10).

[b] Probability of no difference in the number of lung nodules compared to mice that received saline control, as determined using the Mann-Whitney U-test.

[c] qd was daily administration, five days per week.

In other studies, we have found that the timing of the injection of rM CSF-gm prior to irradiation is critical, suggesting that this cytokine may stimulate cells into cycle so that twenty hours later, many are in S- phase, where they are protected or have increased repair mechanisms against irradiation damage. Similar results have been seen for protection/accelerated recovery against lethal doses of cyclophosphamide (CTX) (results not shown). In results similar to those shown in Figure 17.2, we have noted that there is a singificant correlation between the median survival time following lethal irradiation and treatment with rM CSF-gm, PBL number, and bone marrow cell number ten days following irradiation as well as with CFUC frequency and total number of CFUC in the bone marrow. This observation suggests that the action of rM CSF-gm on bone marrow stem cells is the mechanism of activity necessary for prolongation of survival. In contrast to the lack of therapeutic efficacy by rM CSF-gm as a single agent, studies of chemoimmunotherapy—where CTX is administered 15 days following the i.v. injection of tumor cells (this is an animal with a very heavy tumor burden) with subsequent administration of rM IFN-g, rH IL-2, rM CSF-gm or rH CSF-g (generously provided by Amgen) beginning twenty-four hours following CTX—show a significant increase in therapeutic activity of CTX (Table 17.6). Under these conditions, the

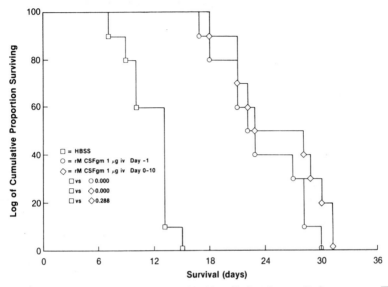

FIG. 17.2. C57BL6 mice received 950 rads of irradiation from a Cesium source. The prior injection (–20 hours) of one µg/animal of rM CSF-gm i.v. or the daily injection of one µg/animal i.v. of rM CSF-gm starting two hours following irradiation for 10 days significantly prolonged the survival of animals receiving lethal irradiation. Ten animals were used per group, and the plot is a Kaplan Meier survival curve. Statistics are the Kurskal Wallis analysis.

BRMs alone do not have any therapeutic activity due to the heavy tumor burden. This observation is based not only on a reduction in the median number of metastases, but also on a significant prolongation in the median survival time. However, similar studies—in which multiple cycles of chemotherapy are given or where BRMs are administered starting approximately four to six hours following CTX administration show no additional therapeutic activity. Under these conditions, the therapeutic activity of CTX itself may be lost. Thus, combination therapy with cytotoxic agents and rM CSF-gm or other cytokines have demonstrated increased therapeutic potential, at least as a myelorestorative measure. The critical nature of the sequence and timing of cytokine administration for chemoimmunotherapy is shown in Table 17.7. In this study, CTX as a single agent had significant therapeutic activity, but when combined with the administration of rH CSF-g starting forty-eight hours following CTX, enhanced therapeutic activity was observed. However, if rH CSF-g was administered beginning four hours or twenty-four hours following CTX, no enhanced activity was

TABLE 17.6. *Chemoimmunotherapy of Experimental B16–BL6 Metastases*[a]

BRM	Dose units/A	CTX	Metastasis Median	(Range)	p versus HBSS[b]	p versus CTX[c]	p versus –CTX[d]
HBSS	—	—	237	40–>300	—	—	—
HBSS	—	+	81	43–192	0.03	—	0.03
rM IFN-g	50,000	—	206	46–>300	0.81	—	—
rM IFN-g	50,000	+	22	12–162	0.00	0.00	0.00
rH IL-2	100,000	—	156	5–>300	0.25	—	—
rH IL-2	100,000	+	58	11–175	0.00	0.07	0.04
rM CSF-gm	50,000	—	221	47–>300	0.82	—	—
rM CSF-gm	50,000	+	38	5–>300	0.00	0.00	0.01
rM IFN-g	50,000	—	133	12–>300	0.17	—	—
rM CSF-gm	50,000	+	22	4–67	0.00	0.00	0.00

[a] Syngeneic mice (C57BL6) received 50,000 B16–BL6 tumor cells by i.v. injection, and chemotherapy (CTX, 300 mg/kg) was administered fourteen days later. Immunotherapy was initiated 24 hours later (day 15) and consisted of tiw, i.p. injection of rM IFN-g or qd, i.p. injection of the other cytokines. Therapy was continued throughout. Necropsies were performed and the extent of experimental metastasis was determined with the aid of a dissecting microscope (N = 10).

[b] Probability of no difference in the number of lung nodules compared to mice that received saline control, as determined using the Mann-Whitney U-test.

[c] Probability of no difference in the number of nodules compared to mice that received CTX, as determined using the Mann-Whitney U-test.

[d] Probability of no difference in the number of nodules compared to mice that received the cytokine alone, as determined using the Mann-Whitney U-test.

observed. Thus, the sequence and timing of cytokine administration is critical, since the cycling stem cells are at increased risk to damage by low levels of non-metabolized CTX.

DISCUSSION

At present, cancer immunotherapy has had relatively limited clinical success. This conclusion is in contradistinction to optimistic and premature reports which have resulted in inflated expectations. Nonetheless, several tumor histiotypes have responded to clinical immunotherapy under specific conditions. Our present understanding of immunoregulation and the mechanisms of immunotherapy suggest that we may be able to develop more effective therapeutic protocols in the future. Many of the preclinical studies discussed in this chapter have lead to the development of hypotheses that can be and have been clinically tested. This strategy differs from more traditional clinical trials, which rely on an empirical approach centered on the MTD. Although

TABLE 17.7. *Chemoimmunotherapy of Experimental B16 Metastases*[a]

CTX[a] mg/kg	rH CSF-g[b] units/A	Time[c] hours	Median No. Mets.	(Range)	p versus HBSS[d]	p versus CTX[e]
—	HBSS	+24	180	37–>300	—	0.047
300	HBSS	+24	75	18–209	0.047	—
—	50,000	+4	192	33–>300	0.546	0.041
300	50,000	+4	71	20–127	0.049	0.714
300	50,000	+24	69	7–161	0.043	0.519
300	50,000	+48	38	11–93	0.021	0.031

[a] Cyclophosamide (CTX) was injected i.p. on day 13 following the i.v. injection of 50,000 B16–BL6 tumor cells.

[b] RH CSF-g was injected i.p., daily (five days per week).

[c] Time following the injection of CTX when immunotherapy was initiated.

[d] Probability of no difference in the median number of nodules compared to mice that received the HBSS control, as determined using the Mann-Whitney U-test.

[e] Probability of no difference in the median number of nodules compared to mice that received the CTX control, as determined using the Mann-Whitney U-test.

such hypothesis-based clinical trials cannot replace the toxicological aspects of phase I clinical trials, they may take the form of phase "Ib", or phase II trials. We must be aware that immunotherapy, particularly with cytokines, which are not potent cytotoxic-cytostatic agents, will not result in a 99.9% reduction in tumor cell number, nor will it reduce a 1cm tumor (10^9 tumor cells) to 10^6 tumor cells. Rather, the therapeutic effects it may have, either directly or indirectly via recovery from myelosuppression or augmentation of effector cell activities, will be slight and will require chronic augmentation-activation to produce significant therapeutic activity. A single injection or a short course of administration will not have any significant activity; rather, as has been observed with hairy cell leukemia, immunotherapy will require long-term treatment.[21,22] Because these are potent immunoregulatory products, they will up-regulate effector cell activity, but they may also down-regulate effector cells at higher doses or produce suppressive effects on other parts of the immunological network. Therefore, one must be aware of the possibility of a bell-shaped immunomodulatory or therapeutic response curve, as shown here in animal studies with rM IFN-g and rH IL-2.

Combination chemoimmunotherapy alone, or in combination with autochthonous bone marrow, has considerable potential for increased therapeutic application. Surprisingly, in addition to the ability of rM CSF-gm to rescue hosts from lethal or high doses of CTX or irradiation, rH IL-2, rH IL-1, and rM IFN-g can significantly prolong survival and/or protect the host during aggressive chemo- or radiotherapy. Thus, combination chemoimmunotherapy protocols with BRMs such as the CSFs, the ILs and the IFNs have considerable potential, hopefully in the near future. This is true not only for the treatment of neoplasia but also for bone marrow transplantation studies.

SUMMARY

It appears that the cytokines have significant therapeutic potential as an adjunct to established therapeutic regimes. As single agents, they will probably have minimal therapeutic activity, although in minimal residual disease settings and/or following debulking regimes by surgery, chemotherapy, or radiotherapy, we might expect significantly increased therapeutic activity by the addition of cytokines to other established treatment protocols. Multiple cycles of chemotherapy will need to be spaced in order to allow the majority of stem cells to return to a non-cycling state. Furthermore, it is unlikely that animal models with different cell kinetic measurements can be used to define human treatment protocols.

REFERENCES

1. Michich, E. and Fefer, A., Biological response modifiers subcommittee report. In: *National Cancer Institute Monograph*, **63**: 1–278, 1983.
2. Talmadge, J. E. and Herberman, R. B., The preclinical screening laboratory: evaluation of immunomodulatory and therapeutic properties of biological response modifiers. *Cancer Treatment Report* **70**: 171–182, 1986.
3. Kleinerman, E. S., Kurzrock, R., Wyatt, D., Quesada, J. R., Gutterman, J. U. and Fidler, I. J., Activation or suppression of the tumoricidal properties of monocytes from cancer patients following treatment with human recombinant gamma-interferon. *Cancer Res.* **46**: 5401–5405, 1986.
4. Maluish, A. E., Urba, W. J., Gordon, K., Overton, W. R., Coggin, D., Crisp, E. R., Williams, R. and Sherwin, S. A., Determination of an optimum biological response modifying (BRM) dose of interferon gamma in melanoma patients. *Proceedings of the American Society of Clinical Oncology*, 1987.
5. Hartmann, D., Adams, J. S., Meeker, A. K., Schneider, M. A., Lenz, B. F. and Talmadge, J. E., Dissociation of therapeutic and toxic effects of poly-inosinic-poly-cytidylic acid admixed with poly-L-lysine and solubilized with carboxy-methyl cellulose in tumor-bearing mice. *Cancer Res.* **46**: 1331–1338, 1986.
6. Black, P. L., Phillips, H., Tribble, H. R., Pennington, R. W., Schneider, M. and Talmadge, J. E., Immune responses in tumor-bearing organs and therapeutic activity of rM IFN-gamma. *Proceedings of the Federation of American Societies for Experimental Biology Meeting* **46**: 1499, 1987.
7. Talmadge, J. E., Tribble, H. R., Pennington, R. W., Phillips, H. and Wiltrout, R. H., Immunomodulatory and immunotherapeutic properties of recombinant gamma interferon and recombinant tumor necrosis factor in mice. *Cancer Res.* in press, 1987.

8. Edwards, B. S., Merritt, J. A., Fuhlbrigge, R. C. and Borden, E. C., Low doses of interferon alpha result in more effective clinical natural killer cell activation. *Journal of Clinical Investigation* 75: 1908, 1985.

9. Ernstoff, M. S., Reich, S., Nishoda, Y. and Kirkwood, J. M., Immunological assessment of melanoma patients treated with recombinant interferon gamma (rIFN-gamma, Biogen, Inc., Cambridge, MA) in a phase I/II trial. *Proceedings of the American Association of Cancer Research Immunology* 26: 280, 1985.

10. Talmadge, J. E., Phillips, H., Schindler, J., Tribble, H. R. and Pennington, R. W., A systematic preclinical study on the therapeutic properties of rH IL-2 for the treatment of metastatic disease. *Cancer Res.*, in press, 1987.

11. West, W. H., Tauer, K. W., Yarnelli, J. R., Marshall, G. L., Orr, D. W., Thurman, G. B. and Oldham, R. K., Constant infusion recombinant interleukin-2 in adoptive immunotherapy of advanced cancer. *New Eng. J. Med.* 316: 898, 1987.

12. Kurnick, J. T., Kradin, R. L., Boyle, L. A. and Burdeshaw, A., Assessment of activation of T lymphocytes infiltrating human lung cancers. *Proceedings of the Federation of American Societies for Experimental Biology* 46: 5979, 1987.

13. Hank, J., Rosenthal, N., Kohler, P., Storer, B. and Sandel, P., Peripheral blood lymphocytes obtained following *in vivo* IL-2 therapy express lymphokine activated killer activity. *Proceedings of the Federation of American Societies for Experimental Biology* 46: 6956, 1987.

14. Creekmore, S. P., Harris, J. E., Ellis, T. M., Braun, D. P., McMannis, J. D., Cohen, I. I., Bhoopalam, N., Jassak, P. F., Cahill, M. A., Canzoneri, C. L. and Fisher, R. I., Phase I/II trial of recombinant interleukin-2 by 24-hour continuous infusion—an Illinois Cancer Council trial. *Proceedings of the American Society of Clinical Oncology*, 1987.

15. McMannis, J. D., Braun, D. P., Fisher, R. I., Creekmore, S. P., Harris, J. E. and Ellis, T. M., Demonstration of circulating lymphokine activated killer (LAK) cells in patients receiving interleukin-2 (IL-2). *Proceedings of the American Association for Cancer Research*, 1987.

16. Cheever, M. A. and Greenberg, P. D., *In vivo* administration of interleukin-2. *Contemporary Topics of Molecular Immunology* 10: 263–282, 1985.

17. Rosenberg, S. A., Lotze, M. T., Muul, L. M., Leitman, S., Chang, A. E., Ettinghausen, S. E., Matory, Y. L. and Skibber, J. M., Observations on the systemic administration of autologous lymphokine-activated killer cells and recombinant interleukin-2 to patients with metastatic cancer. *New Eng. J. Med.* 313: 1485–1492.

18. Rosenberg, S. A., Spiess, P. and Lafreniere, R., A new approach to the adoptive immunotherapy of cancer with tumor-infiltrating lymphocytes. *Science* 233: 1318–1312, 1986.

19. Ellis, T. M., Braun, D. P., Creekmore, S. P., Bhoopalam, N., Harris, J. E. and Fisher, R. I., Appearance and phenotypic characterization of circulating leu 19+ cells in patients receiving recombinant IL-2. *Proceedings of the American Association for Cancer Research*, 1987.

20. Tribble, H., Schneider, M., Bowersox, O. and Talmadge, J. E., Combination immunotherapy with rH TNF and rM IFN-g: Increased therapy and toxicity. *Proceedings of the Federation of American Societies for Experimental Biology* 46: 1430, 1987.

21. Quesda, J. R., Reuben, J., Manning, J. T., Hersh, E. M. and Gutterman, J. V., Alpha interferon for induction of remission in hairy cell leukemia. *New Engl. J. Med.* 310: 15–18, 1984.

22. Thompson, J. A. and Fefer, A., Interferon in the treatment of hairy cell leukemia. *Cancer* 59: 605–609, 1987.

FOOTNOTE.—By acceptance of this article, the publisher or recipient acknowledges the right of the U.S. Government to retain a nonexclusive, royalty-free license in and to any copyright covering the article. This research was supported by the National Cancer Institute, DHHS, under contract No. N01-23910 with Program Resources, Inc. The contents of this publication do not necessarily reflect the views or policies of the Department of Health and Human Services, nor does mention of trade names, commercial products, or organizations imply endorsement by the U.S. Government.

18

Commentary on Part IV:
Tumor Cell Response *In Vivo*

Luka Milas, G. Gordon Steel and Christian Streffer

The posters presented in this session covered a wide range of topics, not all entirely relevant to the subject of the meeting. They can be summarized under the following headings.

DEPENDENCE OF TUMOR RESPONSE ON THE NUMBER OF CLONOGENIC CELLS PER TUMOR

Two presentations, D-5 and D-18, described studies on the relationship between the content of clonogenic cells in murine sarcomas and carcinomas (TD_{50} assay) and the radiocurability of these tumors after single radiation doses (TCD_{50} assay). There was great variability in the TD_{50} values, which extended over four logs, and TCD_{50} values, which extended over 40Gy. Although local tumor irradiation was performed under oxic conditions in one study, D-18, and under hypoxia in the other, D-5, there was a significant inverse relationship between TD_{50} and TCD_{50} values in both studies. Milas *et al.*, (D-18) found evidence that tumor cell clonogenicity was influenced by the macrophage content of tumors. As the number of macrophages in the tumor increased, tumor cells exhibited higher clonogenicity, implying that high macrophage content could be conducive to tumor cell proliferation.

During the subsequent discussion, the relationship between the TD_{50} and the clonogenic fraction was considered. Suit reported that human tumor cells implanted intracranially in nude mice had a TD_{50} usually in excess of 10^4; the number of cells required per colony *in vitro* was much lower. These tumors had an *in vitro* plating efficiency that was much higher. It must be concluded that either the host defence mechanisms inactivate a large proportion of the implanted cells or that the 'true' *in vivo* clonogenic fraction is very low.

255

CELLULAR INTERACTIONS WITHIN TUMORS

Phenotypic heterogeneity within a single tumor is primarily the outcome of genetic instability of tumor cells, but it can also be influenced by the ability of tumor cells to interact with other tumor cells and with normal host cells. These interactions may complicate the prediction of tumor response to treatment. A number of posters considered aspects of cell-to-cell interaction. Miller *et al.* (D-16) isolated several cell lines from a single mouse mammary carcinoma and studied whether cells of two different lines grew independently or influenced each other's growth. The lines varied in their DNA content, enzyme activity, and they produced tumors *in vivo* that grew at different growth rates. These investigators observed that in some combinations, one subpopulation grew at the expense of the other, whereas other combinations resulted in tumors equally composed of the two-cell populations.

Leith and his associates (D-14 and D-15) studied interactions of two cell clones derived from a human colon carcinoma which form tumors upon injection into nude mice. The two clones varied in *in vitro* clonogenicity, in their sensitivity to mitomycin C, and the tumors which they formed had different growth rates. Mixing cells between the two cell lines in varying ratios formed tumors with stable cell proportions. This stability was retained in the face of radiation damage to the tumor bed. Tumor response to mitomycin C could be predicted using a clonogenic assay.

The observations reported here clearly demonstrate that cell subpopulations within a tumor may influence growth behavior and therapeutic sensitivity *in vivo*. In tumors in which cell clones interact with each other, the outcome can influence tumor response to therapy. Tumors may become more sensitive or more resistant to a cytotoxic agent than would be expected on the basis of sensitivities of individual cell clones assayed either *in vitro* or *in vivo*. In these situations, the *in vitro* assessment of drug or radiation sensitivity profiles of individual cell subpopulations will have questionable predictive value.

INITIAL SLOPE OF THE CELL SURVIVAL CURVE

The importance of measuring the initial slope of the oxic cell survival curve was brought out by the work of Fertil and Malaise[1] and Deacon *et al.*,[2] who showed that the surviving fraction at 2Gy of established human tumor cell lines correlates with the clinical radioresponsiveness of corresponding types of tumor. Bristow and Hill (D-6) reported that the *in vitro* sensitivity of cell lines derived from four different murine tumors showed some evidence of correlation with the *in vivo* response of these tumors to 10 doses of 2Gy with four hours between fractions. The correlation with 20Gy single dose was less good.

IN VITRO AND *IN VIVO* ASSAYS

A novel *in vivo* assay, consisting of encapsulation of tumor cells within 1mm diameter globules enclosed by thin semipermeable membranes and implanted into the peritoneal cavity of mice, was described by Gorelik *et al.* (D-9). The semipermeable membrane allows free access of nutrients to tumor cells, but protects them from cytotoxic host cells. The microcapsules containing human tumor cells can therefore be implanted into mice that have an intact immune response. Results of drug testing can be obtained within one or two weeks of the treatment. Fingert *et al.* (D-3) modified the subrenal capsule assay to enable this to be used for the growth of human leukemia cells. The modification consisted of adding fibrinogen and thrombin to leukemia cells, which then grow under the renal capsule as solid tumors. Chemosensitivity of these transplants correlated well with the *in vitro* chemosensitivity of the leukemic cells.

Olive (D-1) described the use of spheroids of Chinese hamster cells implanted into the peritoneal cavity of mice as a method of testing the antitumor activity of cytotoxic agents. Shortly after implantation into the peritoneal cavity, spheroids become totally hypoxic, but one day later the hypoxic fraction decreased to about 30%. Rotman *et al.* (D22) described a method of obtaining cellular clusters composed entirely of viable tumor cells by exposing human tumor specimens to mild mechanical or enzymatic dissociation. Such clusters retained some structural characteristics of the tumor, but were devoid of necrotic tissue and normal cell infiltrates. More than 95% of human tumors of different histologies were amenable to this procedure.

CELLULAR SUBPOPULATIONS AND SAMPLE SELECTION

Chaplin *et al.* (D-2) developed a technique which enables isolation and separation of oxic from hypoxic tumor cells. Following intravenous administration, the fluorochrome Hoechst # 33342 preferentially stains cells that are close to blood vessels. Fluorescence-activated cell sorting then allows the differentially-stained cell population to be separated, and the effects of cytotoxic agents on various subpopulations to be evaluated.

Siemann *et al.* (D-13) assessed total cell recovery, host versus neoplastic cell ratio, plating efficiency, cell cycle distribution, and glutathione levels in multiple biopsies from human tumor xenografts exposed to different enzymatic cell disaggregation procedures. Their results showed that biopsy specimens from the same tumor varied greatly in almost all these parameters, and that different enzymatic procedures generate cell populations with different properties. Thus, neither tumor cell composition nor the cellular characteristics studied were reflective of the tumor as a whole.

IMMUNOLOGICAL INTERACTIONS WITH TUMOR CELLS

Treatment of tumor-bearing hosts with chemotherapeutic agents may alter immune responses to the tumor in a way that is therapeutically deleterious or beneficial. In the Lewis lung carcinoma, Evans *et al.* (D-12) found that recurrent tumors grow faster than did untreated tumors. Although Adriamycin treatment either inhibited or stimulated proliferative activity of a number of immune cell types, its stimulatory action on tumor growth was most likely mediated via the loss of lymphokine production. In contrast to this, low dose cyclophosphamide can increase antitumor immune response either through suppression of suppressor T-cells and/or, as McBride *et al.* (D-21) reported, through its stimulation of, tumor-necrosis factor or interleukin-1 secretion by macrophages. The authors developed a simple assay for assessment of these functions by patients' peripheral blood monocytes. The effects of host cell infiltrates into a rat sarcoma were reported by Afzal *et al.* (D-19). At two to three days following irradiation, there was evidence for significant additional cell kill attributable to specific host response.

HOW LARGE ARE DIFFERENCES IN CLINICAL RESPONSE TO RADIOTHERAPY?

Steel introduced the discussion by inviting comments on what degree of heterogeneity is implied by the steepness of clinical tumor cure curves. Such curves have a maximum steepness that is fixed by Poisson statistics and by the Do value that is associated with fractionated radiotherapy. Figure 18.1 shows three examples of clinical data on the dose-response for local control. The curve for skin tumors obtained by Hliniak *et al.*[3] was extremely steep, and the theoretical Poisson curve is a good fit for it. The cure curves for the other two tumor types[4,5] are much flatter, and typical of a number of other data sets. There are many reasons for the discrepancy between the actual and theoretical curves in this Figure, apart from the fact that data of this type have seldom been accumulated as a result of a controlled clinical trial. These

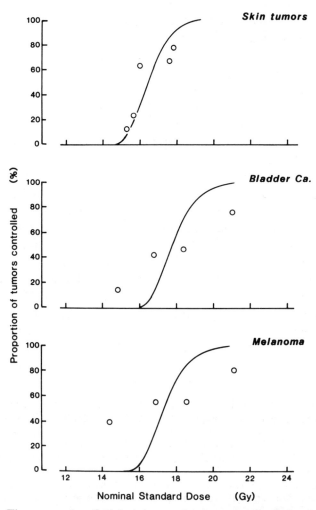

FIG. 18.1. Three examples of clinical data on the dose-response for local control by radiotherapy: (a) squamous cell carcinomas of the skin (Hliniak *et al.*, 1983), bladder carcinomas (Morrison *et al.*, 1975), and (c) melanoma (Trott *et al.*, 1981). The full lines show theoretical curves calculated on the assumption of uniform cellular sensitivity, the steepness of which is determined only by the statistics of survival of one or more clonogenic tumor cells.

reasons include: (a) variations in the quality of the radiotherapy (dose distributions, geographical misses, errors in diagnosis or staging); (b) differences in hypoxia or rates of repopulation, and (c) inter-tumor variations in radiosensitivity.

Clinicians who contributed to the discussion expressed the view that variations included under (a) are fully capable of explaining the observed discrepancies. On the other hand, the range of survival at 2Gy seen by Deacon *et al*[2] within each tumor type category is capable of explaining an even wider variation in radiocurability. The range of radiosensitivities for a group of xenografted melanomas described by Rofstad (Chapter 14) confirms this range. It therefore remains an open question as to what extent a laboratory test of radiosensitivity will be able to predict for radiocurability.

It has been argued that, if the α/β ratio for tumors is greater than for the late-reacting normal tissues that limit radiotherapy, there will be a therapeutic advantage in using a reduced dose per fraction. There was some discussion of the magnitude of the gain that may be expected from this approach. Denekamp had estimated a dose advantage in the tumor (for equal effect on normal tissues) of 8%. Withers thought the value to be nearer 15%. However, in the light of the foregoing discussion about variability in tumor response to radiotherapy, it is clear that these calculations apply to only a selected example of a tumor type that has a fixed α/β ratio (assumed in fact to be around 3Gy). Within any one group of tumors, there will be a range of α/β values, perhaps correlated with low-dose radiosensitivity, and a predictive test may be required to select the best candidates for hyperfractionation.

REFERENCES

1. Fertil, B. and Malaise, E. P., Inherent cellular radiosensitivity as a basic concept for human tumor radiotherapy. *Int. J. Radiat. Oncol. Biol. Phys.* **7**: 621–629 (1981).
2. Deacon, J., Peckham, M. J. and Steel, G. G., The radioresponsiveness of human tumors and the initial slope of the cell survival curve. *Radiotherapy and Oncology* **2**: 317–323 (1984).
3. Hliniak, A. and Trott, K. R., The influence of the number of fractions, overall treatment time, and field size on the local control of cancer of the skin. *B. J. Radiol.* **56**: 596–598 (1983).
4. Morrison, R., The results of treatment of cancer of the bladder—a clinical contribution to radiobiology. *Clin. Radiol.* **26**: 67–75, 1975.
5. Trott, K. R., von Lieven, H., Kummermehr, J., Skopal, D., Lukacs, S., Braun-Falco, O. and Kellerer, A. M., The radiosensitivity of malignant melanomas. Part II: clinical studies. *Int. J. Radiat. Oncol. Biol. Phys.* **7**: 15–20, 1981.

POSTERS

(D-1) Spheroids Implanted in the Peritoneal Cavity of Mice as a Predictive System for Evaluating Drug Activation, Detoxification and Delivery. P. L. Olive. B.C. Cancer Research Centre, Vancouver, British Columbia, Canada V5Z 1L3.

(D-2) Response of Tumor Cells *In Vivo*: Importance of Cell Location. D. J. Chaplin, P. L. Olive, and R. E. Durand. Cancer Research Centre, Vancouver, British Columbia, Canada V5Z 1L3.

(D-3) A Rapid Model for *In Vitro—In Vivo* Correlations of Tumor Cell Response. H. J. Fingert, W. H. Gajewski, N. Mizrahi, P. K. Donahoe and W. C. Wood. Massachusetts General Hospital and Harvard Medical School, Boston, Massachusetts 02114.

(D-4) Number of Clonogenic Cells Required for Recurrence After a Single Radiation Dose. M. Urano. Radiation Medicine, Massachusetts General Hospital, Boston, Massachusetts 02114.

(D-5) The Proportion of Stem Cells in Tumours. R. P. Hill. Physics Division, Ontario Cancer Institute, 500 Sherbourne Street, Toronto, Ontario, Canada M4X 1K9.

(D-6) Intrinsic Radiosensitivity Correlates with Radioresponse *In Vivo* in Murine Tumour Cell Lines. R. G. Bristow and R. P. Hill. Physics Division, Ontario Cancer Institute and Department of Medical Physics, University of Toronto, 500 Sherbourne Street, Toronto, Ontario, Canada M4X 1K9.

(D-7) The Variations in Patient Response Due to Deviations About a Mean Dose. A. M. McDermott and J. F. Dicello, Jr. Clarkson University, Potsdam, New York 13676.

(D-8) Implications of the Linear Quadratic Model for Tumor Control Probability. R. J. Yaes. Department of Radiation Medicine, University of Kentucky Medical Center, Lexington, Kentucky 40536.

(D-9) Prediction of Antitumor Activity of Drugs Using the Novel *In Vivo* Microencapsulated Tumor (MET) Assay. E. Gorelik, A. Ovejera, R. Shoemaker, A. Jarvis and R. Herberman. Pittsburgh Cancer Institute, Pittsburgh, Pennsylvania 15213 and National Cancer Institute, Bethesda, Maryland 20892 and Damon Biotech. Inc., Boston, Massachusetts 02194.

(D-10) Preclinical Studies of the Optimal Therapeutic Protocol (OTP) and Mechanisms of Activity for RH TNF, RM IFN-γ, RH IL-2, and RM CSF as Single Agents and in Combination Chemoimmunotherapy. J. E. Talmadge, H. Tribble, R. Pennington, M. Schneider, H. Phillips, B. Lenz, and P. L. Black. Preclinical Screening Laboratory, Program Resources, Inc., NCI-Frederick Cancer Research Facility, Frederick, Maryland 21701.

(D-11) Effect of Recombinant Cytokines RH TNF, RM IFN-γ, RH IL-2, and RM CSF-GM on Bone Marrow Cellularity and Stem Cell Activity in Mice. J. E. Talmadge, M. Schneider, R. Pennington, J. Keller, and F. Ruscetti. Preclinical Screening Laboratory, Program Resources, Inc. and Biological Response Modifiers Program, DCT, NCI at NCI-Frederick Cancer Research Facility, Frederick, Maryland 21701.

(D-12) Potential Complications of Recurrent Disease Associated with Doxorubicin (AdR) Treatment. M. J. Evans, C. J. Kovacs, and M. Langweiler. East Carolina University School of Medicine, Greenville, North Carolina 27858.

(D-13) Assessing Tumor Properties from Biopsies: Influence of Sample Selection and Enzyme Dissociation Technique. D. W. Siemann, M. J. Allalunis-Turner, P. C. Keng, F. Y. F. Lee, and K. L. Alliet. University of Rochester Cancer Center, Rochester, New York 14642.

(D-14) Compositional Stability of Artificial Heterogeneous Tumors *In Vivo*: Use of Mitomycin C as a Cytotoxic Probe. J. T. Leith, L. E. Faulkner, S. F. Bliven, and S. Michelson. Department of Radiation Medicine and Biology Research, Rhode Island Hospital and Division of Biology and Medicine, Brown University, Providence, Rhode Island 02912.

(D-15) "Thinning the Herd": Modification of Solid Tumor Growth Due to Cell Killing and Changes in the Tumor Microenvironment. S. Michelson, A. S. Glicksman, and J. T. Leith. Department of Radiation Medicine and Biology

Research, Rhode Island Hospital and Division of Biology and Medicine, Brown University, Providence, Rhode Island 02912.

(D-16) Tumor Subpopulation Growth Interactions *In Vivo*: Dominance of One Subpopulation. B. E. Miller, F. R. Miller, and G. H. Heppner. Michigan Cancer Foundation, Detroit, Michigan 48201.

(D-17) Influence of the Tumor Bed Effect on Expression of Intraneoplastic Diversity. J. T. Leith, L. E. Faulkner, S. F. Bliven, and S. Michelson. Department of Radiation Medicine and Biology Research, Rhode Island Hospital and Division of Biology and Medicine, Brown University, Providence, Rhode Island 02912.

(D-18) Tumor Cell Clonogenicity and Tumor Macrophage Content as Parameters in Tumor Radioresponse. L. Milas, J. Wike, N. Hunter, J. Volpe, and I. Basic. M.D. Anderson Hospital and Tumor Institutue, Department of Experimental Radiotherapy, Houston, Texas 77030.

(D-19) Evidence for a Host Immune Response to X-Irradiated Rat Rhabdomyosarcoma Tumors. S. M. Javed Afzal, T. S. Tenforde, K. S. Kavanau, and S. B. Curtis. Lawrence Berkeley Laboratory, University of California, Berkeley, California 94720.

(D-20) The MHC in Tumor-Induced Altered Normal Tissue Tolerance. C. J. Kovacs, M. J. Evans, B. J. Gould, and M. Langweiler. East Carolina University School of Medicine, Greenville, North Carolina 27858.

(D-21) Cyclophosphamide-Induced Alterations in Human Monocyte Functions: W. H. McBride, D. B. Hoon, T. Jung, J. Naungayan, A. Nizze, and D. L. Morton. Radiation Oncology and Division of Surgical Oncology and Jonsson Comprehensive Cancer Center, University of California at Los Angeles, Los Angeles, California 90024.

(D-22) A Micro-Organ Culture for Predicting Individual Tumor Response. B. Rotman, C. Teplitz, and K. Dickinson. Brown University and Rhode Island Hospital, Providence, Rhode Island 02912.

PART V

TUMOR PHYSIOLOGY AND METABOLIC IMAGING

19

Tumor Physiology and Cellular Microenvironments

Wolfgang F. Mueller-Klieser, Stefan M. Walenta, Friedrich
Kallinowski, and Peter W. Vaupel

INTRODUCTION

Heterogeneities in cellular metabolism, proliferation status, and sensitivity to treatment represent crucial problems in non-surgical tumor therapy. These heterogeneities may arise, in part, from inherent genetic properties of cancer cells and, to a certain extent, from epigenetic factors, such as a non-uniform cellular micromilieu in malignant tumors. Heterogeneous distributions of oxygen tensions and of pH have been measured with microelectrodes in C3H mouse mammary carcinomas by Vaupel et al.[1] Non-uniform distributions of oxyhemoglobin saturations have been measured in rodent tumors,[2] and in human tumors[3,4] using a cryophotometric micromethod[5,6] The pronounced variability in the measured values is mainly attributable to inhomogeneities in the tumor microcirculation. The uneven and fluctuating distribution of nutritive blood flow within tumors leads to spatial and temporal heterogeneities in the tumor micromilieu.

This chapter summarizes data on tumor blood flow, oxygenation status, and pH distributions measured in rodent tumor isotransplants, in human tumors xenotransplanted into nude rats, and in tumors in patients. Preliminary results are presented from a novel technique for metabolic imaging using bioluminescence. This method was designed to reveal possible heterogeneities in the spatial distribution of substrates and metabolites—such as glucose, lactate, and ATP—within tumor microregions. Besides the tumor types mentioned above, multicellular tumor spheroids were investigated with the bioluminescence technique.

TUMORS AND SPHEROIDS

Investigations have been carried out on various tumors, including isotransplanted tumors in Sprague-Dawley rats, human tumor xenografts transplanted into immune-deficient rats (WAG/Fra-rnu/rnu), tumors in patients, and multicellular tumor spheroids of rodent or of human origin. Animal tumors have been implanted at various sites using different implantation techniques. The majority of studies has been performed in tissue-isolated preparations obtained by implanting tumor cells into the rat kidney or into a subcutaneous fat pedicle in the inguinal region of nude rats. Using these implantation techniques, tumors were supplied by one artery and drained by one vein only. Further details concerning tissue-isolated human tumor xenografts are published elsewhere.[7,8]

Multicellular spheroids were cultured using a variety of cell lines. These include rodent fibroblasts, cells derived from various rodent tumors, and tumor cells derived from several human colon adenocarcinomas. Spheroid growth was initiated by culturing single cell suspensions in static media on non-adhesive substrates, e.g., on microbiological or agar-coated petri dishes, with subsequent transfer into spinner flasks.[9,10] The cell aggregates that were investigated at various stages of growth were considered model systems for an early, avascular stage of tumor growth and for tumor microregions, i.e., of cells located between tumor microvessels.[11]

TUMOR BLOOD FLOW

The overall tumor blood flow (TBF) was assessed in tissue-isolated tumors by measuring the tumor-venous outflow.[7,8] The use of rats made it possible to perform the experiments at defined systemic parameters, e.g., at constant mean arterial blood pressures. Large differences in TBF values were found among various types of human tumor xenografts of comparable sizes, as indicated in Table 19.1. There was no striking difference between isotransplants in rats and in human tumor xenografts. TBF decreased with increasing tumor wet weight in all tumors investigated. Presumably, the blood supply is unevenly distributed within the tumors. This can be concluded from the applications of the hydrogen clearance technique for local blood flow measurements in C3H mouse mammary carcinomas.[12]

TABLE 19.1. *Blood flow (TBF) in various human tumor xenografts and in isotransplanted rodent tumors at similar sizes (mean tumor wet weight: 3g); values are means from at least 10 experiments*

Tumor type	TBF (ml/g/min)
Medullary breast cancer (xenografts)	0.14
Squamous cell breast carcinoma (xenografts)	0.06
Ovarian carcinomas (xenografts)	0.20
Tumors of the uterus (xenografts)	0.22
DS-carcinosarcoma (isotransplants)	0.25 (see reference 15)

The tissue-isolated tumor model allowed for the determination of numerous overall metabolic rates by measuring the appropriate arteriovenous or venous-arterial concentration differences and by applying Fick's principle using the overall blood flow. These data are published in detail elsewhere[8] and will not be discussed here. A brief review of findings on the oxygenation status of tumors and tumor spheroids is given instead.

OXYGENATION OF TUMORS AND TUMOR SPHEROIDS

The oxygenation status of solid tumors and normal tissues in laboratory animals and in patients was quantified by a cryospectrophotometric micromethod.[5,6] This technique enabled the assessment of oxyhemoglobin saturation (HbO_2) values from single erythrocytes in microvessels using cryostat sections of tissue cryobiopsies. Representative data obtained in human tumors of the oral cavity are shown in Figure 19.1. In general, the HbO_2 values in tumors were considerably lower than those in the adjacent normal tissue (see Figs. 19.1a and 19.1b). Large tumors exhibited low HbO_2 saturations than did smaller tumors. Pronounced regional differences in the measured values were obvious if two biopsies taken from the same tumor were compared (see Figs. 19.1c and 19.1d). Although the tissue oxygen tension is the parameter that is relevant for the metabolism and the sensitivity of tumor cells *in vivo* to cancer treatment, measurements of the HbO_2 saturation in tumor microvessels may provide significant information on the oxygenation status of tumor tissue. This can be concluded from the intercomparison of measured PO_2 and HbO_2 frequency distri-

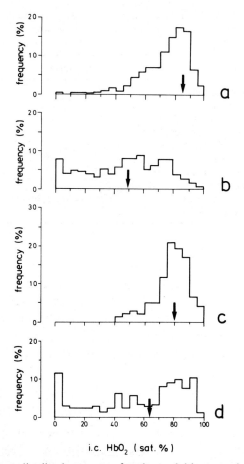

i.c. HbO$_2$ (sat. %)

FIG. 19.1. Frequency distribution curves of oxyhemoglobin saturations (HbO$_2$) values measured in normal tissue and tumors in the oral cavity of patients. Arrows indicate the median saturation values. (a) normal mucosa (n=603); (b) poorly vascularized squamous cell carcinomas (N=4; n=723); (c) and (d) biopsies taken from different locations in the same tumor.

butions and from theoretical considerations regarding inferences drawn from HbO$_2$ values on the intercapillary O$_2$ tension distribution.[13,14]

The peculiarities in tumor tissue oxygenation can be attributed mainly to characteristic properties of the tumor microcirculation.[1,15] A restriction in the nutritive blood flow during tumor progression leads to a "convection-dependent" reduction of the O$_2$ delivery to the cancer cells. The deterioration of the diffusion geometry in tumors, e.g., by enlargement of the intercapillary distances, results in a "diffusion-dependent" restriction in the O$_2$ supply. The significance of diffusion limitation for the oxygenation of tumor microregions was evaluated

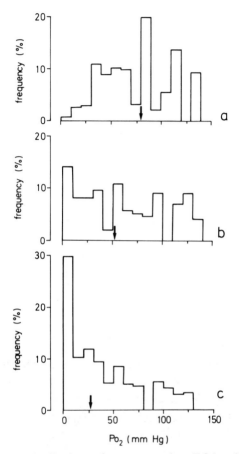

FIG. 19.2. Frequency distributions of oxygen tension (PO_2) values measured in V79–171b spheroids as a function of spheroid size. Mean diameters: (a) 448 μm; (b) 684 μm; (c) 889 μm.

systematically by measurements of oxygen tension (PO_2) with micro-electrodes in multicellular spheroids.[8,16,17] Figure 19.2 demonstrates the frequency distributions of PO_2 values obtained in V79–171b spheroids in three different size ranges. These data represent values that were randomly measured at various locations within the spheroids. Therefore, the histograms may be directly compared with the corresponding frequency distributions of HbO_2 values that were also randomly sampled across the tumors (see Fig. 19.1). It is evident that even at a constant external PO_2 value in the culture medium (corresponding to a constant PO_2 in a tumor microvessel), the O_2 tensions measured are shifted to low values by an increase in spheroid size (corresponding

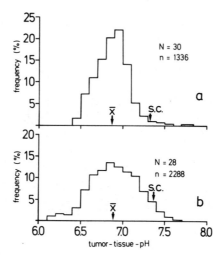

FIG. 19.3. Frequency distributions of tissue pH-values measured in subcutaneous (a) Yoshida sarcomas and (b) xenotransplanted human mammary carcinoma. s.c.: refers to values obtained in normal subcutaneous tissue.

to an increase in the intercapillary distance). The deterioration of spheroid oxygenation would be even more severe, if specific O_2 consumption (Q) would remain constant throughout spheroid growth. However, a marked decrease in Q was observed in V79 spheroids and in other spheroid types as a function of the size of these cell aggregates.[17]

pH-VALUES IN TUMORS

As an approach to further characterizing the interstitial milieu in solid tumors, pH-values were measured in isotransplanted tumors in rats and in human tumor xenotransplants using miniaturized needle pH electrodes.[18] Representative pH-histograms are shown in Figure 19.3a for Yoshida sarcomas and in Figure 19.3b for human mammary carcinomas. It is obvious that tumors are characterized by severe tissue acidosis, with mean pH values 0.4–0.5 units below the average pH measured in subcutaneous tissue. Pronounced spatial heterogeneities in the pH values were found in both tumor types. A close correlation between tissue acidosis and tumor size—similar to that observed for tumor blood flow, tumor oxygenation, and tumor weight—could not be found.

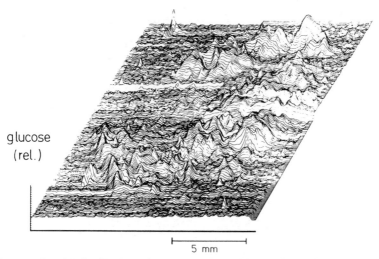

glucose
(rel.)

├──── 5 mm ────┤

FIG. 19.4. Spatial distribution of glucose registered in relative units within a xenotransplanted human mammary adenocarcinoma.

METABOLIC IMAGING

A method for determining the regional distribution of substrates
and metabolites in tissues has been established and modified in our
laboratory for use with tumors and tumor spheroids. The technique,
that was originally designed by Paschen et al.[19,20] for metabolic imaging
in brain tissue, allows for the measurement of glucose, lactate, and
ATP with a spatial resolution of around 50 μm at almost identical
locations in tumor microregions. Measurements were performed on
cryobiopsies from human tumor xenografts and on rapidly-frozen
tumor spheroids of HT 29 colon adenocarcinoma cells. Sequential cryostat sections were made. These sections were freeze-dried and, except
for glucose measurements, were heat-inactivated. Concomitantly, a solution containing enzymes that link the substrate of interest to the luminescence of luciferase via NAD(P)/NAD(P)H was rapidly frozen and
sectioned at −25°C. A sandwich consisting of one frozen section from
the tissue and one from the enzyme cocktail was placed on a photographic film in a darkroom. Upon thawing the sections, the enzymes
diffused into the tissue section and produced a luminescence that was
registered on photographic film. After standard processing, the films
were evaluated by microdensitometry and specific image analysis.

The spatial distribution of glucose in a section through a human
mammary adenocarcinoma xenotransplanted into nude rats is shown
in Figure 19.4. Although the data are plotted in relative units, they
illustrate pronounced heterogeneities in the glucose concentration

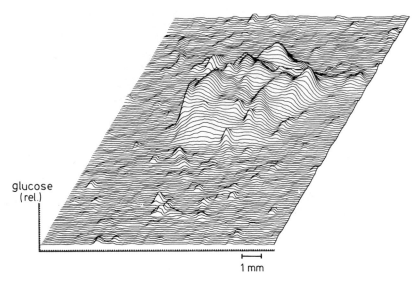

glucose
(rel.)

1 mm

FIG. 19.5. Spatial distribution of glucose registered in relative units within a skeletal muscle of the rat.

within these tumors. Also, an extended area with very low glucose, almost at the background level, was observed. The shape of the substrate distribution was highly reproducible between adjacent sections. Corresponding distribution profiles were obtained for lactate and ATP in adjacent sections, but a direct correlation among the three parameters could not be found. Preliminary data from a limited number of tumors indicate that ATP levels may be less in larger than in smaller tumors. ATP was more evenly distributed than glucose or lactate, although heterogeneities were also present with regard to these parameters. In general, heterogeneities were much less pronounced in normal tissue than in tumors. This is illustrated in Figure 19.5 for the distribution of glucose in the skeletal muscle of the rat. Even if one takes into consideration that the scale is somewhat different in Figures 19.4 and 19.5, there is clear evidence for different degrees of heterogeneities in these two tissue specimens. These data may also illustrate the significance of measuring spatial distributions versus average values for biological parameters, since similar average values may be observed, although they may result from entirely different regional distributions.

As indicated for tumor oxygenation, the heterogeneities in the metabolic milieu in tumors are elicited by a heterogeneous nutrient supply and by a non-uniform removal of metabolic wastes. Thus, the distributions obtained by metabolic imaging using bioluminescence may

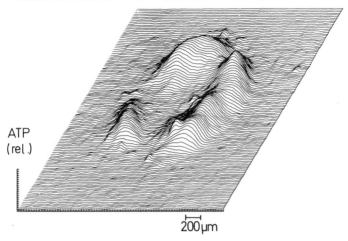

ATP
(rel.)

$\overset{\longmapsto}{200\,\mu m}$

FIG. 19.6. Spatial distribution of ATP registered in relative units in a HT 29 spheroid (diameter: 1590 μm).

reflect convection- and diffusion-dependent heterogeneities. To test whether the diffusion limitation of substances in tumor microregions can be visualized by the bioluminescence technique, the method was applied in multicellular spheroids. Figure 19.6 illustrates the ATP distribution in a central section through an HT 29 spheroid with a diameter of 1590 μm. The data indicate a high ATP level in the viable cell rim and very low levels in the necrotic center. This correlation between the ATP profiles and the histological structure of the spheroids was highly reproducible in all cell aggregates investigated to date. This result was expected, since ubiquitous ATPases, particularly those released upon cell death, rapidly cleave ATP in the extracellular space. Thus, the correlation between the histological structure and the ATP distribution in spheroids may be considered a validation of this imaging procedure. An exclusion of artifacts that may significantly contribute to observed heterogeneities is not possible on the basis of the available data. As in the case of tissue samples, an interrelationship among the distributions of glucose, lactate, and ATP was not found in spheroids.

It may be inferred from the findings on the ATP profiles in spheroids that ATP luminescence may be used for quantifying the amount of necrosis in tumors or for imaging the extent of tumor cell death following a given therapy. Similar considerations may be derived from results of an ATP assay using bioluminescence that was developed by Garewal et al.[21] for discriminating between cytostatic and cytotoxic drug effects in vitro. The in vivo situation may be complicated by the presence of host defense cells in necrotic tissue areas, elevating ATP concentrations

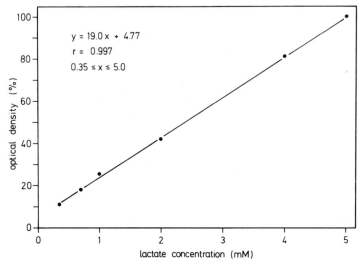

FIG. 19.7. Relative optical density of a photographic film exposed to the bioluminescence in solutions containing various concentrations of lactate.

above the low level found for necrosis in spheroids. Since the imaging bioluminescence technique makes it possible to relate the ATP distribution to the histological structure in serial sections, this potential complication can be evaluated.

Heterogeneities in the metabolic milieu have been demonstrated for glucose, lactate, and ATP in relative units. Preliminary experiments show that these bioluminescence data can be converted to absolute concentrations using calibration curves. As an example, Figure 19.7 demonstrates the optical density of photographic films that measured the bioluminescence from solutions containing various concentrations of lactate. Similar calibration curves have been obtained for glucose and ATP over biologically-relevant concentration ranges. In addition, pilot studies were carried out on spheroids that were inactivated by fixation in formalin and then equalibrated with solutions containing various substrate concentrations. Results from these spheroid studies imply that each substrate distribution can be calibrated in absolute terms. Also, it was demonstrated that this bioluminescence can be detected with an imaging photon-counting system. Therefore, research efforts in the near future will be directed towards the development of a measuring system that allows for the direct measurement and on-line evaluation of bioluminescence that can be directly related to absolute concentrations of these and other substrates. Such a method could supplement investigations in laboratory animals and in patients using non-invasive metabolic imaging procedures, such as positron emission tomography (PET) or nuclear magnetic resonance (NMR).

ACKNOWLEDGMENTS

This work was supported by the Deutsche Forschungsgemeinschaft (Mu 576/2–2, Mu 576/2–3, Va 57/2–4) and by the "Gesellschaft der Gönner und Förderer der Grundlagenforschung des Krebses" (Mainz, W. Germany).

REFERENCES

1. Vaupel, P. W., Frinak, S. and Bicher, H. I., Heterogeneous oxygen partial pressure and pH distribution in C3H mouse mammary adenocarcinoma. *Cancer Res.* **41**: 2008–2013, 1981.
2. Mueller-Klieser, W., Vaupel, P., Manz, R. and Grunewald, W. A., Intracapillary oxyhemoglobin saturation in malignant tumors with central or peripheral blood supply. *Europ. J. Cancer* **16**: 195–201, 1980.
3. Mueller-Klieser, W., Vaupel, P., Manz, R. and Schmidseder, R., Intracapillary oxygemoglobin saturation of malignant tumors in humans. *Int. J. Radiat. Oncol. Biol. Phys.* **7**: 1397–1404, 1981.
4. Wendling, P., Manz, R., Thews, G. and Vaupel, P., Heterogeneous oxygenation of rectal carcinomas in humans—A critical parameter for preoperative irradiation? *Adv. Exp. Med. Biol.* **180**: 293–300, 1984.
5. Grunewald, W. A. and Luebbers, D. W., Cryophotometry as a method for analyzing the intracapillary HbO_2 saturation of organs under different O_2 supply conditions. *Adv. Exp. Med. Biol.* **75**: 55–64, 1976.
6. Vaupel, P., Manz, R., Mueller-Klieser, W. and Grunewald, W. A., Intracapillary HbO_2 saturation in malignant tumors during normoxia and hyperoxia. *Microvasc. Res.* **17**: 181–191, 1979.
7. Vaupel, P., Kallinowski, F., Dave, S., Gabbert, H. and Bastert, G., Human mammary carcinomas in nude rats—a new approach for investigating oxygen transport and substrate utilization in tumor tissues. *Adv. Exp. Med. Biol.* **191**: 737–751, 1985.
8. Vaupel, P., Fortmeyer, H. P., Runkel, S. and Kallinowski, F., Blood flow, oxygen consumption and tissue oxygenation of human breast cancer xenografts in nude rats. *Cancer Res,* **47**: 3496–3503, 1987.
9. Freyer, J. P. and Sutherland, R. M., Selective dissociation and characterization of cells from different regions of multi-cell tumor spheroids. *Cancer Res.* **40**: 3956–3965, 1980.
10. Mueller-Klieser, W. and Sutherland, R. M., Influence of convection in the growth medium on oxygen tensions in multi-cellular tumor spheroids. *Cancer Res.* **42**: 327–342, 1982.
11. Mueller-Klieser, W., Multicellular spheroids—a review on cellular aggregates in cancer research. *J. Cancer Res. Clin. Oncol.* **113**: 101–122, 1987.
12. Vaupel, P., Frinak, S. and Bicher, H. I., Heterogeneous flow and oxygen distribution in microareas of malignant tumors. *Drug Res.* **30**: 15–16, 1980.
13. Vaupel, P., Grunewald, W. A., Manz, R. and Sowa, W., Intracapillary HbO_2 saturation in tumor tissue of DS-carcinosarcoma during normoxia. *Adv. Exp. Med. Biol.* **94**: 367–375, 1978.

14. Mueller-Klieser, W., Vaupel, P. and Manz, R., Tumour oxygenation under normobaric and hyperbaric conditions. *Brit. J. Radiol.* **56**: 559–564, 1983.
15. Vaupel, P., Hypoxia in neoplastic tissue. *Microvasc. Res.* **13**: 399–408, 1977.
16. Mueller-Klieser, W. and Sutherland, R. M., Oxygen tensions in multicell spheroids of two cell lines. *Brit. J. Cancer* **45**: 256–264, 1982.
17. Mueller-Klieser, W., Freyer, J. P. and Sutherland, R. M., Influence of glucose and oxygen supply conditions on the oxygenation of multicellular spheroids. *Brit. J. Cancer* **53**: 345–353, 1986.
18. Kallinowski, F., pH-Verteilung in malignen Tumoren unter Normo- and Hyperthermie-Bedingungen. *Thesis*, University of Mainz, West Germany, 1985.
19. Paschen, W., Niebuhr, I. and Hossmann, K.-A., A bioluminescence method for the demonstration of regional glucose distributions in brain slices. *J. Neurochem.* **367**: 513–517, 1981.
20. Paschen, W., Regional quantitative determination of lactate in brain sections. A bioluminescence approach. J. Cereb. Blood Flow Metabol. **5**: 609–612, 1985.
21. Garewal, H. S., Ahmann, F. R., Schifman, R. B. and Celniker, A., ATP assay: ability to distinguish cytostatic from cytocidal anticancer drug effects. *J. Nat. Cancer Inst.* **77**: 1039–1045, 1986.

20

Positron-Emission Tomography and Predicting Tumor Treatment Response

Alexander J. B. McEwan

INTRODUCTION

The ability of tracer methodology to provide quantifiable data on normal physiological functions, and on those associated with pathology, is well recognized. Where this methodology has been applied to monitoring response to treatment or attempting to provide indicators of tumor behavior, the basic applications have been *in vitro* or animal studies. The ability to perform tracer studies in man has been limited by difficulties in sampling and by the inability to measure *in vivo* the parameters of tumor metabolism in humans.

One step removed from tracer methodology, the discipline of clinical nuclear medicine is recognized as providing indicators of disease states which are based upon physiological principles, rather than those of the radiological sciences, where anatomical information is obtained. The sensitivity of nuclear medicine techniques has long been recognized, for example in the ability of Technetium-99m methylene diphosphonate to image metastatic bone cancer at an earlier stage than is evident on the plain radiograph.

The logical step forward has been the development of *in vivo* assays which will enable us to predict the likely behaviour of a tumor, its probable prognosis and our ability to develop a treatment modality which will, if not cure the patient, provide some significant disease-free interval. This thesis has been developed by Lentle,[1] who has made a plea for the development of imaging procedures which will give prognostic information rather than the simple image based information that is currently available. He has attempted to develop an assay[2] based upon the accumulation of Gallium-67 by small cell lung cancer, and has shown that there is some evidence of gallium uptake being a predictor of response to treatment, and of survival.

The introduction of positron-emission tomography (PET) (with imaging systems capable of a resolution of less than 1 cm) has enabled us to introduce tracer methodology into *in vivo* human imaging. The initial applications of positron tomography were in the neurological sciences, partly because of the fertile ground for research in the diagnosis of a wide range of psychiatric and neurological problems, but also due to the limitations of the early technology, where imaging systems large enough to image the whole body were not available. The development of neuro PET has been reviewed by Phelps *et al.*[3] who describes the development of PET instrumentation and gives an historical and current overview of its use in the determination of cerebral function. Following the development of whole-body systems, the focus of interest moved to the cardiovascular system and a number of elegant studies have now been performed demonstrating the ability of PET to measure subtle changes in myocardial perfusion and myocardial function which appear to have promise in the management of patients with cardiovascular disease.[4,5]

The interest in oncologic applications has, up until now, been limited, and again most of the work that has been published has related to cerebral tumors. Beaney, in an excellent review article, has discussed the possible wide range in applications of PET to oncology.[6]

It is a truism that the response of a tumor to treatment is a complex process, with many factors having to be considered in the development of an *in vivo* predictive assay. The inherent properties of tumor biology are of importance, although there is currently little available evidence on metabolism of tumors in man measured *in vivo*. The degree of hypoxia is clearly an important factor in response to chemotherapy and radiotherapy, and the ability to modify tumor blood flow by, for example, hyperthermia or antihypertensive agents, is an area currently being evaluated empirically. Inherent metabolic properties of the tumor may also be important in determining the histological grade, or more importantly, the behavioral characteristics of the tumor. For example, Patronas *et al.*[7] have reported that the glucose utilization of glioblastoma may be a more important predictor of response to treatment than is histological grading.

However, it is clear that the role of PET in oncology remains to be established, and it is evident that we are now at a stage of knowing how to ask the questions, rather than being able to confidently define the answers. This chapter will describe the ability of PET to measure biochemical and physiological parameters which have oncological importance and which (a) may lead to a clearer understanding of the likelihood of developing *in vivo* predictive assays of tumor response; (b) may develop a greater understanding of the ways in which chemotherapy and radiotherapy schedules work *in vivo*, and (c) may permit the response to therapy to be monitored in such a way that treatment regimes can be modified to achieve a greater therapeutic success. While PET has essentially been a research tool until now and limited in geographical spread, recent advances in cyclotron and scanner technology have made it likely that PET techniques will rapidly straddle the interface between the research laboratory and the clinic. Within the next decade PET could have a clearly defined role in the management of patients with cancer.

BACKGROUND

The principle underlying PET is the ability of opposed radiation detectors to localize, *in vivo*, the origin of annihilation photons following injection of radiotracers and radiopharmaceuticals labeled with positron-emitting radio-nuclides. Annihilation photons are produced by the interaction of a positron and electron with the annihilation of both particles and the emission of two gamma rays of equal energy (511 keV) in directions 180° opposed. A positron is a positive electron which has a range in tissue of approximately 1–2mm before the annihilation interaction. The imaging resolution of current imaging systems is of the order of 8 mm.[8]

POSITRON-EMITTING RADIONUCLIDES

The unique strength of PET lies in the ability of the chemist to label biological compounds with short-lived positron-emitting isotopes of carbon, nitrogen, and oxygen. Fluorine-18 substitutes for the hydroxyl radical in compounds such as fluorodeoxyglucose and fluorinated receptor analogues. The first description of the use of positron emitting radioisotopes for tumor localization was by Wrenn *et al.* in 1951.[9] They discussed the use of positron emitters for coincidence detection and demonstrated localization of the radiopharmaceuticals in 2-D views, using simple gamma-detecting coincidence equipment. The isotopes available for use in PET are listed in Table 20.1. It is evident that their half-lives are short, and so any widescale utilization of these isotopes for labeling compounds requires the onsite presence of a cyclotron for production and rapid utilization in a chemistry facility. Dyson[10] discussed the use of short-lived cyclotron-produced isotopes, and described their application to coincidence counting. From these early descriptions of the use of isotopes has developed an extensive radio-pharmaceutical and radiochemical scientific data base which is now capable of producing not only simple compounds such as radiolabeled water, carbon dioxide, carbon monoxide, and sugars, but also more complex radiotracers. These complex compounds include labeled amino-acids, receptor analogues, and chemotherapy agents which permit the study of fundamental aspects of tumor behaviour and metabolism. Table 20.2[11] lists the principal radiopharmaceuticals used in PET.

TABLE 20.1. *Positron Emitting Radionuclides*

Radionuclide	Half-Life (min)
Carbon – 11	20.4
Nitrogen – 13	10
Oxygen – 15	2.07
Fluorine – 18	109.7
Gallium – 68	68.1
Bromine – 75	101

TABLE 20.2 *PET Radiopharmaceuticals*

Tracer	Measurement
$C^{15}O_2$	blood flow
$H_2^{15}O$	blood flow
$N_2^{15}O$	blood flow
$^{15}O_2$	oxygen utilization
^{11}CO and $C^{15}O$	blood volume
^{11}C-2-deoxyglucose	glucose utilization
^{11}C-aminoacids (e.g., L-methionine)	amino acid uptake/protein synthesis
$^{11}CO_2$	cerebral pH (normal brain)
$^{13}NH_3$	$^{13}NH_3$ uptake (blood flow)
^{13}N amino acids	amino acid uptake/protein synthesis
^{82}Rb Cl	BBB integrity (^{82}Rb uptake) BBB integrity
^{18}F-2-deoxy-D-glucose	glucose utilization
^{68}Ga-EDTA	BBB integrity cerebral blood volume

The ability of any PET system is fundamentally dependent on the production of isotopes, and recent advances in cyclotron technology have considerably simplified the space requirements, the operation, and the manpower required for the use of a combined cyclotron/position tomographic facility. Current cyclotrons[12] are essentially turnkey operations which require no specialized physics support, other than that required in preventive maintenance.

MODELING

Fundamental to the analysis and quantification of uptake of administered activity is the development of an appropriate physiological model.[13,14] PET techniques[15] are unique in their ability to provide data on tumor metabolism and tumor localization which is quantitative; for example, the use of fluorodeoxyglucose allows absolute quantification of glucose utilization in mg per 100 ml of tissue per minute. It may also be semi-quantitative, where ratios of uptake by tumor and normal tissue can be determined to show regional variations of substrate utilization within the tumor and in surrounding structures. Alternatively, the images may be produced on a purely qualitative basis, where tumor-to-background ratios permit visualization of a tumor with no attempt made at quantification. Each of these methods of interpreting data have been described in the literature, and proponents of each method can point to the successful diagnostic utilization of that particular method; Ericson et al.[16] have demonstrated the utility of imaging with $C^{15}O_2$, $^{15}O_2$ and ^{18}FDG to differentiate qualitatively between cavernous hemangioma and cerebral glioma and Fox et al.[17] have described a complex iterative analysis of PET images to improve localization and anatomical correlation of tumor sites with increased sensitivity of primary and metastatic tumor detection.

However, the unique capabilities of PET are in the absolute quantification of data. Where parameters such as tissue blood flow, tissue blood volume, and oxygen and glucose utilization can be quantified, they will provide additional data about tumor metabolism and about possible ways in which treatment may affect tumor behavior or tumor growth.

In the case of amino acid metabolism and utilization by tumors, there is considerable difficulty in developing suitable models, and most of the data that has been produced simply describes semi-quantitatively the uptake of amino acids in tumors and compares that with uptake by normal tissues.

To derive accurate and valid measurements of tissue and tumor utilization of these fundamental biological substrates requires the design of complex models of tracer kinetics.[18] The original description by Sokoloff et al.[19] of a carbon-14 labeled deoxyglucose model based upon autoradiographic studies in rats has led to the beginnings of a fundamental understanding of glucose metabolism by tumors. Further models have been developed for oxygen utilization and for blood volume and blood flow measurements, and the "modeler" is a fundamental component of any PET facility.

To acquire the data for the development of tracer models requires not only a knowledge of absolute uptake of radiopharmaceuticals within the tumor site, but also a knowledge of whole blood or plasma concentration of the tracer in arterial blood. This technique requires multiple arterial blood samples to derive input data. Recent reports suggest that input data may be obtained from "arterialized venous blood" samples. These are drawn while the limb to be sampled is kept in a water bath at a constant temperature of 40°C. This causes shunting of arterial blood into the venous system. The new systems allow assessment of arterial activity by direct measurement of the aortic images. Regional tissue distribution and the regional tissue utilization of the radiopharmaceutical or radiotracer are then displayed as a series of parametric images based upon the data acquired from the tomographic imaging system.[20]

Brooks et al.[21] and Wise et al.[22] have both reviewed the development of tracer models for use in the measurement of metabolism in cerebral tumors and have described ways in which these models may give numerical information which allows comparison of tumor metabolism before and after therapy to assess the relationship to histological grading, tumor behavior and clinical course of treatment.

POSITRON TOMOGRAPHY TECHNIQUE

PET imaging systems are composed of one or more rings of opposed detectors which are capable of measuring activity in multiple axial slices. The patient (source) is positioned in the centre of the ring and data is acquired and stored in computer in digital form for subsequent analysis. Detectors were originally made of sodium iodide crystals, which are the basic detection system used in modern gamma cameras.[23] Pairs of sodium iodide crystals were placed in a ring around the patient, and an area of interest, usually 1 to 2 cm deep, sampled. This technique is slow and enabled only a limited number of sections through the brain to be obtained. Phelps et al.[24] reported the utilization of this technique to measure the distribution of positron-emitting tracers. Technology has now improved and, with the increase in computing and electronics capability, it is now possible to sample up to 15 slices with multiple ring systems with a resolution of 8 mm. This high degree of spatial resolution enables quantification of small areas of tumor and normal tissue to be compared, and for the uptake to be quantified. The detectors most common today are bismuth germanate crystals, first described by Cho and Farukhi.[25] The theoretical limits of resolution with such a system are 3 mm[8].

Lammertsma and Beaney[26] have reviewed the historical development of PET systems. Of considerable importance is a knowledge of the attenuation of the annihilation photons by the intervening tissue. This problem may be solved either by calculations assuming uniform attenuation, or by the use of a fixed ring of positron-emitting radionuclide, which enables the attenuation to be measured directly with the patient in the imaging position. The relative merits of the two techniques have been discussed,[27] but it is clear that in situations outside the CNS, where there is not fixed attenuation in different regions of the body, the direct measurement technique has allowed more accurate quantification.

The final component of any tomographic imaging system is the ability to perform the multiple calculations required for the development of parametric images, for the assessment of absolute uptake, and for the development and presentation of images so that data can be presented in a manner which enables diagnostic and prognostic decisions to be made by the referring clinicians.

It is now evident that developments in cyclotron and imaging technology, and associated advances in the radiopharmacology and radiochemistry of PET agents have brought us to the point where PET is finding a routine clinical use in the neurological sciences and in the cardiological sciences.[28] It is clear that the next major area of development for routine clinical applications will be in the field of oncology. The developmental studies outlining the possibilities of PET in oncology are now being reported. Future studies will be based on, and related directly to, the clinical field, so that the diagnostic and prognostic questions currently being asked of basic and clinical scientists can be answered with in vivo human tumor systems with minimal invasiveness and patient discomfort. It is now possible that clinically-based positron systems will enable us to answer fundamental questions on tumor biology and enable us to derive a treatment protocol with biochemical and physiological understanding of the requirements of tumor treatment, the minimization of normal tissue damage, and the development of entirely new rationally based treatment schedules. The clinical applications of PET will build upon and expand the techniques that are currently available.

CLINICAL APPLICATIONS

The ability of PET not only to image qualitatively, but also to quantify uptake in absolute terms, has enabled a large body of data to be derived on normal tissue metabolism and also on the metabolism of pathophysiological states. These data were originally described in the CNS and latterly in the myocardium. Where oncological data are available, these derive chiefly from studies of CNS tumors.

MEASUREMENT OF TISSUE METABOLISM

Utilizing the technique of sequential steady state inhalation of $C^{15}O_2$, $^{15}O_2$, and ^{11}CO it is possible to quantify regional uptake activities. Arterial activity concentration is used as an input function in the model equations, and absolute values of regional cerebral blood flow (rCBF), regional cerebral metabolic rate of glucose (rCMRO$_2$), regional cerebral blood volume (rCBV), and the regional oxygen extraction ratio (rOER) may be derived. The equations are described by Lammertsma and Beaney[26] and Ackerman et al.[27] have reported values obtained in the normal brain and in patients with cerebrovascular disease. These techniques have now been extensively validated.

An additional metabolic parameter which may be measured using PET is tissue glucose metabolism, using a technique first described by Sokoloff et al.,[19] who validated the model in rat autoradiographic studies using ^{14}C deoxyglucose.[18] Fluorodeoxyglucose (FDG) is the glucose analogue used in patient studies. This compound competes with glucose for transport across both endothelial and cell membranes. Once intracellular, it competes with glucose as the substrate for phosphorylation by hexokinase to FDG-6-PO$_4$. The phosphorylate is not metabolized in the cell, and remains trapped, allowing regional activity to be quantified in tissues with low or negligible levels of glucose 6 phosphatase, such as brain and tumors. The FDG model is thus a simple three-compartment system which allows accurate measurement of regional glucose utilization (rCMR Glu). The measurement of rCMR Glu has been reviewed by Brooks et al.[28]

MEASUREMENT OF TUMOR METABOLISM

The techniques which have been developed to measure CNS metabolism are also valid for the assessment of tumor metabolism. Beaney[6] has reviewed the measurement of rBF, rMRO, OER, and rBV in patients with cerebral tumors and compared values obtained in primary and secondary tumors, edema associated with tumors, and the contralateral cortex. The results are reproduced in Table 20.3, and clearly demonstrate significant variations of metabolic parameters in the area measured.

TABLE 20.3. *Mean Values of Tumor, Edema and Cortical Metabolism in Patients with Primary and Secondary Cerebral Tumors and in Normal Subjects*[6]

	rBF ml/100 l/in)	rOER	rMRO$_2$ (ml O$_2$/100 l/in)	rBV (ml/100 ml)
normal gray matter	45±10	0.4±0.06	3.2±0.3	4.1±0.6
primary tumor	35±35	0.15±0.1	1.0±1.0	4.1±2.3
metastatic tumor	18±13	0.24±0.14	0.9±0.6	2.8±2.3
edema	16±6	0.44±0.09	1.3±0.3	2.2±0.8

Consistent findings in tumor metabolism have shown low oxygen utilization and low oxygen extraction fraction. Blood flow and blood volume are variable, with no consistent pattern demonstrated.

An understanding of tumor metabolism is clearly crucial if optimum therapeutic regimes are to be devised. Tumor hypoxia is often associated with the lack of response to radiotherapeutic protocols, and the opportunity to measure *in vivo* the effects of radiation on normal tissue and tumor metabolism has been described by Brooks *et al.*[28] who have shown clear differences in the behavior of the two issues. In the normal cortex, rBF was shown to increase by the end of a fractionated treatment course, while rCMRO$_2$ remained unchanged. As O$_2$ supply had increased (rBF) and utilization had remained unchanged, the rOER decreased to maintain normal tissue levels. Four months after treatment, rBF was shown to have fallen and rOER to have risen. In tumors, all four parameters were shown to fall progressively, consistent with cellular death. The development of late radiation necrosis[29,30] has been evaluated with FDG and ^{82}Rb to measure cerebral metabolism and blood brain barrier (BBB) integrity.[31] These studies demonstrate a breakdown of the BBB, associated with a fall in glucose utilization.

Metabolism in primary breast tumors has been described by Beaney *et al.*[32] with tumor tissue showing an increase in rBF and MRO^2, compared with normal tissue in the contralateral breast and a significant fall in OER. Animal studies have shown comparable increases for soft tissue sarcomas and using ^{13}NH$_3$, which is not an ideal blood flow tracer as it is partly metabolized, Schelstraete *et al.*[33] have shown an increase in rBF in a variety of human tumors, including breast, sarcoma, and metastatic lymph nodes. However, the metabolic and flow components of NH_3 tissue distribution make it a less than ideal tracer for the measurement of blood flow.

TUMOR GLUCOSE METABOLISM

There is an extensive body of literature on the measurement of rCMR Glu in CNS diseases, and studies of tumor rMR Glu have drawn on the models and values derived for cerebral studies.[34-36] Comparative differences between the metabolism of tumor and normal tissue were examined in 1930 by Dickens and Simer[37] who showed that the respiratory quotient of tumor was below the carbohydrate level and that anaerobic glycolysis was high, associated with respiration comparable to normal tissues. This relationship was further examined by MacBeth and Bekesi,[38] who compared glycolysis and oxygen consumption in freshly-excised tumors and in normal tissue. They confirmed a preponderance of anaerobic glycolysis in breast, colon, and stomach cancers, but not in renal cell carcinoma. Oxygen consumption appeared greater than in normal tissues.

These studies have formed the basis for the extensive interest shown in human tumor glucose utilization. Qualitative and quantitative studies have been reported. Recent reports of non-tomographic imaging have shown increased levels of glucose uptake in a range of primary and metastatic tumors and have shown improved sensitivity when compared with gallium-67 imaging.[39,40] In a limited number of patients when metastatic thyroid cancer, qualitative uptake of FDG in metastases appeared to correlate with a poor prognosis.[41]

The correlation of FDG uptake and prognosis in tumors was first discussed by Patronas et al.[7,42] who proposed that the degree of malignancy was proportional to the glycolytic rate.[43] They subsequently proposed that survival may be predicted in glioma patients by comparing tumor rMR Glu with that of the contralateral cortex in 45 patients.[7] This ratio was consistently high in those patients with limited survival. Median survival time in patients with low ratios was 19 months, compared with median survival in patients with a high ratio of five months. Brook et al.[36] has validated the method reported by Patronas et al., and have shown comparable values in intra patient studies. Support for the relationship of rMR Glu and tumor behavior comes from Minerva et al.[44] who showed that rBF and rBV were unrelated to the degree of malignancy, while rMR Glu in white matter was increased in high grade tumors and was normal in low-grade neoplasms. Hatazawa et al.[45] has suggested that rMR Glu measures the rate of growth in meningiomas, where a rapid doubling time was associated with increased utilization of FDG. Slow-growing tumors showed no comparable focal increase in FDG accumulation. Anaerobic glycolysis by tumors has been confirmed *in vivo* by Rhodes et al.,[46] who found a disproportionate depression of rMRO$_2$ compared with rMR Glu in seven patients with gliomas.

Limitations in the application of FDG uptake analysis in the evaluation of cerebral tumors were suggested by Rhodes et al.[46] and, recently, by Tyler et al.[47] who have shown no correlation between FDG utilization and outcome in patients studied prior to therapy. All studies to this had included patients both before and after radiation and chemotherapy.

It is clear that the quantification of FDG utilization by human tumors is an important analytical tool, which may have considerable value in the *in vivo* assay of tumor behavior. The role of rMR Glu and rMRO$_2$ measurements in the assessment of radiation necrosis has recently been discussed by Doyle et al.[31]

BLOOD BRAIN BARRIER INTEGRITY

The blood brain barrier (BBB) was shown to be disrupted at sites of intracerebral tumors,[48] with the degree being dependent upon changes in the endothelial tight junction. The changes in vessels were found to be more marked with increasing tumor size. The breakdown of the BBB allows access to chemotherapy agents[49] and to blood flow agents, which allow qualitative and semi-quantitative assessment of the degree of BBB disruption. Rubidium-82[50] and ^{68}Ga-EDTA[51] are both positron-emitting tracers, which permit visualization of BBB breakdown. It is possible to define a unidirectional transfer constant[52] which is significantly higher in tumor cells than in normal brain cells. Low-grade astrocytomas were reported to have normal values, while primary and metastatic brain tumors showed greatly increased values although primary tumors had the highest values. This simple measurement demonstrates a potential as an indicator of tumor grading in the CNS.

AMINOISOBUTYRIC ACID (AIB)

The breakdown of the blood brain barrier has been suggested as a mechanism which may be used to allow access of ^{11}C AIB to cerebral tumors for *in vivo* visualization.[53] AIB is a non-metabolized amino acid which is transported into cells—including malignant cells—by the A amino acid transport system. A simple three-compartment model of AIB uptake has been devised,[54] which has permitted comparison of

AIB transfer constant, in small, medium, and large rat gliomas. Uptake as a function of tumor size is described with small tumors ($<$ 2 mm) showing a normal constant, while viable large tumors ($>$ 10 mm) showed a transfer constant an order of magnitude greater than normal gray matter. Outside the CNS, AIB uptake has been shown in a number of spontaneous canine tumors[55] and in nude mice bearing human tumor heterotransplants.[56] Uptake was shown to be a marker of treatment response, with values significantly reduced in the Dunning rat AT and H prostate tumor models following chemotherapy.[57]

AMINO ACID METABOLISM BY TUMORS

Oldendorf[58] originally compared uptake of amino acids in the brain with cerebral blood flow measured by [3]HOH. He was able to devise a brain uptake index, with phenylalanine being taken up with the greatest avidity. He subsequently demonstrated a common transport system for uptake of the basic amino acids.[59] This work has formed the basis for the interest in radiolabeled amino acid uptake by tumors.[60]

The largest series of data is with ^{11}C methionine (Met), where uptake studies have been mainly qualitative, or semi-quantitative. Considerable difficulties exist in modeling amino acid uptake, and it is possible that accurate quantification of amino acid metabolism will not be achieved. Qualitative uptake of [11]C Met was shown in gliomas[61] and in pancreatic cancers.[62] In a series of 16 patients, Ericson et al.[63] showed some correlation with [11]C Met uptake and tumor grade, with high-grade gliomas demonstrating increased uptake. In low-grade gliomas [11]C Met uptake was either normal or reduced, although the extent of [11]C Met uptake was reported to be superior to FDG in defining tumor size and grade. These data have been confirmed for high grade gliomas and for meningiomas.[64] Metastases also appear to show high tumor/non tumor ratios of [11]C Met.[65] There is some correlation between the extent of BBB disruption and [11]C Met uptake,[66] with the suggestion that the amino acid transport mechanism lies at the blood-tissue barrier.

[13]N glutamate was originally suggested as a tumor imaging agent in 1976.[67] Patient studies subsequently confirmed uptake in a series of patients with Ewing's sarcoma[68] who demonstrated uptake in viable tumor. Glutamate uptake decreased following chemotherapy. [13]N glutamate uptake may be related to tumor blood flow,[69] and will also prove difficult to quantify in absolute values. A recent abstract has described the synthesis of ^{11}C labeled tyrosine and demonstrated high concentrations in primary and metastatic tumors.[70]

POLYAMINES

The production of polyamines in cell systems undergoing rapid growth and in cancer[71] has led to the suggestion that measurement of these compounds in blood and in CSF could be used as tumor markers.[72,73] Putrescine is a useful polyamine[74] which can be labeled with carbon-11. In animal studies, it is rapidly taken up in a rat gliosarcoma model, showing uptake 10 times that of normal tissue,[75] and in a rat prostate model.[76] Human tumor studies have recently begun.[77] Uptake is most marked in hypermetabolic tumors, with peak values occurring at fifteen minutes. It may have promise as an agent to define the rate of tumor metabolism and as a marker of response to therapy.

RECEPTOR IMAGING

Considerable interest has been shown in non oncological applications in analogues of neurotransmitters which are capable of defining receptor status in normal and pathophysiological states.[78] A number of models[79] have been defined for quantification of receptor populations for dopamine, serotonin, benzodiazepenes, and opiates.[80-82] Considerable interest has been shown in the development of estrogens radiolabeled with ^{75}Br or ^{18}F[83,84] to demonstrate and quantify receptor status in patients with breast carcinoma, where receptor status has been shown to be an important prognostic indicator.

The ability of radiolabeled monoclonal antibodies (MAbs) to image cancer has been described,[85] and some reports indicate that uptake of some MAbs may have prognostic significance.[86] Developmental studies labeling MAbs with gallium-68 and zirconium-89[87] may allow the introduction of PET imaging with MAbs into the clinic, with an improved understanding of the rate and pattern of uptake as predictive assays of tumor behaviour.

TISSUE HYPOXIA

The importance of tissue hypoxia in the response of tumors to therapy has been discussed extensively in this volume, as has the *in vitro* diagnostic, prognostic, and therapeutic potential of radiosensitizer adducts. Attempts to develop a radiolabeled compound for *in vivo* external imaging of tumor hypoxia have not been successful due to extensive *in vivo* dehalogenation. Considerable efforts have been made to label Misonidazole (MISO) with positron-emitting radionuclides, and Grunbaum *et al.*[88] have recently reported the synthesis of five congeners. The most promising compound appears to be a ^{18}F-fluoromisonidazole, which shows peak uptake at two to four hours. Delayed imaging will not be possible, however, and no patient studies have been reported to date.

CHEMOTHERAPEUTIC AGENTS

Bleomycin, cis-platinum, 5-fluoruracil and BCNU[89-91] have all been labeled with positron-emitting radionuclides and utilized for PET imaging of human cancers. While the initial applications were purely qualitative, Tyler et al.[92] have described the pharmacokinetics of intraarterial and intravenous administration of ^{11}C-BCNU, demonstrating significantly higher tumor concentrations of the drug following arterial route of injection. This study indicates the possibilities of PET analysis of labeled drug kinetics in assessing or predicting response to treatment, and in the development of an understanding of the complex in vivo metabolism of these agents.

SUMMARY

PET is currently able to offer imaging techniques which are able, qualitively or quantitatively, to measure and define parameters which are important in tumor metabolism, in assessment of response to therapy, in assessment of the response of normal tissue to cancer therapy, in demonstration of malignant grading, and in predictions of response to treatment. The data base of these measurements in oncology is small, although it is beginning to expand slowly as the ability of the discipline to image biochemistry in vivo is realized. With the definition of the answers that may be given[93] it remains to the clinicians and clinical scientists to ask the pertinent questions to enable PET to realize its potential in the assessment and prognostic evaluation of human cancers.

REFERENCES

1. Lentle, B. C., Scott, J. R., Schmidt, R. P. et al., The clinical value of direct tumor scintigraphy: A new hypothesis (editorial). J. Nucl. Med. 26: 1215–1217, 1985.
2. Lentle, B. C., Catz, Z., Dierich, H. C. et al., Gallium-67 scintigraphy and non-small-cell bronchogenic carcinoma: A quantitative in vivo predictive assay? C.M.A.J. 137: 815–817, 1987.
3. Phelps, M. E., Maziotta, J. C. and Huang, S. C., Study of cerebral function with positron computed tomography. J. Cereb. Blood Flow Metab. 2: 113–162, 1982.
4. Geltman, E. M., Bergman, S. R. and Sobel, B. E., Cardiac positron emission tomography. In: Positron Emission Tomography, Alan R. Liss, New York, pp. 345–385, 1985.
5. Sobel, B. E., Positron tomography and myocardial metabolism: An overview. Circulation, 72: (suppl. 4) 22-30, 1985.

6. Beaney, R. P., Positron-emission tomography in oncology. *Clin. Oncol.* 5: 199–222 1986.
7. Patronas, J. J., Di Chiro, G., Kufta, C. *et al.*, Prediction of survival in glioma patients by means of positron-emission tomography. *J. Neurosurg.* 62: 816–822, 1985.
8. Ter-Pogossian, M. N., Positron-emission tomography instrumentation. In: *Positron Emission Tomography*, Alan R. Liss, New York, pp. 43–61, 1985.
9. Wrenn, E. R., Good, M. L. and Handler, P., The use of positron-emitting radio-isotopes for the localization of brain tumors. *Science* 113: 525, 1951.
10. Dyson, N. A., The annihilation of coincidence method of localizing positron-emitting isotopes and a comparison with parallel counting. *Phys. Med. Biol.* 4: 376, 1960.
11. Beaney, R. P., Positron-emission tomography in the study of human tumors. *Semin. Nucl. Med.* 14: 24–341, 1986.
12. Hendry, G. O., Straatman, M. G., Carroll, L. R. *et al.*, Design and performance of a compact radioisotope delivery system. C.T.I. Publications, Berkeley, California, 1987.
13. Raichle, M. E., Quantitative *In Vivo* autoradiography with positron-emission tomography. *Brain Res.* 180: 47–68, 1979.
14. Ter-Pogossian, M. N., Raichle, M. E. and Sobel, B. E., Positron-emission tomography. *Sci. Am.* 243: 170–181, 1980.
15. McMillin-Wood, J. B., Biochemical approaches to metabolism: Application to positron-emission tomography. *Circulation* 72: 145–159, 1985.
16. Ericson, L., von Holst, H., Mosskin, M. *et al.*, Positron-emission tomography of cavernous hemangiomas of the brain. *Acta. Radiol. (Diagn.)* 27: 379–383, 1986.
17. Fox, P. T., Perlmutter, J. S. and Raichle, M. E., A sterotactic method of anatomical localization for positron-emission tomography. *J. Comput. Assist. Tomogr.* 9: 141–153, 1985.
18. Alpert, N. M., Ackerman, R. H., Correia, J. A. *et al.*, Measurement of rCBF and $rCMO_2$ by continuous inhalation of ^{15}O labeled CO_2 and O_2. *Acta. Neurol. Scand.* 60 (suppl. 72): 186–197, 1979.
19. Sokoloff, L., Reivich, M., Kennedy, C., *et al.*, The ^{14}C-deoxyglucose method for the measurement of local cerebral glucose utilization: Theory, procedure and normal values in the conscious and anesthetized albino rat. *J. Neurochem.* 28: 897–916, 1977.
20. Phelps, M. and Maziotta, J. C., Positron-emission tomography: Human brain function and biochemistry. *Science* 228: 799–808, 1985.
21. Brooks, D. J., Beaney, R. P. and Thomas, D. G. T., The role of positron-emission tomography in the study of cerebral tumors. *Semin. Oncol.* 13: 83–93, 1986.
22. Wise, R. J. S., Thomas, D. G. T., Lammertsma, A. A. *et al.*, PET scanning of human brain tumors. *Prog. Exp. Tumor Res.* 27: 154–169, 1984.
23. Ter-Pogossian, M. M., Phelps, M. E., Hoffman, E. J. *et al.*, A positron-emission transaxial tomograph for nuclear medicine imaging (PETT). *Radiology* 114: 89, 1975.
24. Phelps, M. E., Hoffman, E. J., Mullani, N. A. *et al.*, Application of annihilation coincidence detection to transaxial reconstruction tomography. *J. Nucl. Med.* 16: 210–224, 1975.
25. Cho, Z. H. and Farukhi, M. R., Bismuth germanate as a potential scintillation detector in positron cameras. *J. Nucl. Med.* 18: 840–844, 1977.
26. Lammertsma, A. A and Beaney, R. P., Positron-emission tomography. *CRC Crit. Rev. Biomed. Eng.* 13: 125–169, 1985.
27. Ackerman, R. H., Correia, J. A., Alpert, N. M. *et al.*, PET studies of stroke. In: *Positron Emission Tomography*, Alan R. Liss, New York, pp. 249–262, 1985.

28. Brooks, D. J., Beaney, R. P. and Thomas, D. G. T., The role of positron-emission tomography in the study of cerebral tumors. *Semin. Nucl. Med.* **13**: 83–93, 1986.
29. Brismar, J., Robertson, G. H. and Davis, K. R., Radiation necrosis of the brain. Neuroradiological consideration with computed tomography. *Neuroradiology* **12**: 109–113, 1976.
30. Salazar, O. M., Rubin, P., Feldstein, M. L. *et al.*, High dose radiation therapy in the treatment of malignant gliomas: Final Report. *In J. Radiat. Oncol. Biol. Phys.* **5**: 1733–1740, 1979.
31. Doyle, W. K., Budinger, T. F., Valk, P. E. *et al.*, Differentiation of cerebral necrosis from tumor recurrence by ^{18}F FDG and [82]Rb positron-emission tomography. *J. Comput. Assist. Tomogr.* **11**: 563–570, 1987.
32. Beaney, R. P., Lammertsma, A. A., Jones, T. *et al.*, Positron-emission tomography for *in vivo* measurement of regional blood flow, oxygen utilization, and blood volume in patients with breast cancer. *Lancet* **1**: 131–134, 1985.
33. Schelstraete, K., Simons, M., Deman, J. *et al.*, Uptake of ^{13}N-ammonia by human tumors as studied by positron-emission tomography. *Br. J. Radiol.* **55**: 797–804, 1982.
34. Miraldi, F., Potential of NMR and PET for determining tumor metabolism. *Int. J. Radiat. Oncol. Biol. Phys.* **12**: 1033–1039, 1986.
35. Jagust, W. J., Budinger, T. F., Huesman, R. F. *et al.*, Methodologic factors affecting PET measurements of cerebral glucose metabolism. *J. Nucl. Med.* **27**: 1358–1361, 1986
36. Brook, R. A., Di Chiro, G., Zukerberg, B. W. *et al.*, Test-retest studies of cerebral glucose metabolism using Fluorine-18 deoxyglucose: Validation of method. *J. Nucl. Med.* **28**: 53–59, 1987.
37. Dickens, F. and Simer, F., The metabolism of normal and tumor tissue: The respiratory quotient and the relationship of respiration to glycolysis. *Biochem. J.* **24**: 1301–1326, 1930.
38. MacBeth, R. A. L. and Bekesi, J. G., Oxygen consumption and anaerobic glycolysis of human malignant and normal tissue. *Cancer Res.* **22**: 244–248, 1962.
39. Paul, R., Roeda, D., Johansson, R. *et al.*, Scintigraphy with (^{18}F)2-Fluoro-2-deoxy-D-glucose of cancer patients. *Int. J. Radiat. Appl. Instrument* **13**: 7–12, 1986.
40. Paul, R., Comparison of fluorine-18-2-fluorodeoxyglucose and gallium-67 citrate imaging for detection of lymphoma. *J. Nucl. Med.* **28**: 288–292, 1987.
41. Joensuu, H. and Ahonen, A., Imaging of metastases of thyroid carcinoma with fluorine-18 fluorodeoxyglucose. *J. Nucl. Med.* **28**: 910–914, 1987.
42. Patronas, N. J., Di Chiro, G., Brooks, R. A. *et al.*, Work in progress: (^{18}F) fluorodeoxyglucose and positron-emission tomography in the evaluation of radiation necrosis of the brain. *Radiology* **144**: 885–889, 1982.
43. Patronas, N. J., Brooks, R. A., De La Paz, R. L. *et al.*, Glycolytic rate (PET) and contrast enhancement in human cerebral gliomas. *A.J.N.R.* **4**: 533–535, 1983.
44. Minerva, K., Yasuda, T., Kowada, M. *et al.*, Positron-emission tomographic evaluation of histological malignancy using oxygen-15 and fluorine-18-fluoro-deoxyglucose. *Neurol. Res.* **8**: 164–168, 1986.
45. Hatazawa, J., Bairamian, D., Fishbein, D. S. *et al.*, Glucose utilization of non-gliomatous cerebral neoplasms as an index of tumor aggressivity. *J. Nucl. Med.* **27**: 104, 1986.
46. Rhodes, C. G., Wise, R. J. S., Gibbs, J. M. *et al.*, *In vivo* disturbance of the oxidate metabolism of glucose in human cerebral gliomas. *Ann. Neurol.* **14**: 614–626, 1983.

47. Tyler, J. L., Diksic, M., Villemure, J. G. *et al.*, Metabolic and haemodynamic evaluation of gliomas using positron-emission tomography. *J. Nucl. Med.* **28**: 1123–1133, 1987.
48. Cox, D. J., Pickington, G. J. and Lantos, P. L., The fine structure of blood vessels in the ethylnitrosourea-induced tumors of the rat nervous system. With special reference to the breakdown of the blood brain barrier. *Br. J. Exp. Pathol.* **57**: 419–430, 1976.
49. Fenstermacher, J. D., Blasberg, R. G. and Patlak, C. S., Methods for quantifying the transport of drugs across brain barrier systems. *Parmacol. Ther.* **14**: 217–248, 1981.
50. Brooks, D. J., Beaney, R. P., Lammertsma, A. A. *et al.*, Quantitative measurement of blood brain barrier permeability using Rubidium-82 and positron-emission tomography. *J. Cereb. Blood Flow Metab.* **4**: 535–545, 1984.
51. Hawkins, R. A., Phelps, M. E., Huang, S. C. *et al.*, A kinetic evaluation of blood brain barrier permeability in human brain tumors with ^{68}Ga EDTA and positron computed tomography. *J. Cereb. Blood Flow Metab.* **4**: 507–515, 1984.
52. Iannotti, F., Fieschi, C., Alfano, B. *et al.*, Simplified, non-*in vivo* PET measurement of blood-brain barrier permeability. *J. Comput. Assist. Tomogr.* **11**: 390–397, 1987.
53. Rapoport, S. I., In: *Blood Brain Barrier in Physiology and Medicine.* Raven Press Books, New York, pp. 177–206, 1976.
54. Yamada, K., Yukitaka, U., Hayakawa, T. *et al.*, Quantitative autoradiographic measurements of blood brain barrier permeability in the rat gliomas model. *J. Neurosurg.* **57**: 394–398, 1982.
55. Bigler, R. E., Zanzonico, P. B., Schmall, B. *et al.*, Evaluation of (1-^{11}C)-α-amino-isobutyric acid for tumor detection and amino acid transport measurement: spontaneous canine tumor studies. *Eur. J. Nucl. Med.* **10**: 48–55, 1985.
56. Conti, P. S., Sordillo, E. M., Sordillo, P. P. *et al.*, Tumor localization of α-aminoisobutyric acid (AIB) in human melanoma heterotransplants. *Eur. J. Nucl. Med.* **10**: 45–47, 1985.
57. Dangendorfer, U., Schmall, B., Bigler, R. E. *et al.*, Synthesis and body distribution of alpha-aminoisobutyric acid-L-^{11}C in normal and prostate cancer-bearing rat after chemotherapy. *Eur. J. Nucl. Med.* **6**: 535–538, 1981.
58. Oldendorf, W. H., Brain uptake of radiolabeled amino acids, amines and hexoses after intra-arterial injection. *Am. J. Physiol.* **221**: 1629–1639, 1971.
59. Oldendorf, W. H. and Szabo, J., Amino acid assignment to one of the three blood-brain barrier amino acid carriers. *Am. J. Physiol.* **230**: 94–98, 1976.
60. Kubota, K., Yamada, K., Fukada, H. *et al.*, Tumor detection with carbon-11 labeled amino acids. *Eur. J. Nucl. Med.* **9**: 136–141, 1984.
61. Hubner, K. F., Purvis, T. J., Mahaley, S. M. *et al.*, Brain tumor imaging by positron-emission computed tomography using ^{11}C labeled amino acids. *J. Comput. Assist. Tomogr.* **6**: 544–550, 1982.
62. Syrota, A., Comar, D., Cerf, M. *et al.*, ^{11}C-methionine pancreatic scanning with positron-emission computed tomography. *J. Nucl. Med.* **20**: 778–782, 1979.
63. Ericson, K., Li, J. A. A., Bergstrom, M. *et al.*, Positron-emission tomography with (^{11}C methyl)-L-methionine, ^{11}C-D-glucose and ^{68}Ga EDTA in supratentorial tumors. *J. Comput. Assist. Tomogr.* **9**: 683–689, 1985.
64. Schober, O., Meyer, G. J., Goab, M. R. *et al.*, Grading brain tumors by C-11-L-methionine PET. *J. Nucl. Med.* **27**: A58, 1986.
65. Schober, O., Duden, C., Meyer, G. J. *et al.*, Non-selective transport of (^{11}C-methyl)-L- and D-methionine into a malignant glioma. *Eur. J. Nucl. Med.* **13**: 103–105, 1987.

66. Bergstrom, M., Ericson, K., Hagenfeldt, L. et al., PET study of methionine accumulation in glioma and normal brain tissue: Competition with branched chain amino acids. J. Comput. Assist. Tomogr. 11: 208–213, 1987.
67. McDonald, J. M., Gelbard, A. S., Clarke, L. D. et al., Imaging of tumors involving bone with ^{13}N glutamic acid. Radiology 120: 623–626, 1976.
68. Reiman, R. E., Rosen, G., Gelbard, A. S. et al., Imaging of primary Ewing sarcoma with ^{13}N-L-glutamate. Radiology 142: 495–500, 1982.
69. Knapp, W. H., Helus, F., Sinn, H. et al., N-13 L-glutamate uptake in malignancy: its relationship to blood flow. J. Nucl. Med. 25: 989–994, 1984.
70. Vaalburg, W., Ishiwata, K., Elsinga, H. et al., L-(1-C-11) tyrosine for the measurement of protein synthesis in tumor and brain with positron-emission tomography. J. Nucl. Med. 27: A711, 1986.
71. Janne, J., Poso, H. and Raina, A., Polyamines in rapid growth and cancer. Biochim. Biophys. Acta. 573: 241–293, 1978.
72. Horn, Y., Beal, S. L., Walach, N. et al., Further evidence for the use of polyamines as biochemical markers of normal and malignant growth. Cancer Res. 42: 3248–3251, 1982.
73. Fulton, D. S., Levin, L. A., Lubich, W. P. et al., Cerebrospinal fluid polyamines in patients with glioblastoma multiforme and anaplastic astrocytoma. Cancer Res. 40: 3293–3296, 1980.
74. Harik, S. L. and Sutton, C. H., Putrescine as a biochemical marker of malignant brain tumors. Cancer Res. 39: 5010–5015, 1979.
75. Volkow, N., Goldman, S. S., Flamm, E. S. et al., Labeled putrescine as a probe in brain tumors. Science 221: 673–675, 1983.
76. Jerabeck, P. A., Dence, C. S. and Kilbourn, M. R., Synthesis and uptake of no carrier added 1-(^{11}C) putrescine into rat prostate. Int. J. Nucl. Med. Biol. 12: 349–352, 1985.
77. Hiesiger, E., Fowler, J. S., Wolf, A. P. et al., Serial studies of human cerebral malignancy with (1-^{11}C) putrescine and (1-^{11}C) 2-deoxy-D-glucose. J. Nucl. Med. 28: 1251–1261, 1987.
78. Kilbourn, M. R. and Zalutsky, M. R., Research and clinical potential of receptor based radiopharmaceuticals. J. Nucl. Med. 26: 655–662, 1985.
79. Perlmutter, J. S., Larson, K. B., Raichle, M. E. et al., Strategies for in vivo measurement of receptor binding using positron-emission tomography. J. Cereb. Blood Flow Metab. 6: 154–169, 1986.
80. Wong, D. F., Wagner, H. N., Dannals, R. F. et al., Effects of age on dopamine and serotin receptors measured by positron tomography in the living human brain. Science 226: 1393–1396, 1984.
81. Charbonnea, P., Syrota, A., Crouzel, C. et al., Peripheral type benzodiazepene receptors in the living heart characterized by positron-emission tomography. Circulation 73: 476–483, 1986.
82. Larson, S. M. and Di Chiro, G., Comparative anatomo-functional imaging of two neuroreceptors and glucose metabolism: A PET study performed in the living baboon. J. Comput. Assist. Tomogr. 9: 676–681, 1985.
83. McElveny, K. D., Carlson, K. E., Velch, M. E. et al., In vivo comparison of 16α – (^{77}Br) bromoestradiol-17β and 16α ^{125}I iodoestradiol-17β. J. Nucl. Med. 23: 420–426, 1982.
84. Brodack, J. W., Kilbourn, M. R., Welch, M. J. et al., Application of robotics to radiopharmaceutical preparation: controlled synthesis of fluorine-18 16α-fluoroestradiol-17β. J. Nucl. Med. 27: 714–721, 1986.
85. Chan, S. Y. and Sikora, K., Monoclonal antibodies in oncology. Radiother. Oncol. 6: 1–14, 1986.

86. Yuan, M., Itzkowitz, S. H. and Boland, S. R., Comparison of T-antigen expression in normal, premalignant and malignant human colonic tissues using lectin and antibody immunohistochemistry. *Cancer Res.* **46**: 4841–4847, 1986.
87. Early, J. F., Link, J. M., Kishore, R. *et al.*, Production of positron-emitting zirconium 89 for antibody imaging by PET. *J. Nucl. Med.* **27**: A437, 1986.
88. Grunbaum, Z., Freauff, S. J., Krohn, K. A. *et al.*, Synthesis and characterization of congeners of misonidazole for imaging hypoxia. *J. Nucl. Med.* **28**: 68–75, 1987.
89. Nieweg, O. E., Beekhuis, H., Spaans, A. M. J. *et al.*, Detection of lung cancer with [55]Co-bleomycin using a positron camera: A comparison with [57]Co-bleomycin and [55]Co-bleomycin single photon scintigraphy. *Eur. J. Nucl. Med.* **7**: 104–109, 1982.
90. Roberts, J. J. and Thomson, A. J., The mechanism of action of antitumor platinum compounds. *Prog. Nucleic Acid Res. Mol. Biol.* **22**: 71–133, 1979.
91. De Spiegeleer, B., Slegers, G. and Vande Casseele, C. *et al.*, Microscale synthesis of N-13 labeled cis-platinum. *J. Nucl. Med.* **27**: 399–403, 1986.
92. Tyler, J. L., Yamamoto, Y. L., Diksic, M. *et al.*, Pharmacokinetics of superselective intra-arterial and intravenous (^{11}C) BCNU evaluated by PET. *J. Nucl. Med.* **27**: 775–780, 1986.
93. Jones, T., The application of positron-emission tomography. In: *Computed Emission Tomography*, Oxford University Press, pp. 221–239, 1982.

21

The Predictive Possibilities for NMR in Oncology

Truman R. Brown

INTRODUCTION

There are many variables which may affect the outcome of a particular treatment regimen in individual patients. What information can we expect to obtain from nuclear magnetic resonance (NMR) that will be helpful in assessing these variables in individual patients? Can NMR be used to predict the effectiveness of a particular regimen? Can it be used to predict the sensitivity of an individual patient to toxic side effects? Can it follow the response of tumors on an individual basis? These are obviously broad questions and it is unlikely that a single technique can hope to answer them all—or even a majority of them—affirmatively. The information provided by NMR is related to the metabolic state of the tissue under study. As these relationships are defined, it is reasonable to expect that some of the above questions will be answered in the affirmative.

Due to the very recent introduction of NMR into clinical medicine, there are no known predictors of tumor treatment response today. This chapter will, therefore, discuss reasonable future expectations which are based upon preliminary studies in both animals and humans, and suggest which possible variables can be measured. The paucity of clinical information is due to the quite recent development of magnets large enough to observe patients at high fields (> 1.5T). This field strength is needed to obtain metabolic information from studies of nuclei other than protons. In fact, it is generally thought that the potential utility of NMR in this area rests on its ability to observe biochemically relevant compounds, non-invasively, in intact tissue. It must be remembered, however, that the NMR relaxation times of water protons are dependent upon tumor properties in a complex way, so that proton images may provide physiological information as well. Considerations like

297

these led to the initial hopes that variations in proton relaxation times might become a diagnostic tool. Unfortunately, no reliable correlation has been established, to date, between a given relaxation time and particular pathology or its progression.

NMR observations can be divided into two broad areas: those related to imaging the anatomy and those related to spectroscopic studies— which rely on the ability of NMR to provide information about the different chemical constituents inside tissue. The physical basis of NMR rests on the fact that many stable nuclei have a magnetic moment which can be made to interact with external magnetic fields at a specific frequency. Obviously, the details of how these interactions occur are beyond the scope of this article. The local environment around the nucleus, the molecule in which it is located, its speed, and the composition of the surrounding solution all contribute to the nature of the signal received. The anatomical information is obtained by observing the signals from protons in water and lipids while varying the strength of the magnetic field across the patient in a controlled way. An image is then reconstructed from the resultant signals. Typically, submillimeter resolution can be obtained. Depending on the details of how the NMR signals are acquired, variations in the relaxation times of the spins (T_1 and T_2) can contribute significantly to the image contrast. These relaxation times are particularly sensitive to the local environment and may provide a way for tumor properties to influence proton images.

Spectroscopic studies can observe biochemical compounds because they resonate at unique frequencies for differing compounds. By observing the variation in levels of metabolites or shifts in their resonant frequencies, information on the metabolic state and ionic composition of the tissue under investigation can be obtained. Because of the non-invasive character of the measurements, they can be repeated and, therefore, the time response of the tissue can be followed as well. Many of the compounds observed, particularly those which contain ^{31}P, are involved in bioenergetic pathways and provide information on how well-energized the tissues are. Because of the differences in concentrations between water and most other biochemically important species, the spatial resolution of the anatomic information is much better than that of metabolic information.

NMR signals thus have the potential to be sensitive to molecular behavior and structure as well as to biochemical and physiological states. It is this sensitivity which raises the expectation that NMR will be useful in distinguishing tumor properties. For example: (1) can the change in proton relaxation times between different classes of tumors be used to predict biological behavior; (2) can the differences observed in the ^{31}P NMR spectra of different tumors be used to determine the response of a particular tumor to therapy; (3) do the metabolic differences observable by ^{13}C NMR indicate different classes of tumor, and (4) is there sufficient information in the NMR measured morphology of a tumor to act as a predictive indicator? The answer to these and similar questions will require considerable research.

IMAGING

Proton imaging techniques produce cross-sectional metabolic maps by applying well-defined magnetic fields across the object being imaged and then untangling the resultant complex frequencies detected from the protons in the object. By varying the details of the excitation and detection, one can develop sensitivity to several different NMR parameters: the proton density, the longitudinal relaxation time (T_1), and the transverse relaxation time (T_2). In addition, the images are sensitive to motion of all sorts, from the molecular to the macroscopic level. In general, these images provide both anatomical information and details about the environment of the water molecules in a given volume. From them, it is possible to determine the relative amounts of fat and water.

The nature of anatomical information is clear. The question is whether images of tumors are likely to be helpful in staging, for example. In certain cases this seems to be true. Studies by McNeal et al.[1] on prostate cancer suggest that high-resolution images of the prostate would be very useful in making diagnoses and in planning treatment strategies. Specially designed coils for prostate examination can acquire images with a few tenths of a millimeter resolution. At this resolution, the anatomical information should be sufficient for classification. In general, however, it is not possible to obtain images with the high resolution needed for histopathology, so expectations that NMR images can provide an *in vivo* pathology examination are unrealistic. Thus, in most cases, an NMR image can localize the tumor, the extent of its spread, and perhaps any lymph node involvement. It will probably be unable, however, to determine cell type, degree of differentiation, and other histopathological information.

In addition to the high quality anatomical images provided by NMR, considerable information about the local distribution of water and lipids can be obtained. Local water relaxation times, T_1's and T_2's, are sensitive to the relative water concentration as well as to the details of the molecular interactions of water with its surroundings, including the local protein and ion concentrations. As is well known, there were early hopes that the T_1's and T_2's would add an additional dimension to imaging and aid in diagnostic studies.[2] This has not been the case to date. In part, this is because the range of parameters which will influence the water relaxation rates is so great that many different phenomena can contribute to the same change in relaxation time, making it difficult to untangle causal connections. In addition, present imaging techniques have a number of artifacts in the measurement of relaxation times. Thus, there is a large body of literature reporting T_1 and T_2 times for various pathologies which, unfortunately, suggests the variability is so large as to make them diagnostically useless. In a comprehensive review of normal and pathological relaxation times, Bottomley et al. [3,4] pointed out numerous reasons for this, concluding that relaxation times could not be viewed as diagnostic at this point in time. However, they also noted that there are a number of important factors which may lead to systematic errors in the measurement of relaxation times, possibly obscuring a genuine difference between normal and pathologic states as well as among different pathologic states. Thus, it is still not clear whether the differences among the relaxation times in a closely grouped set of tumors might be useful, if not for initial staging, then perhaps as a measure of the responsiveness of the tumor to a particular therapy. Here, because each tumor can serve as its own control, it may be possible to see early significant changes. Whether these will correlate with response remains to be determined.

Another important point to consider is whether the difference between normal and pathological tissue in the same individual is a significant predictor. Most of the studies have considered the relaxation times of the tumor alone, rather than comparing it with normal tissue values in the same patient. It may be that ratios or differences will be able to remove some of the present scatter in the data. For example, normal lymph nodes seem to be distinguishable from cancerous ones, at least after surgical removal.[5] If these results can be extended in vivo then they could serve as a clear indicator for the appropriate treatment.

Recent results suggest, at least for certain tumors, a strong correlation between the response of the tumor to radiotherapy and their oxygenation level, as measured by the direct oxygen electrode.[6] Can we determine the local oxygen concentrations or degrees of perfusion in the tumor from changes in relaxation rates? What happens as the oxygen concentration of the air the patient breathes is varied? The development of techniques sensitive to local perfusion would not only aid in this area but could be used to identify ischemic tumors in general.

This information could then be used to select a particular form of therapy optimized to work on an ischemic or non-ischemic tumor, as appropriate. Changes during the course of therapy could also be monitored and appropriate measures taken. More speculative is whether a connection between changes in the relaxation times of protons in a tumor could be correlated with the response of a tumor. Note that this is different from correlating the initial relaxation times with tumor response. Instead, the question is whether measuring changes induced by a particular regimen, either radiotherapeutic or chemotherapeutic, would allow us to predict response earlier than is possible with present techniques.

As stated earlier, we still do not have a firm understanding of the contributing factors which determine the apparent relaxation times. Contributing factors range from local protein concentration, ion composition, degree of perfusion, amount of local perfusion, as well as other parameters which could be affected by the response of a tumor to treatment. In the absence of both a general theory of NMR relaxation and an understanding of the biology of tumor response, it is impossible to make predictions. A series of careful studies will be worthwhile in this area, given both its importance and complexity.

SPECTROSCOPY

In spectroscopic studies, NMR is used to obtain information about the chemical structure and state of intracellular molecules. It should be possible to obtain metabolic information related to the physiological state of the tissue under examination. Unfortunately, because of the low concentration of many of the relevant metabolites—typically 5 to 10 mM—the sensitive volumes which can be examined in humans by this type of NMR must be as large as 5 to 10 ml. The nuclei which can be studied by these techniques are ^{1}H, ^{13}C, ^{19}F, ^{23}Na and ^{31}P. So far, the majority of information has been obtained for ^{31}P—with some preliminary studies measuring ^{1}H, ^{13}C, ^{19}F, and ^{23}Na.

The bulk of NMR spectroscopy, both in humans and animals, has measured ^{31}P as an indicator of the energetic state of the tumor under consideration. [7-15] For the purpose of discussion, assume that it will be possible to obtain ^{31}P spectra of sufficient sensitivity from a 5 to 10 ml region to be able to determine concentrations of ATP to an accuracy of 10% in 30 minutes. This is a difficult experimental problem, but reasonable extrapolations from animal data and the few preliminary human experiments which have been done suggest that this is feasible. Early animal data universally suggest that, given sufficiently strong therapy, the response of the tumor can be followed by examining its energetic state through ^{31}P NMR.[11-13] In most cases the amount of drug used was larger than the standard clinical dose. Thus, changes which may occur in a patient over an extended period have not been observed in animals. This is particularly true of the major changes in phosphorus metabolism which have been observed in rats and mice. Reports of similar behavior[7-11] in humans have been made, although the changes observed are more complex. A recent study by Gademann et al.[14] followed aggressive therapy by isolating the arterial perfusion in a human leg with high concentrations of drug, while simultaneously observing the ^{31}P NMR spectra. The changes observed in the spectrum of the tumor following treatment were similar to what had been observed in animals. Another recent study[15] reported observable differences between adriamycin-sensitive and resistant murine tumors both before and after treatment. If similar measurements can be made with human tumors, spectroscopic observation may be of considerable value in distinguishing between responsive and non-responsive tumors.

An another area of utility of the ^{31}P NMR spectra may be in evaluating normal tissue toxicity. For example, one of the limiting factors in the use of adriamycin is cardiotoxicity. Studies on isolated hearts have observed the effects of both acute and chronic toxicity.[16,17] The ^{31}P NMR spectrum of the myocardium may be able to determine those patients who are more sensitive to adriamycin than the average and modulate their treatment appropriately.

An unexpected finding is that there are high levels of phosphomonoesters (PME) and phosphodiesters (PDE) observed in virtually all tumors.[18,19] The PMEs are generally either phosphorocholine (PC) or phosphoroethylolamine (PE). The PDEs are glycerophosphocholine, glycerophosphoethylolamine, glycerophosphoserine, glycerophosphoglycerol, and glycerophosphoinositol. Whether these observations are relevant to the fundamental biological character of the tumors is unclear at present. However, one possibility is that the high levels of PMEs are due to an increased activity of phospholipase C, which acts to split phospholipids between the glycerol and phosphate moieties, producing a diacylglycerol (DAG) and a phosphomonoester, the exact nature of which depends upon the phospholipid. Since DAG stimulates protein kinase C, a kinase known to be involved in the initiation of cell growth,[20] it may be that at least part of the biochemical defect in these tumors is an active phospholipase which is observed through its effect on the level of PMEs, measurable by NMR. Thus, a knowledge of the levels of these compounds in a particular tumor could very well be related to its biological state. This is clearly very speculative; however, there is no doubt that the metabolism of phosphomono- and diester in tumors is different from normal tissue. Even in the brain, which normally has high levels of these compounds, both PMEs and PDEs are observed to be increased in brain tumors.[11] Since these compounds seem to be present at millimolar levels and can be observed *in vivo* in many circumstances, they have considerable potential for developing into one of the important predictors of tumor response observable by NMR as their metabolism is further elucidated.

Following the *in vivo* metabolism of certain drugs may be possible as well, e.g., a fluorinated drug such as 5FU or a ^{13}C labeled drug. Although it may not be possible to follow the biochemistry of the drug inside the tumor because of size or concentration limitations, the potential exists to determine normal tissue toxicity in a unique way. Several animal studies have been carried out, examining both tumor response and liver toxicity for various levels of drug.[21] Patients tumors and livers have been examined following a 5FU bolus.[22] As yet, there has been insufficient time to determine whether the varying kinetic constants in the disappearance of 5FU and the appearance of its various metabolites can be correlated with response of the patient.

Finally, one must consider the potential for proton spectroscopy in the area of tumor response prediction. The proton spectrum from biological tissue contains a large amount of information. Unfortunately, the presence of the huge water resonance makes it difficult to observe other metabolites at mM concentrations. As has been known for many years, tumors produce substantial amounts of lactic acid. Is it possible to predict, based upon the presence of differing amounts of lactic acid, the behavior of a particular tumor? Can such data predict tumor aggressiveness? Do those tumors which metabolize glucose rapidly grow faster, or is there no correlation between the rate of glucose metabolism and the rate of growth of the tumor? The answers to these questions must await further research.

CONCLUSIONS

It is clear that we are still in a very preliminary stage of understanding the nature of the information which can be obtained from NMR observations of tumors. Not only are we uncertain about the quality of information that can be obtained, we have not yet established its significance to the clinical setting. Over the last ten years, there has been a substantial amount of work with cells, animal tissues and human tissues on the physiological consequences of changes in ATP levels and other high-energy phosphates.[23,24] Most of these studies are based upon the fact that muscle is an energy-transducing machine which is reflected in its levels of ATP and phosphocreatine. Therefore, its operation and many of its diseased states are associated with changes in its energy levels, which can be observed by ^{31}P NMR. Unfortunately, tumors do not have such a simple physiology and have much less clear energetic relationships in terms of input/output. This makes it much more difficult to evaluate and to interpret the ^{31}P spectra which have been obtained. Nevertheless, the unifying characteristic of phosphomonoesters and phosphodiesters which have been observed in virtually all tumors are suggestive, as pointed out above, of the possibility of a common pattern of biochemical and metabolic disorder in these tumors. If this indeed turns out to be correct, then we may have found a window into some of the fundamental processes which underly the disturbance of the cellular proliferative controls that are fundamental to the cause of cancer. It seems likely that NMR measurements of tumor metabolism will be useful in understanding the tumor's response to therapy. To achieve this, we will need to improve our present detection and localization techniques as well as continue with research designed to understand the consequences of variations in the spectroscopic and imaging variables among tumors and following therapy.

ACKNOWLEDGMENT

This work was supported by NIH Grants CA06927 and CA41078.

REFERENCES

1. McNeal *et al.*, this volume.
2. Hazlewood, C. F., Chang, D. C., Medima, D., Cleveland, G. and Nichols, B. L., Distinction between the preneoplastic and neoplastic state of murine mammary glands. *Proc. Natl. Acad. Sci. USA* **69**: 1478–1480, 1972.
3. Bottomley, P. A., Hardy, C. J., Argersinger, R. E. and Allen-Moore, G., A review of ^{1}H nuclear magnetic resonance relaxation in pathology: Are T_1 and T_2 diagnostic? *Med. Phys.* **14**: 1–37, 1987.
4. Bottomley, P. A., Foster, T. H., Argersinger, R. E. and Pfeifer, L. M., Normal tissue hydrogen NMR relaxation times and relaxation mechanisms from 1–100 MHz—dependence on tissue type, NMR frequency, temperature, species, excision and age. *Med. Phys.* **11**: 425–428, 1984.
5. Fossel, E. T., Brodsky, G., DeLayre, J. L. and Wilson, R. E., Nuclear magnetic resonance for the differentiation of benign and malignant breast tissues and axillary lymph nodes. *Ann. Surg.* **198**: 541–545, 1983.
6. Gatenby, R. A., Kessler, H. B., Rosenblum, J. S., Coia, J. A., Moldofsky, P. J., Hartz, W. H. and Broder, G. J., Oxygen distribution in squamous cell carcinoma metastases: Relationship to outcome of radiation therapy. Submitted to *Int. J. Rad. Onc. Biol. Phys.* **14**: 831–838, 1988.

7. Griffiths, J. R., Cady, E., Edwards, R. H. T., McCready, V. R., Wilkie, D. R. and Wiltshaw, E., ^{31}P-NMR studies of a human tumor in situ. *Lancet*, June 25, 1435–1436, 1983.

8. Maris, J. M., Audrey, B. S., Evans, E., McLaughlin, A. C., D'Angio, G. J., Bolinger, L., Manos, H. and Chance, B., [31]P Nuclear magnetic resonance spectroscopic investigation of human neuroblastoma in situ. *New Eng. J. Med.* **312**: 1500–1505, 1985.

9. Ross, B., Marshall, V., Smith, M., Bartlett, S. and Freeman, D., Monitoring response to chemotherapy of intact human tumors by ^{31}P nuclear magnetic resonance. *Lancet* **1**: 641–464, 1984.

10. Segebart, G., Baleriaux, G., Arnold, D. L., Luyten, P. R. and den Hollander, J. A., Image-guided localized ^{31}P MR spectroscopy of human brain tumors in situ: Effect of treatment. *Radiol.* **165**: 215–219, 1987.

11. Oberhaensli, R. D., Bore, P. J., Rampling, R. P., Hilton-Jones, D., Hands, L. J. and Radda, G. K., Biochemical investigation of human tumors *in vivo* with phosphorus-31 magnetic resonance spectroscopy. *Lancet*, **8–11**: 1986.

12. Ng, T. C., Evanochko, W. T., Hiramoto, R. N., *et al.*, ^{31}P NMR spectroscopy of *in vivo* tumors. *J. Mag. Res.* **49**: 271–286, 1982.

13. Naruse, S., Horikawa, Y., Tanaka, C., Higuchi, T., Sekimoto, H., Ueda, S. and Hirakawa, K., Evaluation of the effects of photoradiation therapy on brain tumors with *in vivo* P-31 MR spectroscopy. *Radiol.* **160**: 827–830, 1986.

14. Gademann, G., Semmler, W., Bachert-Baumann, P., Zabel, H. J., van Kaick, G. and W. J. Lorenz, 31-P spectroscopy follow-up studies of human tumors after chemotherapy. *Abstract*, p. 587, S.M.R.M. Meeting, New York, Aug. 17–21, 1987.

15. Evelhoch, J. L., Keller, N. A. and Corbett, T. H., Response-specific Adriamycin sensitivity markers provided by *in vivo* [31]P nuclear magnetic resonance spectroscopy in murine mammary adenocarcinomas. *Can. Res.* **47**: 3396–3401, 1987.

16. Ng, T. C., Daugherty, J. P., Evanochko, W. T., Digerness, S. B., Durant, J. R. and Glickson, J. D., Detection of antineoplastic agent induced cardiotoxicity by ^{31}P NMR of perfused rat hearts. *Biochem. Biophys. Res. Comm.* **110**: 339–347, 1983.

17. Keller, A. M., Jackson, J. A., Peshock, R. M., Rehr, R. B., Willerson, J. T., Nunnally, R. L. and Buja, L., Nuclear magnetic resonance study of high-energy phosphate stores in models of adriamycin cardioxicity. *Mag. Res. Med.* **3**: 834–843, 1986.

18. Evanochko, E. T., Ng, T. C. and Glickson, J. D., Application of *in vivo* NMR spectroscopy of cancer. *J. Mag. Res.* **1**: 508–534, 1984.

19. Brown, T. R., Graham, R. A., Szwergold, B. S., Thoma, W. J. and Meyer, R. A., Phosphorylated metabolites in tumors, tissues and cell lines. Annals. New York Academy of Sciences, **508**: 229–240, 1987.

20. Kikkawa, U. and Nishizuka, Y., The role of protein kinase C in transmembrane signaling. *Ann. Rev. Cell Biol.* **2**: 149–178, 1986.

21. Stevens, A. N., Morris, P. G., Iles, R. A., Sheldon, P. W. and Griffiths, J. R., 5-Fluorouracil metabolism monitored *in vivo* by ^{19}F NMR. *Br. J. Can.* **50**: 113–117, 1984.

22. Wolf, W., Albright, M. J., Silver, M. S., Webber, H., Reichardt, U. and Sauer, R., Fluorine-19 NMR spectroscopic studies of the metabolism of 5-Fluorouracil in the liver of patients undergoing chemotherapy. *Mag. Res. Imag.* **5**: 165–169, 1987.

23. Meyer, R. A., Kushmerick, M. J. and Brown, T. R., Application of [31] P-NMR spectroscopy to the study of striated muscle metabolism. *Am. J. Physiol.* **242**: C1–C11, 1982.

24. Shulman, R. G., Brown, T. R., Ugurbil, K., Ogawa, S., Cohen, S. M. and den Hollander, J. A., Cellular applications of ^{31}P and ^{13}C nuclear magnetic resonance. *Science* **205**: 160–166, 1979.

22

Commentary on Part V: Tumor Physiology and Metabolic Imaging

Robert M. Sutherland, Gordon, F. Whitmore, and Kenneth A. Krohn

The outcome of non-surgical regimens for the treatment of malignancy depends primarily on two factors: effective delivery of the toxic agent(s) and the response of both tumor and normal cells to the agent(s). It is becoming increasingly clear that tumor tissues are heterogeneous. In addition to intertumor variations which may be largely under genetic control, there are intratumor heterogeneities which arise as a result of physiological variations, such as cellular metabolism, proliferation state, and drug exposure, in microenvironments within a single tumor.

The concept of intratumor heterogeneity necessitates the measurement of cell subpopulations which may play a major role in determining long-term outcome, even if they play a relatively small role in determining short-term response. In the evaluation of any predictive assay, it is therefore important to consider whether it is a predictor of short-term response or long-term outcome. The distinction is important.

A great deal of current interest relates to the potential use of non-invasive techniques, such as nuclear medicine, positron-emission tomography (PET), magnetic resonance imaging (MRI), and magnetic resonance spectroscopy (MRS) as predictors of tumor physiology, optimum treatment protocols and, ultimately, of outcome. Many of these approaches are new and must be evaluated in model systems where the underlying biology is reasonably well-understood and where the non-invasive approach can be validated.

Since the discovery that nitro aromatic radiosensitizer are preferentially toxic to hypoxic cells, some research has focused on their potential use as detectors of hypoxic cell populations which are likely to be critical determinants of the long-term outcome of radiation therapy and which, for other reasons, may be resistant to conventional chemotherapy. Evidence was presented by Rasey et al. (E-1) and Raleigh et al. (E-2) that fluorinated derivatives of 2-nitroimidazoles preferentially localized in hypoxic regions of animal tumors and that these adducts could be detected by either Anger camera or MRI. Attempts to use bromine substituted 2-nitroimidazoles (King and Bolomey, E-4) have been less successful.

In a study of thirteen patients, Urtasun et al. (E-3) showed that ^{3}H misonidazole could label human tumors in vivo and be detected after surgical excision by autoradiography. None of the five high grade sarcomas exhibited significant labeling, but six of six small cell lung carcinomas and one melanoma all exhibited significant labeling, presumably indicating hypoxic cells. In one squamous cell carcinoma of the tongue, the tumor failed to exhibit significant labeling, but there was labeling of adjacent normal epithelial tissue.

While the use of labeled sensitizers to identify hypoxic cell fractions appears potentially useful, several questions remain to be answered. Are experimental animal tumors typical of human tumors? Is labeling specific to hypoxic cells and are labeled cells viable? In this connection, the observation by Hlatky and Sachs (E-21) that aerobic cells which have been previously exposed to hypoxia will continue to localize 2-nitroimidazoles, is of concern. Does the observed binding of sensitizers to normal tissues predict possible sensitization of normal tissue response by sensitizers? Can one hope to detect the oxygenation state of viable cells following treatment? Can simplified methods such as biopsy, PET or MRI detect the presence of minority hypoxic cell fractions?

With respect to the latter question, radiobiological studies of the RIF-1 and SCK tumors (Song et al. E-9) have indicated hypoxic cell fractions of 8% and 40%, respectively. However, repeated oxygen probe measurements yielded essentially identical average values of PO_2 for the two tumors. Since the average PO_2 is essentially a bulk measure, similar to what might be obtained by low resolution PET or MRI approaches, these observations suggest limitations to the usefulness of noninvasive approaches for the determination of hypoxic cell fractions within tumors.

The advent of PET scanning has increased interest in the use of labeled compounds such as thymidine, glucose, and deoxyglucose as indicators of tumor physiology. While it is commonly assumed that thymidine labeling is a measure of DNA synthesis, a recent study of thymidine utilization in heart, liver, and spleen by Shields *et al.* (E-6) points out a variety of possible confounding effects. These include: (1) competition by endogenous synthesis, (2) differential uptakes of $_3$H– and ^{14}C–thymidine and (3) reutilization of thymidine and its breakdown products. Presumably, as a result of the latter, while spleen shows approximately 85% of label incorporated into DNA, liver shows less than 15% of incorporated thymidine localized to DNA. Although it is not clear to what extent the observations of thymidine uptake in relatively slowly metabolizing normal tissues are typical of more rapidly dividing tumor tissue, the observations suggest that care must be exercised in the interpretation of thymidine uptake studies.

The Sokoloff deoxyglucose method is often used to measure glucose metabolism in brain and tumor tissue. It is often assumed that the rate constants involved in the determination are similar for all components of brain and also for normal tissue. Recent studies by Graham *et al.* (E-8), show significant differences between various components of brain and also between tumor and normal brain. Such differences could markedly affect the interpretation and the authors suggest that the determination of separate constants for normal and tumor tissue should be made and perhaps the necessity to revise these values during the course of therapy would follow.

Tumor blood flow may play a role in determining the outcome of radiation therapy, chemotherapy, and hyperthermia. Because many of the higher energy radiations used for radiation therapy can induce the production of short-lived positron-emitting isotopes, it was suggested by Roberts *et al.* (E-5) that this activity might be used to estimate tissue mass, and composition, blood volume, and blood flow within the irradiated volume. Preliminary tests have been carried out in rodents and in man but, given the inherent logistical problems—the necessity to analyze complex buildup and decay curves and the mixed physiology within the irradiated volume—it seems unlikely that the approach will gain wide applicability.

Combinations of chemotherapeutic agents and radiation are often used in the treatment of brain malignancies, posing the question of whether radiation might affect drug delivery either because of effects on blood flow or vascular permeability. In a preliminary study, Spence *et al.* (E-7) showed that 20 Gy of photon radiation has no effect on blood flow within the first twenty-four hours, but may cause a transient decrease in the transport of water soluble agents to brain tumors. Whether such an effect would be detected following a conventional fractionated radiation exposure and whether it would affect conventional chemotherapeutic regimens has not been established.

Several laboratories have investigated ^{31}P magnetic resonance spectroscopy (MRS) as a method to evaluate tumor energy status as a reflection of oxygenation and blood flow. As tumors in rodents increase in size, NTP, PCr and pH decrease while Pi increases (Sutherland et al. (E-11), Stein et al. (E-15), Rajan et al. (E-14), and Okunieff et al. (E-13)). The effect of 100% inspired oxygen on in vivo tumor metabolism was also examined by Okunieff et al. (E-13). This increases the PCr/Pi ratio while breathing 10% oxygen, decreases PCr and ATP, and increases Pi. Interestingly, no changes in these parameters were observed in resting skeletal muscle and brain. It appears that the fractional increase in PCr/Pi which occurs after breathing 100% oxygen is a sensitive, non-invasive method of detecting tissue metabolic deficiency.

Responses to therapy have also been measured with ^{31}P MRS. After BCNU treatment of 9L gliosarcomas, tumor cells appeared to be in a more energized state (Steen et al. E-15) the PCr/NTP nearly doubled and Pi/PME decreased by day four post-treatment in tumors which regressed in size. These changes suggest that the surviving cells are more highly energized and the tumor contains a lower proportion of hypoxic or necrotic tissue. Similar observations were made by Rajan et al. (E-14) after radiation treatment of the RIF-1 fibrosarcoma. The ratios of Pi/ATP, PME/ATP, and Pi/PCr decreased significantly by day three post-irradiation, and the pH became more alkaline by day four. There was a dose-dependent rate of recovery of these parameters. These changes reflect the combined effects of cell death, reoxygenation kinetics, and proliferation after irradiation of the tumors.

In a related study of radiation response of human tumors in the clinic, it has been found by Ng et al. (E-12) that squamous cell carcinoma and non-Hodgkin's lymphoma generally do not show the acid pH shift observed by many investigators for tumor growth in rodents. There was a sensitive decrease in PDE after radiation therapy, which was interpreted as effects on cell membranes. During therapy, PDE/ATP continually decreased in some patients but not in others, and was related to response. The pH often became more alkaline after radiation.

Although these studies of ^{31}P MRS have begun to establish the sensitivities of the parameters measured in relation to oxygenation and the dose dependencies for radiation and drugs, they have also raised some questions requiring further consideration. Are human tumors different from rodent tumors in regard to their ability to regulate intracellular pH? The acidic pH values which have been measured in human tumors with microelectrodes may reflect extracellular pH, while nuclear magnetic resonance (NMR) measures may reflect intracellular pH. The location of the Pi compartment in tumors upon which the pH shift is based is not known.

There is no consensus at this time as to which ^{31}P species (or ratios) are most sensitive for following changes in energy status (oxygenation) or responses to therapy. Improvements in ability to detect minor peaks, especially those associated with cellular lipid metabolism, may greatly increase sensitivity and provide important additional information.

There is often considerable scatter in the data obtained. Does this indicate real biological inter-tumor heterogeneity, or does it reflect methodological problems? Certainly, variability in control of physiological factors (such as body temperature) in mice affected by anesthetics or possible problems with positioning of coils for measuring the signals need to be evaluated. Since investigators are beginning to collect spectroscopy and imagining data from tumors in patients, it is time to consider designing controlled clinical trials on selected groups of patients. Such pilot studies should be designed and conducted in close collaboration with oncologists.

Compared with ^{31}P MRS, studies of ^1H have the advantage of sensitivity, since protons and water are present in high concentrations. Relatively small volumes can be studied spectroscopically and also imaged. Tissue factors which are of physiologic and pathologic origin influence the relaxation characteristics (T_1 and T_2) of water protons. Thus, to the extent that such factors are perturbed by therapy and related to certain pathophysiological states, magnetic resonance imaging (MRI) may be used to predict therapeutic effectiveness. Factors which may significantly influence T_1 and T_2 are cell-cycle stage, quiescence, necrosis, and edema (Ngo et al. E-19, and Braunschweiger et al. E-18).

Other basic characteristics of tumor cells associated with the capacity to metastasize are being studied to determine whether they can be measured by ^1H MRS. Decay rates of spin-lattice ($1/T_1$) and spin-spin ($1/T_2$) relaxation times in primary and metastatic disease have been measured (Schmidt et al. E-20). Correlation of decay rates with parameters of malignancy such as survival time and tumor mass have been established.

In other studies using the RIF-1 fibrosarcoma in mice, Braunschweiger et al. (E-18) have investigated effects on T_1 and T_2 associated with cytotoxic tumor reduction with cyclophosphamide. Alterations in factors such as tumor water distribution, blood flow, vascular patency and capillary permeability would be expected to alter T_1 and T_2. These pathophysiological parameters were measured in order to relate them to the MRS measurements. Shortening of T_1 and T_2 was seen as early as twenty-four hours after drug treatment. T_1 shortening and recovery kinetics for T_1 and T_2 were correlated with cytotoxic tumor reduction with cyclophosphamide. Alterations in factors such as tumor water distribution, blood flow, vascular patency, and capillary permeability would be expected to alter T_1 and T_2. These pathophysiological parameters were measured in order to relate them to the MRS measurements. Shortening of T_1 and T_2 was seen as early as twenty-four hours after drug treatment. T_1 shortening and recovery kinetics for T_1 and T_2 were dose-dependent. T_2 recovery preceded T_1 recovery and was temporarily related to recovery of cell proliferation. T_1 recovery preceded tumor growth and was temporarily related to the vascular responses which were associated with the expansion of the surviving cell population and the re-establishment of pretreatment tissue water distribution. Gd-DTPA-dimethyl glucamine enhancement of T_1 relaxation in drug-treated tumors reflected the early increases in tumor extra-cellular water distribution attributable to cell kill and lysis. These interesting data indicate the potential for MRI techniques and paramagnetic contrast enhancers to measure early changes in tissue water distribution as a consequence of therapy, induced cell kill and lysis. It appears that proton MR techniques may provide a useful non-invasive way to serially monitor the changes in tissue water mobility, secondary to physiologic responses to cytotoxic therapy.

In another study of chemotherapeutic response, ^{1}H MRS spectral changes were measured in human ovarian carcinoma cells *in vitro* after treatment with cisplatin. Using 500 MHz high resolution and water suppression methods, Wenger *et al.* (E-17) showed that spectra from poorly viable drug-treated cells differed from untreated controls at nine spectral peak positions. One of these positions (1.17–1.25 ppm) was reduced as early as one hour after exposure to a relatively low dose of drug, which was later determined to reduce clonogenic efficiency by 80%.

The resolution of MRI is high, as demonstrated by the ability to image and discriminate the viable rims (200mm) and necrotic centers of multicell spheroids (Freyer *et al.* E-16, and Sutherland *et al.* E-11). It appears that even greater refinements of resolution are possible using newly developed high resolution MR imaging equipment.

Although these investigators have begun to obtain data required to interpret the biological bases of these results, much more research is required. What is the biological relevance of T_1 and T_2? Increases in

T_1 associated with increase of tumor size may be related to increased or redistributed water compartments. It is possible that poor oxygenation may also affect this parameter. Researchers at this conference have suggested that the changes in T_2 may be more closely related to alterations in cell cycle or growth fractions.

It would be important to continue the studies relating differences in T_2 to metastatic potential in order to determine whether metastatic potential among tumors of similar size can be distinguished. It also appears that there would be significant advantages to combining imaging with spectroscopy of the same tumors. It may be possible, for example, to observe multifocal necrosis, indicative of heterogeneous microenvironments. These techniques should also be actively pursued in order to monitor normal tissue changes induced by therapy. In addition to predicting relative responses of different tumors to therapy, MRS and MRI could be valuable as monitoring techniques during therapy in order to determine scheduling; for example, reoxygenation kinetics could be measured.

Several new methods are being developed which show promise for providing important supplemental data which will be helpful in interpreting some of the ^{31}P MRS studies. ^{13}C MRS studies of chemical probes containing a sulfur atom of phosphorothioates indicate that these probes are sensitive to redox state (Golden *et al.* E-10). There is a chemical shift of the ^{13}C next to the sulfur, depending upon whether it is reduced or oxidized. It appears possible to measure the redox state in volumes as small as 1 cm^3.

Directions to be pursued related to these methods include studies of the specificity of redox probes for S-S/SH (GSH) and the *in vivo* applicability in different tissues. The possibilities for high resolution imaging to reveal other substrates also requires further investigation. These methods, in association with new paramagnetic probes to increase sensitivity and discrimination, may prove very powerful tools.

Other methods discussed at this meeting, such as cryospectrophotometry (Sutherland *et al.* E-11 and Mueller-Klieser *et al.* Chapter 19) and bioluminescence (Mueller-Klieser *et al.* Chapter 19) provide detailed information on microregional distribution of important substrates. These and other quantitative computer-interfaced methods to study metabolites in tumor cell microenvironments, including necrosis before, during and after therapy, will provide critical data to assist interpretation of other non-invasive methods such as MRS and MRI.

Positron-emission tomography (PET) can provide quantitative dynamic information on tumor functional metabolism using various substrates labeled with positron emitters such as ^{15}O, ^{13}N, ^{11}C, and ^{18}F (see Chapter 20). Specific functional differences between tumors and surrounding normal tissues are being identified. These include blood flow, fractional extraction of oxygen, glycolytic activity, and uptake of amino acids and drugs such as FdUrd and BCNU. Data for uptake and retention of BCNU provide some prediction of how tumors will respond. One limitation of PET is its resolution, at best—5–8mm. However, integration of this technique with some of the others should provide very powerful predictive potential for tumor response to therapy.

It is apparent that there is a great deal of current interest in the development of non-invasive approaches for determining tumor physiology with the ultimate aim of altering the outcome of treatment. At the present time most of these approaches are in the experimental stage, and a great deal of both basic science and clinical evaluation remains to be done. As these developments proceed, there will need to be cross-comparisons between clinical laboratory measurements, and it will be important throughout that we do not lose sight of what is already known about tumor biology, in particular the potential problem of intratumor heterogeneity resulting from microenvironments.

POSTERS

(E-1) Tumor Hypoxia Imaging with F-18 Fluoromisonidazole. J. S. Rasey, E. G. Shankland, Z. Grunbaum, A. M. Spence, K. A. Krohn, G. V. Martin, J. H. Caldwell, C. A. Mathis, Y. Yano and T. F. Budinger. University of Washington, Seattle, Washington and Seattle VAH Medical Center, Seattle, Washington and Lawrence Berkeley Laboratory, Berkeley, California.

(E-2) F-19 Magnetic Resonance Spectroscopic Detection of Hypoxic Cells in Experimental Tumors: Correlation with Fluorescence Immunohistochemistry, Autoradiography and Scintillation Counting. J. A. Raleigh, A. J. Franko, G. G. Miller, P. S. Allen, L. Trimble and D. A. Kelly. Cross Cancer Institute and University of Alberta, 11560 University Avenue, Edmonton, Alberta, Canada T6G 1Z2.

(E-3) The Measurement of Hypoxic Cells in Solid Human Tumors by the "Misonidazole Binding" Technique. R. C. Urtasun, J. D. Chapman, J. A. Raleigh, A. J. Franko, C. J. Koch and S. McKinnon. Department of Radiation Oncology, Cross Cancer Institute and the Department of Radiology and Diagnostic Imaging, University of Alberta, Edmonton, Alberta, Canada T6G 1Z2.

(E-4) The Synthesis and Evaluation of Radiobromine Labeled Misonidazole Analogs as Hypoxic Tumor Imaging Agents. A. J. Kolar, R. S. Tilbury, G. K. King and L. A. Bolomey. University of Texas System Cancer Center and Medical School, Houston, Texas.

(E-5) A Modified Oxygen-15 Washout Method Applied to Fast Neutron Therapy. W. K. Roberts, J. W. Blue and F.Q.H. Ngo. Cleveland Clinic Foundation, Cleveland, Ohio 44106.

(E-6) Approaches to Measuring Tumor Growth *in vivo* using C-11 Thymidine and PET. A. F. Shields, R. C. Quackenbush, D. V. Coonrod, L. E. Lingren, J. M. Link, K. A. Krohn and M. M. Graham. Fred Hutchinson Cancer Center and University of Washington, Seattle, Washington.

(E-7) Regional Blood-To-Tissue Transport and Flow in an Irradiated Rat Glioma Model. A. M. Spence, M. M. Graham, G. L. Abbott, M. Muzi, L. A. O'Gorman and T. K. Lewellen. Departments of Medicine and Radiology, University of Washington, Seattle, Washington 98195.

(E-8) Limitations of the Deoxyglucose Method for the Measurement of Glucose Metabolic Rates in Brain Tumors. M. M. Graham, A. M. Spence, M. Muzi and G. L. Abbott. Departments of Radiology and Neurology, University of Washington, Seattle, Washington 98195.

(E-9) Relationship Between the Radiation Response of Tumors and Physiological Factors. C. W. Song, J. G. Rhee, I. Lee, L. M. Chelstrom and S. H. Levitt. University of Minnesota Medical School, Department of Therapeutic Radiology, Box 494, UMHC, Minneapolis, Minnesota 55455.

(E-10) Measurement of Tissue Redox State with C-13 NMR. R. N. Golden, E. G. Shankland, Z. Grunbaum, J. C. Livesey, T. L. Richards, R. A. Wade and K. A. Krohn. Imaging Research Laboratory, Department of Radiology, University of Washington, Seattle, Washington 98195.

(E-11) Measurement of Tumor Oxygenation and Energy Status Using Cryospectrophotometry and ^{31}P Magnetic Resonance Spectroscopy. R. M. Sutherland, F. L. Degner, E. K. Rofstad, R. L. Howell, R. G. Bryant, T. L. Ceckler, B. M. Fenton and T. E. J. Gayeski. University of Rochester, Rochester, New York 14642.

(E-12) Predicting and Measuring the Response of Human Neoplasms to Radiation Therapy Using Phosphorous MRS in situ. T. C. Ng, S. Vijayakumar, A. W. Majors, F. J. Thomas, T. F. Meaney, N. J. Baldwin and I. Koumoundouros. Division of Radiology, Cleveland Clinic, 9500 Euclid Avenue, Cleveland, Ohio 44106.

(E-13) Effects of Oxygen on the Metabolism of Murine Tumors Using *In Vivo* Phosphorous-31 NMR. P. Okunieff, E. McFarland, E. Rummeny, C. Willett, B. Hitzig, L. Neuringer and H. Suit. Massachusetts General Hospital, Harvard Medical School, Department of Radiation Medicine, and Department of Radiology and Department of Pulmonary Medicine and Massachusetts Institute of Technology, Francis Bitter National Magnet Laboratory and Harvard Medical School.

(E-14) The Response of RIF-1 Murine Tumor to Gamma Irradiation: 31-P NMR Study. S. S. Rajan, S. J. Li, R. G. Steen, J. P. Wehrle, L. Dillehay, J. Williams and J. D. Glickson. Department of Radiology and the Oncology Center, Johns Hopkins School of Medicine, Baltimore, Maryland 21205.

(E-15) *In Vivo* ^{31}P NMR Detects the Response of 9L Gliosarcoma to Chemotherapy with BCNU. R. G. Steen, R. J. Tamargo, S. Rajan, K. McGovern, H. Brem, J. P. Wehrle and J. D. Glickson. Departments of Radiology and Neurological Surgery, Johns Hopkins University School of Medicine, Baltimore, Maryland 21205.

(E-16) High-Resolution NMR Imaging Inside an Intact Multicellular Tumor Spheroid. J. P. Freyer, L. O. Sillerud and M. Mattingly. Toxicology and Neurobiology Groups, Los Alamos National Laboratory, Los Alamos, New Mexico 87545 and Bruker Instruments, Billerica, Massachusetts 01821.

(E-17) Cisplatin-Induced ^{1}H-NMR Spectral Changes in Human Ovarian Carcinoma Cells. G. D. Wenger, C. E. Cottrell, C. Roll, S. P. Balcerzak and B. C. Behrens. Division of Hematology/Oncology, Department of Internal Medicine and Campus Chemical Instrument Center, The Ohio State University, Columbus, Ohio 43210.

(E-18) Proton Relation Times in Cyclophosphamide (Cp) Treated RIF-1 Tumors. P. G. Braunschweiger, K. L. Reynolds and E. G. Maring. AMC Cancer Research Center, 1600 Pierce Street, Denver, Colorado 80214.

(E-19) Biological Factors that Affect NMR Relaxation Rates of Tumors. F. Q. H. Ngo and C. A. Belfi. Laboratory of Radiobiology and NMR Research, Research Institute, The Cleveland Clinic Foundation, Cleveland, Ohio 44106.

(E-20) Functional Tumor Staging: *In Vivo* NMR Assay. R. P. Schmidt, H. R. Hooper, P. S. Allen, B. C. Lentle, J. D. Chapman and A. Kanclerz. Cross Cancer Institute and University of Alberta, Edmonton, Alberta, Canada T6G 1Z2.

(E-21) Hypoxia and Glucose Deprivation in a Tumor Analog. L. Hlatky and R. Sachs. University of California, Berkeley, California 94706.

23

Conclusions: Prediction of Tumor Treatment Response

Lester J. Peters, J. Donald Chapman and H. Rodney Withers

This monograph is the proceedings of a Conference organized to provide a multidisciplinary forum for one of the most important current research topics in oncology: the ability to predict treatment outcome. Because no single treatment is uniformly successful nor free of morbidity for any cancer, various therapeutic options exist. Thus, the most fundamental skill of an oncologist (surgical, radiation, or medical) is his ability to select the most appropriate treatment option for each individual patient, regardless of modality.

There are two separate elements in deciding how to manage a patient with cancer. First is the assessment of the natural history of the disease, including the likely patterns of growth and spread, and the probability of controlling the disease with any treatment. This assessment determines the basic strategy of therapy, e.g., curative or palliative, regional or systemic. To a large extent, decisions of this type are mandated by the disease and are beyond the control of the physician. The second element in the management decision is to decide on a specific treatment option within the basic strategy chosen. When several options of comparable efficacy exist, this is often a subjective decision reflecting the prejudices and biases of the oncologist. To make these decisions more objective is the goal of research into prediction tumor treatment response.

Although many chapters of this volume did not specifically address the aspect of selecting between treatment options, one of the undoubted successes of the Banff Conference was to draw into sharp relief the distinction between predicting the natural history of disease and predicting the response to a particular treatment. In Table 23.1, the major parameters proposed as potential predictors are listed along with our assessment of their intrinsic ability to predict the natural history of disease and/or response to treatment. In this table, a (+) designation refers only to the rationale underlying the parameters as predictors. It

317

TABLE 23.1. *Potential Predictors of Natural History and Treatment Response*

Parameters	Predictor of	
	Natural History	Treatment Response
Tumor Regression/Necrosis	?	+
Intrinsic Cell Sensitivity	−	+
Proliferation Kinetics	+	+
Ploidy/Cytogenetics	+	?
Surface Receptors/Antigens	+	?
Proto-Oncogene Expression	+	?
Host Cell Infiltrates	?	+
NK Cell Activity	+	−
pO_2/pH	−	+
O_2 and Heat-Regulated Proteins	−	+
Endogenous Thiols	−	+
P-Glycoprotein	−	+
DNA-Drug Adducts	−	+
DNA Repair Enzymes	−	+
MRS/MRI ^{31}P	?	+
^{1}H	?	?
PET Metabolism	?	?
(^{11}C, ^{13}N, ^{15}O, ^{18}F) Receptors/Markers	?	?
Pharmacokinetics	−	?

+ = probable; ? = possible; − = unlikely

does not imply independently valid predictive ability, for this remains to be proven.

What reasonable expectation can one have that any potential predictive assay of tumor treatment response will have clinical utility? Some chapters in this monograph and much discussion at the Conference addressed the problems and pitfalls associated with this goal. The criteria of an ideal predictor of treatment outcome were easily agreed upon (Table 23.2), but equally easily, it was acknowledged that no potential predictor could achieve this ideal. Paramount among the obstacles to achieving this ideal are those listed in Table 23.3. These are indeed formidable obstacles, and provide the stimulus for many years of research effort. However, it is important that recognition of the obstacles should not paralyze us into inactivity. Sufficient rationale and technologic development exist for at least some of the assays listed in

TABLE 23.2. *Criteria of Ideal Predictor of Treatment Outcome*

Correlate specifically with treatment outcome independently of other known parameters

Be measurable precisely and rapidly

Have a low susceptibility to sampling error

Have low risk of false negativity

Be harmless and inexpensive

Table 23.1 to begin prospective clinical testing, especially assays of *in vitro* tumor cell sensitivity, *in vivo* cell proliferation kinetics, and *in vivo* metabolic parameters, particularly hypoxia. With regard to the pervading concern about intra-tumoral heterogeneity and the hazards involved in interpreting the results obtained from biopsy samples, the analogy can be made with anatomic and surgical pathology. All pathological diagnoses are subject to sampling error, yet the implicit recognition of this fact does not prevent us from accepting the powerful but not infallible information so derived. Furthermore, as long as the magnitude of inter-tumoral heterogeneity exceeds that of intra-tumoral heterogeneity, (as appears to be the case) there is no reason why biopsy samples should not provide sufficient discrimination for useful predictive assays.

Clinical testing of a putative predictor of tumor treatment response must be done in a disciplined, prospectively controlled fashion in order to assess its value along rigorous guidelines. The steps involved are set out in Table 23.4. The first requirement is to identify a cohort of patients with specified stages of disease and to treat them according to a well-defined protocol. Strict quality assurance is mandatory, since no predictive assay of treatment response can have validity if treatment is inadequate. Multivariate analysis of the factors influencing treatment outcomes should then be performed. The simple demonstration of a

TABLE 23.3. *Problem Areas*

How to define and quantitate tumor stem cells

Heterogeneity: Clonal (including interactions)
Spatial
Metabolic

Accuracy and reproductibility of assay technique

TABLE 23.4. *Steps in Development of a Predictive Assay*

Clinical Testing
Selection of patient cohort for study
Treatment by defined protocol
Strict quality control
Multivariate analysis of treatment outcome
Weight of assay data in prognostic equation
Accept or reject for routine use

correlation between an assay result and an observed treatment response does not, in itself, constitute validation of the clinical utility of the assay, since it may merely reflect other established prognostic indicators. The preferred way to test independent significance of the assay data is to construct a prognostic equation based on known variables and then to see if the accuracy of the equation is significantly improved by addition of the assay data. If it is, the weight of the new term in the prognostic equation in relation to the cost and difficulty of the assay will ultimately determine whether it achieves clinical acceptance.

There is no question that clinical oncologists need more refined predictors of treatment outcome in order to best serve their patients and to avoid unnecessary treatment-related morbidity. The interest shown in the Banff Conference, both in terms of the diverse disciplines represented, and in the quality of the scientific contributions and discussions, are evidence of the recognition of this need by the scientific community. Difficulties and problems undoubtedly exist, and it would be naive to anticipate imminent dramatic advances. However, research momentum is strong and growing, and we have every reason to believe that the next Conference on Prediction of Tumor Treatment Response will be even more productive and exciting than this one has been.

Index